Anxiety: Neurobiology, Clinic and Therapeutic Perspectives

Anxiété : Neurobiologie, Clinique et Perspectives Thérapeutiques

British Library Cataloguing in Publication Data
A catalogue record for this book
is available from the British Library

ISBN 2-7420-0018-6
ISSN 0768-3154

First published in 1993 by

Editions John Libbey Eurotext
6 rue Blanche, 92120 Montrouge, France. (33) (1) 47 35 85 52
ISBN 2-7420-0018-6

John Libbey and Company Ltd
13 Smiths Yard, Summerley Street, London SW18 4HR,
England.
(44) (81) 947 27 77

Institut National de la Santé et de la Recherche Médicale
101 rue de Tolbiac, 75654 Paris Cedex 13, France.
(33) (1) 44 23 60 00
ISBN 2-85598-544-7

ISSN 0768-3154

© 1993 Colloques INSERM/John Libbey Eurotext Ltd,
All rights reserved
Unauthorized publication contravenes applicable laws

Anxiety : Neurobiology, Clinic and Therapeutic Perspectives

Anxiété : Neurobiologie, Clinique et Perspectives Thérapeutiques

A Symposium (Colloque Thématique) of the Société des Neurosciences (France)

Proceedings of an International Meeting held in Dinard (France), 20-21 September 1993
Comptes rendus d'un Colloque International qui s'est tenu à Dinard (France) les 20 et 21 Septembre 1993

Subventionné par l'Institut National de la Santé et de la Recherche Médicale, l'Association pour la Neuro-Psycho-Pharmacologie, la Société des Neurosciences, l'Institut de Recherches Internationales Servier et la Direction des Recherches, Etudes et Techniques de la Délégation Générale pour l'Armement

Edited by

**Michel Hamon
Hélène Ollat
Marie-Hélène Thiébot**

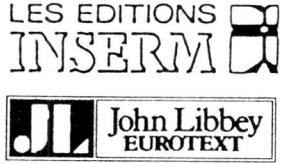

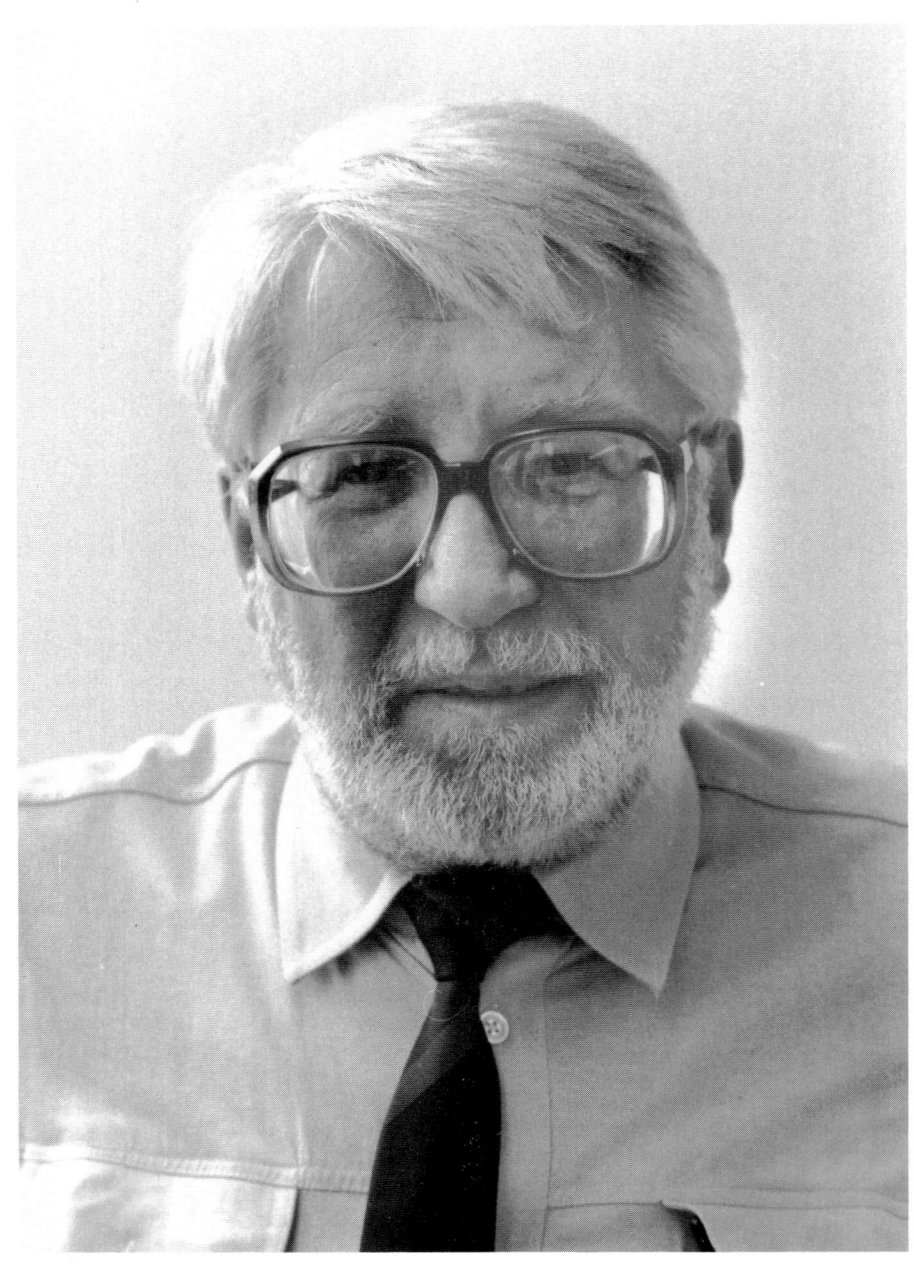

Professor Willy E. HAEFELY

Avant-propos

Bien que l'anxiété constitue une réaction émotionnelle normale, que tout le monde éprouve à un moment ou à un autre dans la vie courante, elle peut aussi revêtir, de par sa fréquence, son intensité, etc, des caractères pathologiques (anxiété généralisée, agoraphobie, sociophobie, attaques de panique, etc). Le développement des benzodiazépines en tant qu'anxiolytiques au début des années soixante a été la première étape, à la fois dans le traitement (au moins de certaines formes) de l'anxiété pathologique, et dans la découverte des mécanismes biologiques qui la sous-tendent. Récemment, de nouveaux composés ont été décrits comme possédant des potentialités anxiolytiques dans les situations modèles chez l'animal. Ces observations laissent à penser que de nouveaux anxiolytiques, sans les effets secondaires des benzodiazépines (sédation, relaxation musculaire, amnésie antérograde, tolérance et dépendance) seront prochainement disponibles. Notre but, en organisant ce Symposium, a été de faire le point des connaissances sur - les mécanismes neurobiologiques impliqués dans l'anxiété, - les perturbations des systèmes endocrines et immunitaires qui lui sont associées, - les mécanismes d'action des benzodiazépines et d'autres composés anxiolytiques, et, enfin, d'évaluer la pertinence des directions de recherche actuelles pour le développement de nouveaux anxiolytiques.

La première partie de ces comptes rendus présente les aspects cliniques de l'anxiété pathologique, et analyse en détail les situations expérimentales qui sont utilisées chez l'animal pour induire des comportements anxieux. L'intérêt de ces modèles animaux pour à la fois étudier les modifications biologiques associées à l'anxiété et prédire les potentialités anxiolytiques des agents pharmacologiques, est également évalué dans ce chapitre.

La deuxième partie est consacrée aux mécanismes neurobiologiques du stress et de l'anxiété, avec une attention particulière pour les neuromédiateurs majeurs du système nerveux central que sont le GABA, les catécholamines et la sérotonine. En outre, les perturbations des systèmes endocrines et immunitaires associées au stress et à l'anxiété y sont également analysées.

La troisième partie présente les données les plus récentes sur les cibles moléculaires des anxiolytiques, à savoir les récepteurs du GABA et de la sérotonine.

Enfin, la dernière partie de ce livre est consacrée aux nouvelles directions de recherche, notamment celles qui laissent à penser que le développement de nouveaux anxiolytiques sera possible à partir de l'étude des systèmes sérotoninergiques, cholécystokininergiques et à acides aminés excitateurs au niveau cérébral.

Nous dédions cet ouvrage au Pr Willy Haefely, qui, en 1974, a découvert le rôle clé du GABA dans les mécanismes d'action des benzodiazépines. C'est avec sa gentillesse coutumière qu'il avait accepté de nous faire l'honneur de participer à ce Symposium. Sa disparition brutale en avril dernier est une perte immense pour nous.

Le Comité d'Organisation
Michel Hamon
Hélène Ollat
Marie-Hélène Thiébot

Foreword

Although everybody had and will experience anxiety, its intensity, frequency and characteristics may vary from what can be considered as "normal" to pathological, with disorders such as generalized anxiety, agoraphobia, sociophobia, panic attacks, etc. The development of benzodiazepines as anxiolytics in the early sixties has been a major step firstly in the treatment of (at least some forms of) pathological anxiety, and secondly in the understanding of the associated biological mechanisms. Recently, new drugs have been developed which also exert anxiolytic-like effects in relevant animal models, leading to the proposal, and hope, that novel anxiolytics without the secondary effects of benzodiazepines (sedation, myorelaxation, anterograde amnesia, tolerance and dependence) will be available as therapeutic anti-anxiety agents. The goal of this Symposium was to take stock of the present knowledge of - the neurobiological mechanisms of anxiety, - the associated endocrine and immune alterations, - the mechanisms of actions of benzodiazepines and other anxiolytics, and - to critically assess the relevance of new directions in the search of potential anxiolytics.

The first section of these proceedings presents the clinical aspects of pathological anxiety, and carefully analyzes the experimental situations that are used in animal models to induce anxiety-like behaviours, and thus to explore the associated biological mechanisms and potential anxiolytic properties of drugs.

The second section deals with the neurobiological mechanisms associated with stress and anxiety-like behaviours in animals, with special attention to the major brain neurotransmitters GABA, catecholamines and serotonin. In addition, the endocrine and immune changes associated with stress and anxiety are also critically analyzed.

The third section is devoted to the present knowledge of the molecular targets of potent anxiolytic drugs, i.e. mainly the receptors for GABA and serotonin.

In the last section, new issues and directions are presented. In particular, the potential therapeutic interest of new drugs acting at receptors for serotonin, cholecystokinin or excitatory aminoacids is critically analyzed in light of the most recent data from relevant animal studies.

We would like to dedicate this book to our friend Pr Willy Haefely, who made, in 1974, the cardinal discovery of the pivotal role of GABA in the mechanism of action of benzodiazepines as anxiolytics, and kindly accepted to participate in this Symposium. His sudden death in April this year was a great loss for all of us.

The Organizing Committee
Michel Hamon
Hélène Ollat
Marie-Hélène Thiébot

Remerciements

Nous remercions tous les collègues qui ont contribué au succès de ce Colloque par leur participation au travers de conférences, de présentations affichées et de discussions.

Nous sommes très reconnaissants à Mesdames Sylvie Larvor et Claude Sais pour leur participation décisive, efficace et souriante à l'organisation du Colloque. La qualité de leur accueil à Dinard a été unanimement appréciée.

Nous remercions aussi les organisations publiques et privées qui ont subventionné et rendu possible ce Colloque:

- l'Association pour la Neuro-Psycho-Pharmacologie,
- l'Institut de Recherches Internationales Servier,
- l'Institut National de la Santé et de la Recherche Médicale (INSERM), qui a financé également la publication de ce livre,
- la Société des Neurosciences,
- la Direction des Recherches, Etudes et Techniques (DRET) de la Délégation Générale pour l'Armement (DGA), sous le contrat n°93-1062.

Acknowledgements

We wish to thank our colleagues who contributed to the success of this meeting by their participation through lectures, poster presentations and discussions.

We direct our thanks to Mrs Sylvie Larvor and Claude Sais who contributed so kindly and efficiently to the organization of the meeting, and serve as secretaries and hostesses.

We also thank the following public organizations and private companies whose support made this Symposium possible:

- the "Association pour la Neuro-Psycho-Pharmacologie"
- the "Institut de Recherches Internationales Servier"
- the "Institut National de la Santé et de la Recherche Médicale" (INSERM), which is also sponsoring the publication of this book
- the French "Société des Neurosciences"
- the research organization of the French Army, the "Direction des Recherches, Etudes et Techniques" (DRET), a division of the "Délégation Générale pour l'Armement" (DGA), under grant # 93-1062.

List and address of contributors
Liste et adresse des intervenants

Abadie P., INSERM U.320, Centre Cycéron, Université de Caen, boulevard Henri Becquerel, 14021 Caen, France

Adelbrecht C., Génétique, Neurogénétique et Comportement, URA CNRS 1294, UFR Biomédicale, Université Paris V-René Descartes, 45, rue des Saints-Pères, 75270 Paris cedex 06, France

Bailly D., Centre d'Information et de Traitement des Dépendances, Laboratoire de recherche sur l'Anxiété, C.H.R.U., 57, boulevard de Metz, 59037 Lille cedex, France

Balster R.L., Medical College of Virginia, Department of Pharmacology and Toxicology, MCV Station, Box 613, Richmond, Virginia 23298-0613, États-Unis

Barbaccia M.L., Department of Experimental Medicine, University of Rome «Tor Vergata», Rome, Italie

Baron J.-C., INSERM U.320, Centre Cycéron, Université de Caen, Boulevard Henri Becquerel, 14021 Caen, France

Baulieu E.-E., INSERM U.33, Communications Hormonales, 80, avenue du Général Leclerc, 94276 Le Kremlin-Bicêtre, France

Belotti M., Laboratoire de Neurosciences Comportementales et Cognitives, URA CNRS 339, Université de Bordeaux 1, avenue des Facultés, 33045 Talence cedex, France

Belzung C., Laboratoire d'Ethologie et de Psychophysiologie, Parc de Grandmont, 37200 Tours, France

Béracochéa D.J., Laboratoire de Neurosciences Cognitives et Comportementales, URA CNRS 339, Université de Bordeaux 1, avenue des Facultés, 33405 Talence cedex, France

Beuscart R., Centre d'Information et de Traitement des Dépendances, Laboratoire de recherche sur l'Anxiété, C.H.R.U., 57, boulevard de Metz, 59037 Lille cedex, France

Beuzen A., Laboratoire d'Ethologie et de Psychophysiologie, Parc de Grandmont, 37200 Tours, France

Bickerdike M., Department of Physiology and Pharmacology, Nottingham University Medical School, Queen's Medical Centre, Nottingham NG7 2UH, Grande-Bretagne

Biggio G., Department of Experimental Biology, University of Cagliari, Via Palabanda, 12, 09123 Cagliari, Italie

Bontempi B., Laboratoire de Neurosciences Cognitives et Comportementales, URA CNRS 339, Université de Bordeaux 1, avenue des Facultés, 33405 Talence cedex, France

Bouhou E., Laboratoire d'Ethologie et de Psychophysiologie, Parc de Grandmont, 37200 Tours, France

Boulenger J.-P., Département de Psychiatrie, CHUS, 3001, 12e Avenue Nord, Sherbrooke, Québec JIH 5N4, Canada

Bourin M., GIS Médicament, Faculté de Médecine, 44035 Nantes cedex 01, France

Bradwejn J., St-Mary's Hospital Centre, Mc Gill University, 3820 Lacombe Avenue, Montréal H3T1M5, Canada

Brocco M., Institut de Recherches Servier (I.D.R.S.), 7, rue Ampère, 92800 Puteaux, France

Buhot M.-C., CNRS, Laboratoire de Neurobiologie, E6, B.P. 71, 31, chemin Joseph-Aiguier, 13402 Marseille cedex 20, France

Cadogan A-K., Department of Physiology and Pharmacology, Nottingham University Medical School, Queen's Medical Centre, Nottingham NG7 2UH, Grande-Bretagne

Chapouthier G., Génétique, Neurogénétique et Comportement, URA CNRS 1294, UFR Biomédicale, Université Paris V-René Descartes, 45, rue des Saints-Pères, 75270 Paris cedex 06, France

Clément Y., Génétique, Neurogénétique et Comportement, URA CNRS 1294, UFR Biomédicale, Université Paris V-René Descartes, 45, rue des Saints-Pères, 75270 Paris cedex 06, France

Concas A., Department of Experimental Biology, University of Cagliari, Via Palabanda, 12, 09123 Cagliari, Italie

Costentin J., Unité de Neuropsychopharmacologie Expérimentale, CNRS URA 1170, Faculté de Médecine et Pharmacie de Rouen, B.P. 97, 76803 Saint-Etienne-du-Rouvray, France

Cuccheddu T., Department of Experimental Biology, University of Cagliari, Via Palabanda, 12, 09123 Cagliari, Italie

Dantzer R., INRA-INSERM U.176, Laboratoire de Neurobiologie Intégrative, Rue Camille Saint-Saëns, 33077 Bordeaux cedex, France

Daugé V., Département de Pharmacochimie Moléculaire et Structurale, INSERM U.266 - CNRS URA D1500, Université René Descartes, 4, avenue de l'Observatoire, 75270 Paris cedex 06, France

Dekeyne A., Centre de Recherche Roussel-Uclaf, Pharmacologie-Neurobiologie, 111, route de Noisy, 93230 Romainville, France

Depaulis A., Laboratoire de Neurophysiologie et Biologie des Comportements, Centre de Neurochimie du CNRS, 5, rue Blaise Pascal, 67084 Strasbourg cedex, France

Derrien M., Département de Pharmacochimie Moléculaire et Structurale, INSERM U.266 - CNRS URA D1500, Université René Descartes, 4, avenue de l'Observatoire, 75270 Paris cedex 06, France

Destrade C., Laboratoire de Neurosciences Cognitives et Comportementales, URA CNRS 339, Université de Bordeaux 1, avenue des Facultés, 33405 Talence cedex, France

Dewailly D., Centre d'Information et de Traitement des Dépendances, Laboratoire de recherche sur l'Anxiété, C.H.R.U., 57, boulevard de Metz, 59037 Lille cedex, France

Durieux C., Département de Pharmacochimie Moléculaire et Structurale, INSERM U.266 - CNRS URA D1500, Université René Descartes, 4, avenue de l'Observatoire, 75270 Paris cedex 06, France

Fink H., Institute of Pharmacology and Toxicology, Humboldt University of Berlin, PF 140, 10117 Berlin, Allemagne

Floris S., Department of Experimental Biology, University of Cagliari, Via Palabanda, 12, 09123 Cagliari, Italie

François-Bellan A.-M., INSERM U.297, Laboratoire de Neuro-Endocrinologie Expérimentale, Faculté de Médecine secteur Nord, Boulevard Pierre Dramard, 13916 Marseille cedex 20, France

Galey D., Laboratoire de Neurosciences Comportementales et Cognitives, URA CNRS 339, Université de Bordeaux 1, avenue des Facultés, 33045 Talence cedex, France

Gozlan H., INSERM U.288, Faculté de Médecine Pitié-Salpêtrière, 91, boulevard de l'Hôpital, 75634 Paris Cedex 13, France

Griebel G., Laboratoire de Psychophysiologie, 7 rue de l'Université, 67000 Strasbourg, France

Grino M., INSERM U.297, Laboratoire de Neuro-Endocrinologie Expérimentale, Faculté de Médecine secteur Nord, Boulevard Pierre Dramard, 13916 Marseille cedex 20, France

Guernier M., Centre de Recherche Roussel-Uclaf, Pharmacologie-Neurobiologie, 111, route de Noisy, 93230 Romainville, France

Hamon M., INSERM U.288, Faculté de Médecine Pitié-Salpêtrière, 91, boulevard de l'Hôpital, 75634 Paris Cedex 13, France

Haug M., Université Louis Pasteur, Laboratoire de Psychophysiologie, CNRS URA 1295, 7, rue de l'Université, 67000 Strasbourg, France

Héry F., INSERM U.297, Laboratoire de Neuro-Endocrinologie Expérimentale, Faculté de Médecine secteur Nord, Boulevard Pierre Dramard, 13916 Marseille cedex 20, France

Héry M., INSERM U.297, Laboratoire de Neuro-Endocrinologie Expérimentale, Faculté de Médecine secteur Nord, Boulevard Pierre Dramard, 13916 Marseille cedex 20, France

Jaffard R., Laboratoire de Neurosciences Cognitives et Comportementales, URA CNRS 339, Université de Bordeaux 1, avenue des Facultés, 33405 Talence cedex, France

Joly D., Département de Biologie, Synthélabo Recherche (L.E.R.S.), 31, avenue Paul Vaillant-Couturier, B.P. 110, 92225 Bagneux cedex, France

Krazem A., Laboratoire de Neurosciences Cognitives et Comportementales, URA CNRS 339, Université de Bordeaux 1, avenue des Facultés, 33405 Talence cedex, France

Ladurelle N., Département de Pharmacochimie Moléculaire et Structurale, INSERM U.266 - CNRS URA D1500, Université René Descartes, 4, avenue de l'Observatoire, 75270 Paris cedex 06, France

Lavallée Y.-J., Département de Psychiatrie, CHUS, 3001, 12e Avenue Nord, Sherbrooke, Québec JIH 5N4, Canada

Lüddens H., Laboratory for Molecular Neuroendocrinology, Center for Molecular Biology, Im Neuenheimer Feld 282, D-69120 Heidelberg, Allemagne

Mano M.-P., Laboratoire de Neurosciences Comportementales et Cognitives, URA CNRS 339, Université de Bordeaux 1, avenue des Facultés, 33045 Talence cedex, France

Marsden C.A., Department of Physiology and Pharmacology, Nottingham University Medical School, Queen's Medical Centre, Nottingham NG7 2UH, Grande-Bretagne

Martin B., Génétique, Neurogénétique et Comportement, URA CNRS 1294, UFR Biomédicale, Université Paris V-René Descartes, 45, rue des Saints-Pères, 75270 Paris cedex 06, France

Martin P., Groupe de Recherche AMC, 70, boulevard Bessières, 75017 Paris, France

Miachon S., Laboratoire de Neurochimie Fonctionnelle, INSERM U.171 et CNRS URA 1195, Centre Hospitalier Lyon-Sud, 69310 Pierre-Bénite, France

Millan M.J., Institut de Recherches Servier (I.D.R.S.), 7, rue Ampère, 92800 Puteaux, France

Misslin R., Laboratoire de Psychophysiologie, 7, rue de l'Université, 67000 Strasbourg, France

Naïli S., CNRS, Laboratoire de Neurobiologie, E6, B.P. 71, 31, chemin Joseph-Aiguier, 13402 Marseille cedex 20, France

Nixon M.K., GIS Médicament, Faculté de Médecine, 44035 Nantes cedex 01, France

Oberlander C., Centre de Recherche Roussel-Uclaf, Pharmacologie-Neurobiologie, 111, route de Noisy, 93230 Romainville, France

Oliver C., INSERM U.297, Laboratoire de Neuro-Endocrinologie Expérimentale, Faculté de Médecine secteur Nord, Boulevard Pierre Dramard, 13916 Marseille Cedex 20, France

Ollat H., Association pour la Neuro-Psycho-Pharmacologie, 25, rue de la Plaine, 75020 Paris, France

Parquet P.-J., Centre d'Information et de Traitement des Dépendances, Laboratoire de recherche sur l'Anxiété, C.H.R.U., 57, boulevard de Metz, 59037 Lille cedex, France

Patra S.K., Centre for Advanced Study in Psychology, UTKAL University, Bhubaneswar 751 004, Orissa, Inde

Perche F. , Université Louis Pasteur, Laboratoire de Psychophysiologie, CNRS URA 1295, 7 rue de l'Université, 67000 Strasbourg, France

Pineau N., Laboratoire d'Ethologie et de Psychophysiologie, Parc de Grandmont, 37200 Tours, France

Rex A., Institute of Pharmacology and Toxicology, Humboldt University of Berlin, PF 140, 10117 Berlin, Allemagne

Robel P., INSERM U.33, Communications Hormonales, 80, avenue du Général Leclerc, 94276 Le Kremlin-Bicêtre, France

Roques B.-P., Département de Pharmacochimie Moléculaire et Structurale, INSERM U.266 - CNRS URA D1500, Université René Descartes, 4, avenue de l'Observatoire, 75270 Paris cedex 06, France

Roscetti G., Department of Experimental Medicine, University of Rome «Tor Vergata», Rome, Italie

Sanger D.J., Département de Biologie, Synthélabo Recherche (L.E.R.S.), 31, avenue Paul Vaillant-Couturier, B.P. 110, 92225 Bagneux cedex, France

Sanna E., Department of Experimental Biology, University of Cagliari, Via Palabanda, 12, 09123 Cagliari, Italie

Serra M., Department of Experimental Biology, University of Cagliari, Via Palabanda, 12, 09123 Cagliari, Italie

Servant D., Centre d'Information et de Traitement des Dépendances, Laboratoire de recherche sur l'Anxiété, C.H.R.U., 57, boulevard de Metz, 59037 Lille cedex, France

Simon P., Unité de Neuropsychopharmacologie Expérimentale, CNRS URA 1170, Faculté de Médecine et Pharmacie de Rouen, B.P. 97, 76803 Saint-Etienne-du-Rouvray, France

Tassin J.-P., Chaire de Neuropharmacologie, Collège de France, INSERM U.114, 11, place Marcelin-Berthelot, 75231 Paris cedex 05, France

Thiébot M.-H., INSERM U.288, Faculté de Médecine Pitié-Salpêtrière, 91, boulevard de l'Hôpital, 75634 Paris Cedex 13, France

Venault P., Génétique, Neurogénétique et Comportement, URA CNRS 1294, UFR Biomédicale, Université Paris V-René Descartes, 45, rue des Saints-Pères, 75270 Paris cedex 06, France

Vogel E., Laboratoire de Psychophysiologie, 7, rue de l'Université, 67000 Strasbourg, France

Weibel L., Laboratoire de Psychophysiologie, 7, rue de l'Université, 67000 Strasbourg, France

Wiley J.L., Medical College of Virginia, Department of Pharmacology and Toxicology, MCV Station, Box 613, Richmond, Virginia 23298-0613, États-Unis

Wright I., Department of Physiology and Pharmacology, Nottingham University Medical School, Queen's Medical Centre, Nottingham NG7 2UH, Grande-Bretagne

Young J., INSERM U.33, Communications Hormonales, 80, avenue du Général Leclerc, 94276 Le Kremlin-Bicêtre, France

Zivkovic B., Département de Biologie, Synthélabo Recherche (L.E.R.S.), 31, avenue Paul Vaillant-Couturier, B.P. 110, 92225 Bagneux cedex, France

Contents
Sommaire

V Foreword
VI *Avant-propos*

VII Acknowledgements
VIII *Remerciements*

IX List and address of contributors
Liste et adresse des intervenants

I. CLINICAL ASPECTS AND ANIMAL MODELS
I. ASPECTS CLINIQUES ET MODÈLES COMPORTEMENTAUX CHEZ L'ANIMAL

3 **J.-P. Boulenger, Y.-J. Lavallée**
Pathological anxiety: clinical and theoretical aspects
L'anxiété pathologique : aspects cliniques et théoriques

15 **M. Bourin, J. Bradwejn, M.K. Nixon**
Provocative agents and the biology of panic attacks
Agents inducteurs et biologie des attaques de panique

25 **M.-H. Thiébot**
Current behavioural models of anxiety in animals: how predictive are they for anxiolytic activity?
Modèles animaux pour l'étude de l'anxiété : quelle est leur valeur prédictive dans le développement des anxiolytiques ?

39 **A. Depaulis**
Neurobiology of defensive reactions in animals as an approach to human anxiety
Neurobiologie des réactions de défense chez l'animal - Intérêt par rapport à l'anxiété chez l'homme

II. BIOLOGICAL ASPECTS OF STRESS AND ANXIETY
II. ASPECTS BIOLOGIQUES DU STRESS ET DE L'ANXIÉTÉ

53 G. Biggio, T. Cuccheddu, S. Floris, E. Sanna, M.L. Barbaccia, G. Roscetti, M. Serra, A. Concas
Stress and GABAergic transmission in the rat brain: the effect of carbon dioxide inhalation
Stress et transmission GABAergique dans le cerveau du rat : effet d'une inhalation de dioxyde de carbone

65 J.-P. Tassin
Stress and catecholamines: similarities and differences between NA and DA systems
Stress et catécholamines: similitudes et différences entre les systèmes NA et DA

75 C.A. Marsden, M. Bickerdike, A-K. Cadogan, I. Wright, A. Rex, H. Fink
Serotonergic mechanisms and animal models of anxiety
Mécanismes sérotoninergiques et modèles animaux d'anxiété

83 F. Héry, A.-M. François-Bellan, M. Grino, M. Héry, C. Oliver
Stress and neuroendocrine systems
Stress et systèmes neuro-endocrines

97 R. Dantzer
Stress, anxiety and immunity
Stress, anxiété et immunité

III. NEUROPHARMACOLOGICAL ASPECTS - MOLECULAR TARGETS OF ANXIOLYTIC DRUGS
III. ASPECTS NEUROPHARMACOLOGIQUES - LES CIBLES MOLÉCULAIRES DES ANXIOLYTIQUES

107 H. Lüddens
$GABA_A$/BZ receptors: recent advances in molecular biology
Récepteurs $GABA_A$/BZ : les données récentes de la biologie moléculaire

119 D.J. Sanger, D. Joly, B. Zivkovic
Anxiolytic drugs and cognitive function
Agents anxiolytiques et fonctions cognitives

129 J.-C. Baron, P. Abadie
In vivo study of central-type benzodiazepine receptors in humans by means of positron emission tomography
Etudes in vivo des récepteurs centraux des benzodiazépines chez l'homme par tomographie d'émission de positons

141 H. Gozlan, M. Hamon
Pharmacology and molecular biology of central 5-HT receptors
Pharmacologie et biologie moléculaire des récepteurs centraux de la sérotonine

IV. POTENTIAL ANXIOLYTIC DRUGS - THERAPEUTIC PERSPECTIVES
IV. ANXIOLYTIQUES POTENTIELS - PERSPECTIVES THÉRAPEUTIQUES

153 M.J. Millan, M. Brocco
Serotonin and anxiety: mixed $5-HT_{1A}$ agonists - $5-HT_{1C/2}$ antagonists as potential anxiolytic agents
Sérotonine et anxiété : potentialités anxiolytiques des composés mixtes agonistes $5-HT_{1A}$ et antagonistes $5-HT_{1C/2}$

167 V. Daugé, N. Ladurelle, M. Derrien, C. Durieux, B.-P. Roques
Potential therapeutic applications of CCK antagonists in anxiety and panic disorders
Applications thérapeutiques potentielles des antagonistes de la CCK dans le traitement de l'anxiété et des attaques de panique

177 J.L. Wiley, R.L. Balster
NMDA antagonists: a novel class of anxiolytics ?
Les antagonistes NMDA : une nouvelle classe d'anxiolytiques ?

Poster presentations
Communications affichées

187 D. Bailly, D. Servant, D. Dewailly, R. Beuscart, P.-J. Parquet
Plasma cortisol and ACTH responses to o-CRF stimulation in patients with obsessive compulsive disorder
Réponses du cortisol et de l'ACTH plasmatiques à la stimulation par le CRF ovin chez des patients présentant un trouble obsessionnel-compulsif

189 M. Belotti, M.-P. Mano, D. Galey
Effects of specific modulation of neurotransmitter systems in the septal region on anxiety level and working memory performance in C57BL/6
Effets de modulations spécifiques de systèmes de neurotransmission dans la région septale sur le niveau d'anxiété et les performances mnésiques chez la souris C57BL/6

191 D.J. Béracochéa, B. Bontempi, A. Krazem, C. Destrade, R. Jaffard
Effects of methyl-beta-carboline-3-carboxylate (βCCM) on emotional and memory disorders resulting from experimental mamillary bodies lesions and chronic alcohol consumption in Balb/c mice
Effets du méthyl-bêta-carboline-3-carboxylate (βCCM) sur les troubles émotionnels et mnésiques induits par des lésions des corps mamillaires et la prise chronique d'alcool chez les souris BALB/c

193 A. Beuzen, C. Belzung, N. Pineau, E. Bouhou
Link between anxiety and memory: behavioural and pharmacological study in the mouse
Lien entre anxiété et mémoire : étude comportementale et pharmacologique chez la souris

195 M.-C. Buhot, S.K. Patra, S. Naïli
Role of serotonin 1 receptors in hippocampal functions: a psychopharmacological study in the rat
Rôle des récepteurs de la sérotonine de type $5\text{-}HT_1$ dans les fonctions hippocampiques : étude psychopharmacologique chez le rat

197 Y. Clément, B. Martin, C. Adelbrecht, P. Venault, G. Chapouthier
Implication of an autosomal locus in the activity in open-field by the analysis of two inbred strains of mice and their segregating populations
Mise en évidence de l'implication d'un locus autosomal dans l'activité en «open-field» par l'analyse de deux lignées consanguines de souris et leurs populations ségrégeantes

198 A. Dekeyne, M. Guernier, C. Oberlander
Effects of alpha-2 adrenoceptor agonist and antagonists in the safety signal withdrawal paradigm
Effet d'un agoniste et de divers antagonistes des adrénocepteurs alpha-2 dans le test de disparition du signal de sécurité

200 G. Griebel, R. Misslin, L. Weibel, E. Vogel
The free exploratory paradigm: an effective method for measuring neophobia behavior in mice and testing potential neophobia reducing drugs
L'exploration libre : un test efficace pour étudier un comportement néophobique chez la souris et apprécier les potentialités anti-néophobiques des agents pharmacologiques

201 M. Haug, F. Perche, J. Young, E.-E. Baulieu, P. Robel
Brain neurosteroids: dehydroepiandrosterone reduces aggression in mice
Les neurostéroïdes du cerveau : la déhydro-épiandrostérone diminue l'agressivité chez la souris

203 P. Martin
Effects of anxiolytic and antidepressant drugs in an animal model of panic
Effets des anxiolytiques et des antidépresseurs dans un modèle animal de l'attaque de panique

205 B. Martin, Y. Clément, P. Venault, G. Chapouthier
A gene on mouse chromosome 4 is involved in anxiogenic processes
Un gène sur le chromosome 4 est impliqué dans les processus anxiogènes chez la souris

206 S. Miachon
Isolation and ACTH induced muricidal behavior in male Wistar rats
Comportement muricide induit par l'isolement et l'ACTH chez le rat mâle Wistar

207 A. Rex, H. Fink, C.A. Marsden
The effect of CCK-4 and L 365.260 on cortical extracellular 5-HT release on exposure on the elevated Plus maze
Effets du CCK-4 et du L 365-260 sur les taux de 5-HT extracellulaire dans le cortex au cours du test du labyrinthe en croix surélevé

209 D. Servant, D. Bailly, D. Dewailly, R. Beuscart, P.-J. Parquet
Recent life stress and the corticotropin releasing factor test in panic disorder
Test au CRF et trouble panique - Rôle des événements de vie stressants

211 P. Simon, J. Costentin
Dopamine transmission and anxiety in mice
Transmission dopaminergique et anxiété chez la souris

213 Author index
Index des auteurs

I. Clinical aspects and animal models

I. *Aspects cliniques et modèles comportementaux chez l'animal*

Pathological anxiety:
clinical and theoretical aspects

Jean-Philippe Boulenger and Yvon-Jacques Lavallée

Anxiety Clinic, Département de Psychiatrie, Centre Hospitalier Universitaire de Sherbrooke, Fleurimont (Québec) J1H 5N4, Canada

SUMMARY

Modern diagnostic systems distinguish several subcategories of anxiety disorders. Clinical features including symptoms, time-course and possible complications contribute to differentiate diagnostic entities such as panic disorders, phobic disorders, obsessive-compulsive disorders and generalized anxiety disorders. The definition of specific criteria for each of these categories has been a major step in the evolution of psychiatric research allowing a better reliability of clinical evaluations and the development of structured diagnostic questionnaires. These questionnaires have contributed to a large extent to the tremendous increase of epidemiological research in the field of mental health over the last decade. These diagnostic systems are submitted to a regular review process taking into account the outcome of recent clinical research related to these disorders. In the field of anxiety preliminary evidence suggest that common underlying mechanisms may exist in several anxiety disorders as well as between anxiety and depressive disorders. Though these findings are unlikely to change the existing diagnostic categories in the near future they are nevertheless important to consider for a better understanding and treatment of these frequent and sometimes disabling psychiatric disorders.

INTRODUCTION

Anxiety is an emotional phenomenon which is both frequent and ubiquitous. As a necessary part of the response to various stressful stimuli anxiety is related to the normal psychological functioning of humans but may also appear as a reaction to various medical or psychiatric conditions. However, in some individuals, after a careful evaluation ruling out such medical conditions or the recent occurence of major life-events, anxiety symptoms will appear as the center of the patient's suffering and the major

feature of a clinical state labelled as "pathological anxiety" or "anxiety disorder".
Despite its frequency, pathological anxiety remains ill-defined. Theoretically, this label characterizes clinical states where anxiety is not provoked by a real threat, is out of proportion to the degree of danger, persists beyond the threat or becomes maladaptive for a given individual (Marks, 1987). At the end of the last century, these states were described as "neuroses" by Freud who viewed them as the result of unconscious conflicts originating in childhood. Another psychiatrist, Janet called them "psychasthenia" and suggested that they were related to a decrease of psychological tension leading to a lack of adaptation to reality. However, rather than focussing on common denominators of pathological anxiety, recent research has put more emphasis on defining the differences existing between its various clinical expressions. This evolution was due in part to the development of behavioural and cognitive approaches which distinguish between three major components in the expression of pathological anxiety: cognitive (psychological), somatic (physiological) and behavioural. These distinctions have contributed immensely to better definition, understanding and treatment of the various clinical expressions of pathological anxiety. Among these components, the cognitive aspect remains essential for the diagnosis of anxiety disorders in general; furthermore, its qualitative features are essential in defining the major subcategories of these disorders. The somatic dimension is also always present but to various degrees; most clinical studies however have failed to demonstrate significant correlations between the intensity of the subjective experience of anxiety and that of its physiological components. The behavioural component, eg avoidance or compulsion, is not always associated with the two previous ones; when present its evolution over time does not always parallel that of the other components. Such discordance has been well documented in studies on the efficacy of cognitive-behavioural therapies and has lead to the concept of "desynchrony" between the various components of anxiety (Rachman and Hodgson, 1974). It is also noteworthy that the behavioural component of anxiety is the only one that can be assessed through animal models while in clinical experience behavioural modifications are not always present and most of the time not specific for the diagnosis of a given disorder. Furthermore, the behavioural modifications elicited in numerous animal paradigms by objectively painful and/or stressful stimuli may be difficult to compare to the complex association of cognitive, somatic and behavioural consequences of stimuli that are neutral for the majority of humans but stressful for a minority of them due to their subjective and/or irrational evaluation of a given situation (Boulenger, 1991). Such discrepancies do not exist however in other paradigms, such as the conditioned emotional response (CER), where animals are made to respond adversely to stimuli that are neutral to others.

ANXIETY DISORDERS: PRESENT CLASSIFICATIONS

The 10th edition of the International Classification of Diseases (ICD-10) of the World Health Organization (1992) and the 4th edition of the Diagnostic and Statistical Manual (DSM-IV) of the American Psychiatric Association (1993) show a wide overlap in the nomenclature of anxiety disorders (Table I).

TABLE I: CURRENT CLASSIFICATIONS OF ANXIETY DISORDERS

DSM-IV	ICD-10

Panic disorders
  - with agoraphobia
  - without agoraphobia
Agoraphobia
Specific phobia
Social phobia
Obsessive-compulsive disorder
Post-traumatic stress disorder
Acute stress disorder
Generalized anxiety disorder
	Panic disorder
	Agoraphobia
	  - without panic disorder
	  - with panic disorder
	Specific phobia
	Social phobia
	Obsessive-compulsive disorder
	Post-traumatic stress disorder
	Acute stress reaction
	Generalized anxiety disorder
	Mixed anxiety and depressive disorder
	Neurasthenia

Though the main clinical features of these disorders appear very similar in both diagnostic systems, it is however noteworthy that the criteria necessary to fulfill specific diagnoses may differ between them leading sometimes to diagnostic discrepancies for the same patients. Nevertheless, the use of diagnostic systems and criteria have led to the development of structured diagnostic questionnaires that have considerably increased the validity and reliability of psychiatric diagnoses. They have also allowed a precise assessment of the extent of anxiety disorders and other psychiatric problems in the general population with a very good agreement between epidemiological studies done in Europe and in the United States (Lépine et al, 1993). In both continents, the life-time prevalence of anxiety disorders is about 15 % in the general population, phobic disorders being the most frequent; however, this prevalence rate increases to 30-40 % when surveys are done in primary care settings, a fact probably due to the frequent physical complaints that usually accompany these disorders and lead the patients to seek medical evaluations. The main clinical syndromes recognized by both classifications are panic disorders and agoraphobia, obsessive-compulsive disorders, phobic disorders and generalized anxiety disorders.

1) Panic disorders and agoraphobia

Though the life-time prevalence of panic disorders ranges from 1-2 % in the general population, it is certainly the most frequent diagnostic category encountered in medical or psychiatric settings. This frequency is related to the high level of physical distress experienced by these patients and also to the frequent complications occuring in the course of this disorder, both reasons also leading to a socio-economic burden which is the highest among all psychiatric disorders (Klerman et al, 1991). Though the concept of panic disorders has been challenged by several European authors, it is now widely accepted that the repeated occurence of sudden, unexpected episodes of severe anxiety (panic attacks) may lead to the developement of more chronic forms of anxiety: anticipatory anxiety and/or situational anxiety (agoraphobia). Anticipatory anxiety relates to the permanent apprehension that panic may reoccur unexpectedly inducing a state of hyperarousal and increased reactivity often described by patients as the "fear of fear". In contrast with the ethymological meaning of the word (fear of public places), agoraphobia relates to the fear of various situations in which the occurence of panic attacks could be embarassing or distressing for the patient. The most common situations inducing distress and/or avoidance in agoraphobic patients are: driving a car, waiting in line, shopping, crowded places, bridges, tunnels, elevators, public transportations... sometimes leading to major limitations in social or professional occupations. The first panic attacks usually occur without immediate reasons but secondarily to various stressful life-events (surgery, loss of relatives or friends, delivery, divorce...) to sleep deprivation, to drug withdrawal or intoxication (caffeine, cocaïne, marijuana). They are associated with intense physical symptoms, probably reflecting a sudden autonomic dysfunction, to the fear of an impending doom: dying, loosing control, fainting, falling, becoming mad... According to recent research, this fear is related to a cognitive bias leading these patients to interpret sudden physiological symptoms as the precursors of a possible catastrophy. However, it is not known if this "catastrophic interpretation" bias preceeds the first panic attacks or is secondary to their sudden and unexpected onset (Barlow, 1988). The fact that panic attacks may awaken patients from their sleep suggests that biological mechanisms also play a major role in the occurence of these episodes. These biological mechanisms probably involve a dysregulation of the central noradrenergic system but might implicate other neurotransmitter systems as well. Clinical research has shown that these patients have an increased response compared to normal controls when challenged with anxiogenic agents other than those affecting the noradrenergic system: caffeine, sodium lactate, CO_2, cholecystokinin, methyl-chlorophenylpiperazine (mCPP),... However, the frightening effect of any sudden physiological symptom in these patients costs doubts about the specificity of these challenges: up to now the increased psychological response to anxiogenic agents reported in panic disorder was rarely accompanied with modifications of biological markers that would confirm the would confirm the existence of a biological dysfunction in these patients.

Though panic attacks are frequent during adolescence, panic disorders usually begins during early adulthood. The evolution of the disorder is irregular: in about one third of the patients symptoms will abate spontaneously after a few month, while in another third anxiety symptoms will become chronic symptoms. Furthermore, several kinds of psychiatric complications are likely to happen in the course of panic disorder, especially alcoholism, depression and suicide attempts; an increased risk for cardio-vascular complications has also been suggested in a limited number of studies (Sims, 1984).

2) <u>Obsessive-compulsive disorders</u>

The life-time prevalence of obsessive-compulsive disorders in the general population is similar to that of panic disorders but its frequency as a reason of consultation is about 10 times lower. This is probably due to the chronic evolution of this disorder which, in contrast to panic disorders, rarely brings the patient in the medical system in relation to physical complaints. In obsessive-compulsive disorders, the main clinical feature is the occurence of intrusive ideas or images (obsessions) that are both senseless and unacceptable, thus inducing discomfort and anxiety and an active struggle in order to get rid of them. For example, ideas of contamination will induce severe anxiety that will be relieved through compulsive washing; in other patients, anxiety will be relieved through avoidance or other compulsions like counting or checking repeatedly. Usually starting during adolescence or early adulthood, obsessive-compulsive disorders progress most of the time slowly and rarely come to physician's attention before several years of evolution leading sometimes to a major handicap related to the extent of compulsive rituals. Some cases are so severe and resistant to usual treatments that neurosurgery is still performed in some countries for intractable cases of obsessive compulsive disorders. Cognitive-behavioural approaches have been successful in explaining and treating some of the key-features of this disorder (Marks, 1987). However, studies focusing on possible biological mechanisms involved in obsessive-compulsive disorders have yieldied information challenging the classification of this disorder among other anxiety disorders. Case-reports have suggested that obsessive-compulsive symptoms are more frequent in neurological disorders affecting the striatum, eg Tourette's disease, Huntington chorea and Parkinson's disease. Brain imaging studies also strongly suggest that a neuroanatomical network involving the prefrontal cortex, the striatum and the thalamus is implicated in the expression of obsessive-compulsive symptoms (Insel, 1992). This network could be affected both by neurosurgical procedures known to be useful in the treatment of this disorder and by serotonergic influences at the striatum level: in contrast to panic disorders patients who are sensitive to different kinds of antidepressants, patients with obsessive-compulsive disorders are known to respond specifically to serotonin reuptake inhibitors and not to MAOIs or noradrenaline reuptake inhibitors. However, up to now, clinical research have failed to demonstrate the existence of a serotonergic dysfunction in these patients; furthermore, the existence of similar brain imaging patterns in both obsessive-compulsive disorders and depression suggest that the specificity of these findings also remain to be demonstrated.

3) <u>Phobic disorders</u>

Phobic disorders have a life-time prevalence of 5-10 % in the general population, but rarely bring the patients to medical attention. In phobic disorders, the main clinical feature is that anxiety is related to a specific object or situation; when confronted with the stimulus patients will systematically experience a high level of discomfort or a panic attack. In many patients, avoidance behaviors will thus prevent the experience of painful anxiety symptoms. According to the nature of the stimuli feared by the patients, several kinds of phobic disorders have been described: 1) simple phobias most often related to heights, animals, insects or blood and injuries; 2) social phobias related to situations where the patient interacts with others, eg social gatherings and public speaking; 3) agoraphobia where situations feared by the patients are similar to those mentioned previously but not related to the occurence of unexpected panic attacks. It is noteworthy that specific phobias have different ages of onset, animal phobias beginning in early childhood, blood phobia in late childhood, social phobia in adolescence and agoraphobia in early adulthood. Usually, the course of phobic disorders is quite stable and is rarely associated with the bad prognosis observed in a fair number of panic disorders and obsessive-compulsive patients. Though phobic disorders are best explained in terms of psychological mechanisms, the "preparedness" theory of phobia suggests that genetic factors may explain why fears develop specifically towards stimuli that were probably meaningful in the evolution of mankind (stangers, animals) (Marks, 1987). It is also interesting that heredity also plays a role in the transmission of blood phobia, a fear characterized by a vagal reaction rather than the adrenergic symptoms usually observed with other phobic stimuli. Recent clinical research showing that MAOIs antidepressants may be specifically active in social phobics also suggest that biological factors may be involved in the pathogenesis of at least some these disorders (Boulenger, 1991).

4) <u>Generalized anxiety</u>

The life-time prevalence of generalized anxiety disorder is estimated to be between 4-6 % in the general population according to criteria requesting at least a 6 month duration to diagnose this condition. However, the amount of research concerning this disorder is limited due to the vagueness of its diagnostic criteria. Within anxiety disorders generalized anxiety is the diagnostic category with the lowest inter-rater reliability and its very existence is still a matter of controversy. Cognitive psychologists suggest that this disorder is characterized by excessive worrying concerning daily-life events and the overestimation of future possible problems (Barlow, 1988). On the other hand, psychiatrists believe that generalized anxiety is most of the time the consequence of other psychiatric problems, representing a residual symptomatology and/or a predisposing factor for depression or other anxiety disorders. Due to its chronicity, this condition is also difficult to distinguish from personality disorders and/or "trait anxiety". As opposed to "state anxiety" that is felt at a moment in time, "trait anxiety" refers to a habitual tendency to be anxious in general, a personality trait making a subject more likely to present anxiety symptoms in stressful situations; such a predisposing factor is very often found in patients with panic disorders or depression, prior to the onset of their symptoms. In generalized anxiety disorders, worrying is often associated with physical symptoms but rarely with behavioural ones. These patients usually benefit from non pharmacological treatments: relaxation, supportive therapy, cognitive therapy. However, it is noteworthy that in addition to benzodiazepines, antidepressant drugs may also be used successfully in patients requiring pharmacological treatment (Boulenger, 1991).

5) <u>Other anxiety disorders</u>

Other anxiety disorders include excessive reactions to stressful life-events, post-traumatic disorders being related to major stresses like natural catastrophy, agressions, serious accidents involving casualties... Though neurasthenia only appear in ICD-10, this syndrome is interesting in relation to the recent discussions surrounding the specificity of the concept of "chronic fatigue" syndrome (Schluederberg et al, 1992). At last, mixed anxiety-depression is a new diagnostic category introduced in the ICD-10 for the many patients seen in primary care settings and suffering brom both anxiety and depressive symptoms but not severe enough to fulfill criteria for specific anxiety or depressive disorders (Boulenger and Lavallée, 1993). As discussed later in this chapter, this concept also recognizes the intimate relationship existing between anxiety and depression symptoms in most patients suffering from psychiatric problems.

ANXIETY DISORDERS: ONE OR DIVISIBLE?

Though present classifications focus on clinical differences in the expression of anxiety disorders, it is also important to mention the wide overlap existing in the symptomatology, the evolution and the treatment of these disorders. Diagnostic comorbidity between anxiety disorders is frequent as well as their comorbidity with depressive disorders; furthermore, the presence of depressive symptoms (not fulfilling diagnostic criteria for major depressive disorders) is also frequent in the course of most anxiety disorders as well as the presence of symptoms belonging to other anxiety syndromes (Boulenger and Lavallée, 1993). Another difficulty existing in the diagnosis of these conditions is that the high comorbidity between symptoms, syndromes and/or diagnoses also exist when the evolution of these disorders is considered. For example, patients with phobic disorders may develop panic disorders and agoraphobia then depression, then generalized anxiety disorders, with a more or less complete disappearance of their previous symptoms. Taking into account this transversal as well as longitudinal comorbidity, authors like Tyrer (1989) proposed the identification of a "general neurotic syndrome" lumping together clinical entities that may have been abusively separated in current classifications. This syndrome would also include a background of common personality disturbances (anxious predisposition) and the association with a positive history family of similar conditions, i.e. anxiety and/or depressive disorders. Though the validity of this concept remains to be demonstrated, the hypothesis of a general neurotic syndrome is consistent with clinical research findings suggesting that common etiopathological factors underlie the expression of various symptoms of anxiety and depression. In a sample of 3798 pairs of unselected twins, Kendler et al (1987) have shown that traditional factor analysis of self-reported symptoms indicate that depression and anxiety tend to form separate symptom clusters, but that multivariate genetic analysis showed that genes act largely in a non specific way to influence the overall level of psychiatric symptomatology; in contrast, environmental factors appeared largely responsible for the separation between anxiety and depression symptom clusters. The hypothesis of a common genetic predisposition to various anxiety disorders and depression is also supported by family studies, showing that relatives of patients with a specific disorder show higher rates of depression and anxiety disorders in general that relatives of normal controls. Finally, an extensive review of psychometric studies also suggest that a common general distress factor characterized by feelings of inferiority and rejection, demoralization, self-consciousness and general affective distress exist in patients with depression or anxiety disorders as well as in subjects with sub-syndromal levels of these symptoms; numerous studies have confirmed that this "neurotic" factor was stable as a personality trait and showed a significant heritability (Clark and Watson, 1991).These various findings suggesting the existence of a pathogenic factor common to several anxiety disorders and depression are also supported by the common efficacy of cognitive-behavioural approaches in these patients, a fact that led J. Wolpe (1988) - one of the father of behaviour therapy - to call for a renascence of the concept of neurosis. Furthermore, these concepts are also supported by the efficacy of antidepressant drugs over a wide spectrum of syndromes including depression, panic disorders, obsessive-compulsive disorders, phobic disorders and generalized anxiety disorders (Boulenger, 1991). This efficacy is not related to the level of depression experienced by these patients and develops progressively over time without major differences in the doses necessary to obtain relief of the different target-symptoms i.e. depression, obsessions-compulsions, panic attacks or general anxiety, suggesting a common mode of action across these disorders. Hudson and Hope (1990) have even suggested that the therapeutic spectrum of antidepressants may also include other disorders such as boulimia, enuresis, chronic pain, that could also belong to a wide spectrum of "affective disorders" sharing a common pathophysiology.

CONCLUSION

Recent clinical research support Freud's and Janet's opinion that common etiopathogenic factors may exist among anxiety disorders and between anxiety and depressive disorders. This hypothesis should be kept in mind when studying anxiety disorders which are considered in most patients as the result of three major influences: 1) predisposing factors; 2) precipitating factors; 3) factors involved in the expression and the maintenance of emotional symptoms. Diagnostic classifications are important to operationalize clinical research in these areas and their introduction has spurred a major progress in the field of psychiatry. However, one should be aware of their limitations. As stated by the DSM-IV task force (American Psychiatric Association, 1993): "In DSM-IV, there is no assumption that each category of mental disorder is a completely discrete entity with absolute boundaries dividing it from other mental disorders or from no mental disorder. There is also no assumption that all people described as having the same mental disorder are alike in all important ways. This outlook allows greater flexibility in the use of the system, encourages more specific attention to boundary cases, and emphasized the need to capture additional clinical information that goes beyond diagnosis."

REFERENCES

American Psychiatric Association (1993): DSM-IV draft criteria. Washington: *American Psychiatric Press*.
Barlow, D.H. (1988): Anxiety and its disorders: the nature and treatment of anxiety and panic. New York, London: *The Guilford Press*.
Boulenger, J.P. (1991): Animal models of anxiety: what do they mean? In *Animal models of psychiatric disorders. Vol. 3*. ed. P. Soubrié, pp. 20-23. Basel: *Karger*.
Boulenger, J.P. (1991): Role of antidepressants in anxiety disorders. In *Current practices and future developments in the pharmacotherapy of mental disorders*, ed. H.Y. Meltzer and D. Nerozzi, pp. 183-190. Amsterdam: *Excerpta Medica*.

Boulenger, J.P., and Lavallée, Y.J.(1993): Mixed anxiety and depression: diagnostic issues. *J. Clin. Psychiatry* 54 (1, suppl.):3-8.

Clark, L.A., and Watson, D. (1991): Tripartite model of anxiety and depression: psychometric evidence and taxonomic implications. *J. Abnorm. Psychol.* 100: 316-336.

Hudson, J.I., and Hope, H.G. (1990): Affective spectrum disorder: does antidepressant response identify a family of disorders with a common pathophysiology? *Am. J. Psychiatry* 147: 552-564.

Insel, T.R. (1992): Toward a neuroanatomy of obsessive-compulsive disorder. *Arch. Gen. Psychiatry*, 49: 739-744.

Kendler, K.S, Heath, A.C. et al (1987): Symptoms of anxiety and symptoms of depression: same genes, different environment? *Arch. Gen. Psychiatry* 44: 451-457.

Klerman, G.L., Weissman, M.M. et al (1991): Panic Attacks in the Community: Social Morbidity and Health Care Utilization. *JAMA* 265:742-746.

Lépine, J.P., Wittchen, H.U. et al (1993): Lifetime and current comorbidity of anxiety and affective disorders: Results from the International WHO/ADAMHA CIDI field trials. *Int. J. Methods Psychiatr. Res.* (in press)

Marks, I.M. (1987).: Fears, phobias and rituals: panic, anxiety and their disorders. New York: *Oxford University Press*.

Rachman, S.J., and Hodgson, R.S. (1974): Synchrony and desynchrony in fear and avoidance. *Behav. Res. Ther.* 12: 311-318.

Schluederberg, A., Straus, S.E. et al (1992): Chronic Fatigue Syndrome Research: Definition and Medical Outcome Assessment. *Ann. Int. Med.* 117:325-331.

Sims, A. (1984): Neurosis and mortality: investigation and association. *J. Psychosom. Res.* 28:353-362.

Tyrer, P. (1989): Classification of neurosis. Chichester, New York: *John Wiley*.

Wolpe, J. (1988): The renascence of neurotic depression: its varied dynamics and implications for outcome research. *J. Nerv. Ment. Dis.* 176: 607-613.

World Health Organization (1992): The ICD-10 classification of mental and behavioural disorders: clinical and diagnostic guidelines. Geneva: *WHO*.

Résumé

Les systèmes modernes de classification distinguent plusieurs sous-catégories au sein des troubles anxieux. Des caractéristiques cliniques comme les symptômes, l'évolution et les complications possibles permettent de différencier plusieurs entités diagnostiques telles que les troubles panique, les troubles phobiques, les troubles obsessifs-compulsifs et l'anxiété généralisée. La définition de critères spécifiques à chacune de ces catégories a représenté une étape majeure pour l'évolution de la recherche psychiatrique en permettant une meilleure fiabilité des évaluations cliniques et le développement de questionnaires diagnostiques structurés qui ont largement contribué à l'augmentation importante des recherches épidémiologiques en santé mentale au cours de la dernière décennie. Les systèmes diagnostiques sont soumis à un processus de révision régulier, tenant compte des résultats des recherches cliniques les plus récentes. Dans le domaine de l'anxiété, les résultats préliminaires de ces dernières suggèrent que des mécanismes étiologiques communs rattachent plusieurs types de troubles anxieux et certains troubles dépressifs. Bien que ces données soient peu susceptibles de modifier à brève échéance les systèmes de classification existants, elles sont néanmoins importantes pour améliorer notre compréhension et notre traitement de ces troubles psychiatriques fréquents et souvent invalidants.

Anxiety: Neurobiology, Clinic and Therapeutic Perspectives. Eds M. Hamon, H. Ollat, M.-H. Thiébot. Colloque INSERM/ John Libbey Eurotext Ltd. © 1993, Vol. 232, pp. 15-23.

Provocative agents and the biology of panic attacks

Michel Bourin*, Jacques Bradwejn**, Mary Kay Nixon*

*GIS Médicament, Faculté de Médecine, 44035 Nantes Cedex 01, France; ** St-Mary's Hospital Centre, Mc Gill University, 3820 Lacombe Avenue, Montréal H3T1M5, Canada*

SUMMARY

The use of provocative agents has greatly helped in the under standing of the neurobiological mechanisms of panic attacks. Various agents such as sodium lactate, carbon dioxide (CO_2), caffeine, yohimbine, isoproterenol and cholecystokinin (CCK) have been utilized as panicogenes in healthy volunteers as well as panic patients. In the same manner, different neurotransmitter systems, have been explored in an attempt to understand the etiology of panic disorder. Generally most provocative agents lack in specificity, limiting their use in identifying neurotransmitter systems involved in panic attacks. On the other hand, CCK appears to offer several advantages over other challenge strategies such as lactate, CO_2, or caffeine. It exists as a neurotransmitter in the human CNS, with its own neuronal pathways and receptors. In high incidence, it reliably provokes panic attacks in a dose dependent manner. In general, it is considered more physiologically compatible when used in humans in panic disorder research. What now remains to be clarified is the relationship between CCK and noradrenergic and serotoninergic systems in the understanding of the neurobiology os panic attacks.

INTRODUCTION

The neurobiology of panic disorders has been the subject of exhaustive research. Some authors have suggested that panic attacks may be triggered by a central nervous system dysfunction in mid-brain structures that involve noradrenergic and serotoninergic neurotransmitter systems. Exhaustive reviews of these theories appear in several publications (GORMAN and coll. 1989, REDMOND 1987).
Studies of cerebral disorders underlying panic attacks have developed rapidly over the last decade. Two main research approaches have been adopted.
The first relates to laboratory studies using panicogenes such as lactate, carbon dioxide (CO_2), caffeine, yohimbine, isoproterenol and cholecystokinin (CCK). The second relates to understanding the mechanism of action of antipanic agents. The use of these two approaches has helped in identifying neurotransmitter systems which may be involved in panic attacks.

I - STUDIES WITH SODIUM LACTATE

Intravenous perfusions of sodium lactate, 0.5 to 1 M, induced panic attacks in 26 to 100% of patients presenting with panic disorder (PD). This is in opposition to healthy volunteers in which IV sodium lactate induced panic attacks in only 0 to 30% of cases (MARGRAF et al. 1986). It must be noted however that there is an overlap between results obtained from PD patients and those from healthy volunteers. Patients with major depression, presenting with secondary panic attacks have a response to I.V. sodium lactate which is similar to PD patients (COWLEY et al. 1986) while patients with major depression without panic attacks have panic responses similar to normal controls (Mc GRATH et al. 1988). There seems to be no difference in response however with patients who have occasional panic attacks and those with more persistant panic attacks. These studies suggest that the panicogenic response to lactate is related to panic attacks more than to PD.

The same patients without panic attack, however, respond to lactate like patients presenting with PD. For example, generalized anxiety patients respond with a similar increase in anxiety as those patients presenting with PD. On the other hand, the amount of lactate that induced panic attacks in patients with social phobia resembles that which was also observed in patients with PD (LIEBOWITZ et al. 1985). Although the initial report suggested that social phobics did not panic with lactate, later studies by the same group of researchers found that they did. It seems that instead of being related to a history of panic attacks, a panicogenic response to lactate is associated with the pre-test level of anxiety. Significant anxiety before the test is a major predictor of a panic response to lactate in patients presenting with PD as well as with normal subjects (YERAGANI et al. 1987).

In spite of twenty years of study, the mechanism that underlies panic attacks induced by lactate remains unknown. Blood levels of norepinephrine or epinephrine are not elevated when panic is induced by lactate, suggesting that panic is not related to an increase in norepinephrine function (GAFFNEY et al. 1988). Also, an elevation of central norepinephrine function does not appear to explain the action of sodium lactate (POHL et al 1987, CARN et al. 1986). Panic attacks induced by lactate are not associated with increased concentrations of norepinephrine metabolites such as 3-methoxy-4-hydroxyphenylglycol (MHPG). On the other hand, metabolic alkalosis is probably not the mechanism of action. Considering that sodium lactate and sodium bicarbonate induce panic attacks and increase concentrations of CO_2, this increase in CO_2 has been proposed as a mechanism of action. It was suggested that patients presenting with PD are hypersensitive to CO_2 and that chronically they hyperventilate to reduce their blood concentration of CO_2 (GORMAN et al. 1989b) when CO_2 concentrations increase. It was hypothesized that CO_2 induced panic attacks, based on studies where the inhalation of CO_2 induced panic attacks in patients with PD but not in normal subjects.

II - STUDIES WITH CARBON DIOXIDE

Inhalation of air containing 4 to 7.5 per cent carbon dioxide clearly induced panic attacks in patients with panic disorder and a single inhalation of 35 per cent CO_2 in O_2 induced panic attacks in patients with PD but not with controls (GRIEZ et al. 1987, FYER et al. 1987). The percentage of patients and healthy subjects that panic with CO_2 differ according to studies. This could be due to different criteria used to define panic attacks or the various methods used to administer CO_2. Nevertheless, the results generally indicate that panic disorder patients are hypersensitive to the effects of CO_2 inhalation. As with lactate, the specificity of the diagnosis of anxiety induced by CO_2 is contestable in that 64% of women with premenstruel tension and without a previous history of panic can experience panic attack after a single administration of 35 per cent CO_2 in O_2. Psychological factors play an important role in those who experience panic induced by CO_2. SANDERSON et al. 1989 found that when patients who presented with panic attacks had the illusion of controlling the quantity of CO_2 inhaled they panicked much less than when they did not have this illusion. As previously stated, the hypothesis was made that CO_2 and lactate, after being metabolized to CO_2, induced panic attacks by stimulation of respiratory centers which are more likely hypersensitive in this type of patient. Nevertheless, it is not easy to understand what causes panic attacks. KLEIN and GORMAN 1987 have proposed that CO_2 stimulates the locus coeruleus, the most important cortical cell group where norepinephrine is localized. These authors believe that CO_2 is able to induce panic attacks by augmenting norepinephrine activity. The link between panicogenic effects of CO_2 and stimulation of the locus coeruleus is interesting, however, this is not in agreement with the noradrenergic theory of PD. Panic disorder and panic attacks induced by CO_2 do not appear to be associated with an elevation of norepinephrine. As well, panic attacks induced by CO_2 do not augment blood levels of MHPG.

III - STUDIES WITH CAFFEINE

It has been demonstrated that caffeine can cause anxiety and a review by UHDE 1988 addresses this association. Anecdotal reports have put forth evidence suggesting that caffeine intoxication can at times mimic panic attacks and generalized anxiety. Direct evidence of the action of caffeine was obtained by studying its effects in a double blind placebo controlled study with both panic disorder patients and normal subjects. Results indicated that patients with panic disorder were more sensitive to the panicogenic effects of caffeine than normal controls (BOULENGER and UHDE, 1982). In an initial study, UHDE and coll. 1984, compared various doses of caffeine 240, 450 and 720 mg of caffeine base and placebo were administered orally to eight healthy volunteers. Even with this small dose range it was demonstrated that a dose-effect relationship exists between the amount of caffeine administered and anxiety as measured by the Zung scale. Two of the eight volunteers presented with characteristic panic attacks after receiving 720 mg of caffeine. This suggests that caffeine, at high enough doses, can be anxiogenic and even panicogenic in normal subjects. In order to study differential effects of caffeine in panic disorder patients and healthy volunteers, the authors chose to use 480 mg of caffeine, which caused moderate anxiogenic effects but did not induce panic attacks in control subjects. Thus, a dose of 480 mg was chosen in the later study involving 24 panic disorder patients and 16 normal controls. Subjects received either placebo or 480 mg of caffeine in this second study. Nine of 24 patients (37,5%) and none of 14 healthy volunteers exhibited panic attacks after administration of caffeine. Those who panicked presented with symptoms very similar to that of a normal panic attack. None of the patients in the study nor the normal controls presented with panic attacks when receiving placebo.

These preliminary results suggest that patients presenting with panic disorder were more sensitive to the panicogenic effects of caffeine than normal controls. In an identical study, CHARNEY et al. 1985, used a caffeine model in which 10 mg/kg of caffeine citrate was given to patients with PD and normal controls. Twenty one patients presenting with DSMIII criterea for panic disorder or agoraphobia with panic attacks and seventeen normal controls participated in the study. Fifteen of the twenty one patients (71%) had panic attacks while none of the controls experienced panic attacks in response to caffeine.
In the two studies discussed panic attacks induced by caffeine were considered very similar to spontaneous panic attacks. Several patients did though have vague symptoms of panic attack after caffeine.
The dose of caffeine used by UHDE and coll. 1984 is not comparable to that of CHARNEY and coll. 1985. For example, the latter used caffeine citrate of which there is only 50 % caffeine as compared to the molecular weight of caffeine base. The difference in results could however be easily explained by the fact that caffeine base is considered to have less bioavailability than caffeine citrate.

IV - STUDIES WITH CHOLECYSTOKININ

Cholecystokinin (CCK) is the most abundant neuropeptide in the mammalian cerebral cortex and limbic system (CRAWLEY, 1985). CCK is evident in significant quantities in regions known to be important in the mediation of panic disorder, including the cerebral cortex, striatum, amygdala, hippocampus and brainstem nuclei where it is believed to function as a neurotransmitter or neuromodulator. Specific CCK recognition sites, presently divided into CCK-A and CCK-B subtypes, have been characterized and drugs selectively active on these receptor subtypes have been synthetized (WOODRUFF and HUGHES, 1991)
Interest in the role of CCK in anxiety and panic stems from a microiontophoretic experiment which showed that benzodiazepines selectively attenuated the excitatory action of $CCK-8_S$ on hippocampal pyramidal neurons in rats (BRADWEJN and MONTIGNY, 1984).

The electrophysiological studies mentioned above used $CCK-8_S$ but evidence suggested that this form did not cross the mammalian blood-brain barrier, therefore the tetrapeptide form (CCK-4) was used for human administration.
In a pilot study, the behavioral effects of CCK-4 were evaluated in patients with panic disorder (BRADWEJN et al., 1990). Eleven untreated patients ranging in age from 20 to 51 years participated in the study. Using a double-blind methodology patients were challenged with CCK-4 (50 µg) and placebo on two separate days. All 11 patients panicked with CCK-4 while none of the patients panicked with placebo. The patients clearly indicated that the CCK-4 induced attacks were phenomenologically very similar or identical to their usual panic attacks. The only obvious difference was that the onset of the attacks was more abrupt with the peptide.
These preliminary reports indicated that CCK-4 was panicogenic in man and could provide a pharmacologic model of panic attacks. To further establish the relevance of CCK-4 as a specific biological challenge strategy, our group set out to establish whether this neuropeptide possessed other characteristics of a panicogenic agents (BRADWEJN et al., 1991b). The seven criteria for an "ideal" challenge agent proposed by GUTTMACHER et al. (1983) and GORMAN et al. (1987) were considered in evaluating CCK-4.
So far, we have demonstrated that CCK-4 satisfies six of the seven criteria (BRADWEJN et al. 1993, BRADWEJN et al., 1991a,c): (1) it is safe for use in humans; > 400 subjects have received CCK-4 without any significant adverse effects being observed: (2) it reliably reproduces the emotional and somatic symptoms that accompany panic attacks (3) patients equate the induced attacks to their usual attacks (4) panic patients show an enhanced sensitivity to the panicogenic effects of CCK-4 compared with subjects with no personal or family history of panic attacks: (5) the effects of CCK-4 are consistent and reproducible (BRADWEJN et al.); and behave in a dose-related manner, (6) the effects of CCK-4 are antagonized by imipramine (7) the effects of CCK-4 are not antagonized by non antipanic agents .
In addition to satisfying most criteria for an ideal challenge agent, we have also shown that the behavioral effects of CCK-4 are similar to those produced by CO_2 (BRADWEJN and KOSZYCKI, 1991; KOSZYCKI et al., 1991). In one study (BRADWEJN and KOSZYCKI, 1991b), 22 panic disorder patients received either 25 µg of CCK-4 or a single inhalation of 35% CO_2 in oxygen. Although there was a tendency for more patients to panic with CCK-4 than with CO_2, the panic attacks induced with either agent were quantitatively and qualitatively similar. In a second study (KOSZYCKI et al., 1991) with 26 healthy volunteers, we found that the panic rate was similar for 25 µg of CCK-4 (17%) and 35% CO_2 (21%). These findings indicated that CCK-4 is at least as potent as CO_2 in provoking panic attacks and raises the possibility that both agents might act on the same neurobiological system or on separate

systems with a final common pathway. The comparison of CCK-4 with other provocation agents, particularly sodium lactate which is the most extensively studied agent, might shed light on whether panic attacks stem from anomalies in a single chain of events and may also help identify specific neurotransmitter systems which might be involved.

Considering that benzodiazepinzes (BZD) receptor agonists antagonise CCK induced excitation of rat hippocampal neurons, a study was performed to determine whether CCK-4 might act as an inverse agonist of BZD receptors. Healthy volunteers (20 M; 10 F) were pre-treated with flumazenil (2 mg i.v.), the BZD receptor antagonist, or placebo (0,9 % NaCl i.v.) 15 mins before CCK challenge (50 mg i.v.), in a randomized, double-bind, crossover design. Responses were evaluated with the Panic Symptom Scale DSM III-R criteria, including moderate to severe anxiety, were used to judge the occurence of a panic attack. The panic rate following CCK-4 was similar for flumazenil (13/30) and placebo (14/30). Treatment effects and treatment by injection period interactions were not statistically significant for the number, sum intensity and duration of symptoms. Mean (± SD) scores for flumazenil and placebo respectively were 10.57 ± 3.3 and 10.87 ± 3.3 for the number of symptoms, 24.03 ± 11.6 and 23.80 ± 11.9 for the sum intensity of symptoms and 111.57 ± 37.7 and 123.23 ± 47.5 seconds for the duration of symptoms. These findings do not support the hypothesis that CCK-4 acts as a BZD receptor inverse agonist in inducing panic in normals (BRADWEJN et al., in press).

The effect of L-365, 260, a CCK_B antagonist was investigated on CCK-4 induced panic attacks in panic disorder (PD) was investigated. Patients were treated with L-365,260 (10 or 50 mg PO) or placebo 90 minutes before a challenge with a submaximal dose of I.V. CCK-4 (20 µg). Twenty four patients were entered; 3 patients received a single challenge and 21 patients were challenged on two occasions according to a double blind, incomplete block design. The panic rate following challenge with CCK-4 was as follows: 13/15 (placebo), 5/15 (10 mg), and 0/15 (50 mg); $p < 0.01$ for 10 mg and 50 mg against placebo. The adjusted mean (± SD) sum intensity scores on the Panic Symptom Scale were 37.2 ± 15.6 (placebo) 25.7 ± 16.3 (10 mg) and 12.4 ± 15.9 (50 mg). Differences between 50 mg and placebo were statiscally significant ($p < 0.01$) and differences between 10 mg and placebo approached significance ($p = 0.07$). These data demonstrate that L-365,260 can block CCK-4-induced panic

Cholecystokinin tetrapeptide (CCK-4) given i.v. to African green monkeys, has profound and dose-related effects on behaviors thought to reflect anxiety and panic (ERVIN et al., 1991).

These behaviors are potently and dose-responsively reduced by non-peptide CCK-B antagonists of several pharmacological classes. They are incompletely, or less potently blocked by non-peptide CCK-A antagonists. Analysis of the effects of putative "central" and "peripheral" antagonists has not been completed.

In monkeys the effects of CCK-4 are also potently antagonized by adenosine A2 agonists and by anxiolytics derived from benzodiazepines. Adenosine A1 agonists such as cyclopropyladenosine fail to block CCK-4 induced behaviors, and when given alone, elicit behaviors characteristic of anxiety. In rodents, adenosine A2 agonists elevate brain serotonin and reduce brain norepinephrine, while adenosine A1 agonists produce the reverse profile. These and other data form the basis for a hypothesis stating that the anxiogenic effects of CCK-4 can be reduced by noradrenergic blockade and or adrenergic depletion and exacerbated by noradrenergic agonists. Preliminary results suggest that propranolol, but not atenolol, incompletely reduces CCK-4 behaviors in African green monkeys, and that short-term depletion of catecholamine precursors via amino acid loading likewise reduces the anxiogenic effects of CCK-4.

In previous studies it was found that the intraventricular administration of cholecystokinin tetrapeptide (CCK-4, 200 ng), a selective agonist at CCK_B receptors, significantly potentiated the defensive agressiveness in male Wistar rats, whereas caerulein (200 ng), an nonselective CCK agonist, decreased the number of fights between animals. Intraventricular injection of pentagastrin, an agonist of CCK_B receptors, at high doses (CCK-5, 5-10 mg) when combined with provocations (slight blowing on the rat) induced behaviour which could be considered panic-like. Namely, rats shrieked, jumped suddenly out of the test box, and moved with long jumps into the corner of the experimental room where they stayed completely notioneless for several minutes.

Various CCK agonists (caerulein, CCK-8, CCK-5, CCK-4) induced the anxiogenic-like effect in the elevated plus-maze test. This anxiogenic-like effect of CCK agonists was correlated with their affinity for CCK_B receptors in the cerebral cortex, but not CCK_A receptors in the pancreas (table 1).

Table 1

THE CORRELATION BETWEEN ANXIOGENIC-LIKE EFFECT OF CCK AGONISTS AND THEIR AFFINITY AT CCK RECEPTORS IN THE RAT CEREBRAL CORTEX AND PANCREAS

CCK agonist	Anti-exploratory effect in plus-maze (pmol/kg)	IC50 values against 3H-pCCK-8	
		cerebral cortex	pancreas
		(nM)	(nM)
Caerulein	0.074	1.1	0.6
Pentagastrin	0.670	10	6200
CCK-4	17.3	411	> 10000
Pearson's		0.9999	0.808
		$p = 0.008$	$p > 0.4$

The nonselective CCK agonist, caerulein, reduced exploratory activity of rats after systemic (VASAR et al., 1993) as well as intraventricular administration (SINGH et al., 1991). Comparison of doses of caerulein, affecting the exploratory activity of rats after the intraventricular (minimal effective dose 1.3 mg per rat) (SINGH et al., 1991) and subcutaneous treatment with caerulein (minimal effective dose 0.0425 mg per rat) (VASAR et al., 1993), does not support the idea that forebrain CCK_B receptors are involved in the action of peripherally injected CCK agonist. However, subdiaphragmatic vagotomy, which antagonized the motor depressant effect of caerulein, did not affect the anti-exploratory action of CCK agonist. Therefore, it is very unlikely that the anxiogenic-like action of caerulein is located in the gastrointestinal tract. Pretreatment of rats with devazepide (1 mg/kg), a preferential antagonist at CCK_A receptors, potentiated that anti-exploratory action of caerulein. By contrast, CCK_B antagonists LY 288513 (1 mg/kg) and L-365,260 (10 mg/kg) completely reversed this of CCK agonist effect.

In conclusion, it seems most likely that CCK_B receptors located in brainstem structures are responsible for the proagressive and anxiogenic-like effects of CCK agonists in the rat. Moreover, an obvious antagonism exists between CCK_A and CCK_B receptors in the regulation of emotional behaviour.

V - THE NORADRENERGIC SYSTEM

REDMOND and HUANG (1979) were the first to propose that hyperactivity of the locus coeruleus (LC) is linked with anxiety. Their theory was based partially on the observation that stimulation of the locus coeruleus induced fear in monkeys. This behavior appeared after electrical stimulation of the LC as well as after chemical stimulation with alpha 2 adrenergic receptor antagonists such as yohimbine. Yohimbine acts by blocking the presynaptic alpha 2 receptor, thereby augmenting the amount of norepinephrine available to stimulate the locus coeruleus. This hypothesis appeared to be confirmed when it was found that yohimbine induced more anxiety and panic attacks in panic patients when compared to normal subjects. Patients who panicked with yohimbine had MHPG plasma concentrations higher that those who did not panic. Clonidine, on the other hand, diminishes noradrenergic function via stimulation of alpha 2 pre-synaptic receptors, reduces anxiety in panic patients, and induces significant decreases in MHPG compared to patient controls. These results strongly suggest that the sensitivity of pre-synaptic alpha 2 receptors is increased in panic patients.

Another point to be raised is regarding the post-synaptic function of alpha 2 receptors and the measurement of human growth hormone (GH) in response to clonidine stimulation. In effect, release of GH probably depends on stimulation of alpha 2 post synaptic receptors, for example with clonidine. Many researchers have found that the release of GH is altered in panic patients. This suggests that the reduction of sensitivity of post-synaptic receptors in panic patients could be explained by a compensatory mechanism augmenting the availability of norepinephrine at the post synaptic receptor level.

However, the exaggerated reduction in arterial pressure with clonidine indicates an augmented sensitivity of alpha 2 post synaptic receptors.

Even if this hypothesis is true, many of the results of studies described above have not been reproduced. For example, UHDE et al., 1989 found an equal reduction in arterial pressure after clonidine in panic patients and normal subjects. Other researchers have found normal GH release in panic patients after clonidine administration. In the same manner, the cortisol response to clonidine was shown to be equivalent in panic patients and normal subjects. If panic attacks are correlated with an increase in norepinephrine function, one would predict that MHPG concentrations (CHARNEY and coll., 1983) would be elevated during panic attacks. This however was not found. The single proven fact remains the association between yohimbine and elevated MHPG concentrations.

The anxiogenic effect of yohimbine, however, does not seem to correlate with elevated noradrenergic function. In a study of 10 normal volunteers, 10 mg per os of diazepam antagonized anxiety induced by 30 mg per os of yohimbine but did not antagonize the elevation of MHPLG levels. It may be that the increase in MHPG induced by yohimbine does not reflect increases which may occur during spontaneous attacks. It should also be noted that naturally occuring panic attacks (ie those not induced by a pharmacological agent) do not elevate MHPG levels either.

Therapeutic studies with panic disorder also tend to argue against the role of alpha 2 receptor abnormalities in panic. If norepinephrine hyperactivity is implicated in panic states, one would expect that agents which diminish noradrenergic activity could be therapeutically active.

Long term antipanic effects of clonidine were examined in two studies. One placebo controlled study lasting 4 weeks used on average 2.7 mg/day of clonidine in 23 patients of which 14 had a history of panic disorder. Only three panic disorder patients improved significantly while 3 had their condition aggravated.

In another placebo controlled study involving 18 panic patients over a 10 week period, clonidine at doses > 2 mg/day was not effective in antagonizing spontaneous panic attacks. Additionally, propranolol displays a weak therapeutic action in P.D.

VI - THE SEROTONINERGIC SYSTEM

Much of the evidence from animal studies shows that a decrease in serotoninergic function causes a reduction in anxiety while an elevation of this function can induce anxiety (for a review, see KAHN et al., 1988). Recent studies in humans indicate that serotonin, in the regulation of anxiety, acts on three types of receptors, that is 5 HT1a, 5 HT2, and 5 HT3 receptors. In man, M-chloro-phenyl-piperazine (MCPP), which is a direct 5 HT agonist at 5 HT1 and 5 HT2 receptors, induces anxiety. MCPP injected intravenously at a dose of 0.1 mg/kg induced anxiety and panic attacks in panic patients and normal subjects. This effect appears to be linked to dose and route of administration. Other researchers used MCPP orally at a dose of 0.5 mg/kg, and did not demonstrate anxiety in normal subjects. Using a smaller dose orally, 0.25 mg/kg, it was shown that MCPP could augment anxiety and panic attacks in panic patients but not in normal subjects.

Based on these last results it was hypothesized that panic patients are hypersensitive to the anxiogenic effects of MCPP, likely due to increased sensitivity of post-synaptic 5 HT receptors. Hormonal responses to MCPP appear to corroborate this hypothesis. While a weak dose of MCPP, 0.25 mg/kg orally, causes increased release of cortisol only in panic patients, larger doses, eg. 0.1 mg/kg, this time given intravenously, increased cortisol levels in panic patients as well as controls. Administration of 60 mg fenfluramine, a 5 HT agonist, orally provides further evidence to complement the hypothesis of hypersensitive receptors. Fenfluramine induced anxiety and panic attacks and elevated release of cortisol and prolactin in female panic patients, in contrast with normal subjects and patients presenting with major depression. DEN BOER and WESTENBERG (1990), however using 5 hydroxy-tryptophan (5 HTP) as a stimulating agent, found a similar release of cortisol in panic patients and normal subjects. The majority of normal subjects and 10 out of 20 patients vomitted during the test, making interpretation of results difficult.

In a study using tryptophan, the precursor of serotonin, it was demonstrated that prolactin levels were normal in panic patients. More interesting is that fenfluramine and MCPP, in opposition to tryptophan, induced exaggerated behavioral responses in panic patients suggesting that the 5 HT deficit is presynaptic. Another explanation is that the effects of MCPP might be on other neurotransmitter systems. Therapeutic studies with panic patients and indirect serotonin agonists such as 5 HTP, as well as clomipramine and fluvoxamine which are inhibitors of serotonin reuptake, have demonstrated biphasic responses, that is an initial exacerbation of symptoms followed by an amelioration of symptoms. This phenomenon has not frequently been described in the many studies using 5 HT agonists in depression. 5 HT has effects on the noradrenergic system and the principal metabolite of clomipramine (desmethyl-clomipramine) possesses NA uptake inhibition properties. Therefore, initial aggravation of symptoms could be attributed to increased noradrenergic activity. It might also be explained by the initial decrease in 5 HT neurotransmission which eventually leads to enhanced 5 HT transmission.

CONCLUSION

The use of provocative agents has greatly helped in the understanding of neurobiological mechanisms of panic attacks. However, the lack of specificity of many provocative agents has limited their use in the identification of neurotransmitter systems which might be involved in panic attacks.

It has been demonstrated that CCK-4 possesses panicogenic activity in man and animals and that it may represent an important research tool to study the neurobiological underpinnings of panic disorder. We believe that CCK-4 offers several advantages over other challenge strategies such as lactate, CO_2 or caffeine. Unlike other challenge agents, CCK-4 is a neurotransmitter present in human CNS for which neuronal pathways and receptors have been identified. It reliably provokes panic attacks, with a high incidence, and in a dose-dependent manner.

Also, rapid i.v. infusion of CCK-4 is technically simple, requiring only a small volume of saline. This mode of administration has an advantage over the slow infusion procedures necessary for other provocative agents such a lactate. Lactate infusion has been associated with non-specific physiologic factors such a volume overload or metabolic changes which can introduce non-specific psychological effects (MARGRAF et al., 1986). The technical advantage of CCK-4 administration, in addition to its presence in the mammalian CNS, renders it more suitable for research in panic disorder. We have now to understand the relationship between CCK and noradrenergic and serotoninergic systems. Initial results support the idea that there is a strong connection between CCK anxiogenic activity and 5 HT3 receptors (VASAR et al, 1993, MALINGE et al, 1992).

REFERENCES

BOULENGER JP, UHDE TW. Caffeine consumption and anxiety : Preliminary results of a survey comparing patients with anxiety disorders and normal controls. Psychopharmacol Bull, 1982, 18, 53-57.

BRADWEJN J, de MONTIGNY C. Benzodiazepines antagonize cholecystokinin-induced activation of rat hippocampal neurons. Nature, 1984, 312, 363-364.

BRADWEJN J, KOSZYCKI D. Comparison of CO_2 induced panic attacks with cholecystokinin-induced panic attacks in panic disorder. Prog Neuro-Psychoparmacol Biol Psychiatr, 1991b, 15, 237-239.

BRADWEJN J., KOSZYCKI D, METERISSIAN G. Cholecystokinin-tetrapeptide induced panic attacks in patients with panic disorder. Can J Psychiatr, 1990, 35, 83-85.

BRADWEJN J, KOSZYCKI D, BOURIN M. Dose ranging study of the effect of CCK-4 in healthy volunteers. J Psychiatr Neurosci 1991a, 16, 260-264.

BRADWEJN J, KOSZYCKI D, PAYEUR R. Cholecystokinin-tetrapeptide: A provocation agent for research in panic disorders? *In* Briley M, File S (eds), New concepts in anxiety. Mac Millan Press, London, 313-319, 1991b.

BRADWEJN J, KOSZYCKI D, SHRIQUI C. Enhanced sensitivity to cholecystokin-tetrapeptide in panic disorder: Clinical and behavioural findings. Arch Gen Psychiatr 1991c, 48, 603-607.

BRADWEJN J, KOSZYCKI D, PAYEUR R., BOURIN M, BORTHWICK H. Replication of action of cholecystokinin tetrapeptide in panic disorder: clinical and behavioral findings. Am J Psychiatr, 1992, 149, 962-964.

BRADWEJN J, KOSZYCKI D, PAYEUR R, BOURIN M. CCK-4 and panic disorder. *In* Psychoparmacology of panic, SA Montgomery Ed, 110-117, Oxford University Press, 1993.

BRADWEJN J, COUETOUX du TERTRE A, KOSZYCKI D, BOURIN M. Flumazenil does not antagonise CCK-4 induced panic in healthy volunteers. Psychopharmacology (in press).

CARR DB, SHEEHAN DV, SURMAN OS et al. Neuroendocrine correlates of lactate-induced anxiety and their response to chronic alprazolam therapy. Am J Psychiatry, 1986, 143, 483-494.

CHARNEY DS, REDMOND DE Jr. Neurobiological mechanisms in human anxiety. Evidence supporting central noradrenergic hyperactivity. Neuropharmacology, 1983, 22, 1531-1536.

CHARNEY DS, HENINGER GR, JALLON PI. Increased anxiogenic effects of caffeine in panic disorder. Arch Gen Psychiatr, 1985, 42, 233-243.

COWLEY DS, DAGER SR, DUNNER DL. Lactate induced panic in primary affective disorder Am J Psychiatry, 1986, 143, 646-648.

CRAWLEY JN. Comparative distribution of cholecystokinin and other neuropeptides. Ann NY Acad Sci, 1985, 448, 1-8.

DEN BOER JA, WESTENBERG HGM. Behavioral neuroendocrine and biochemical effects of 5-hydroxy-tryptophan administration in panic disorder. Psychiatry Res, 1990, 31, 267-278.

ERVIN F, PALMOUR R, BRADWEJN J. A new primate model for panic disorder. New research program and abstracts. 144th Meeting of the American Psychiatric Association, New-Orleans, May 14, 1991, NR 216, p. 100.

FYER AJ, UY J, MARTINEZ J, GOETZ R et al. CO_2 challenge of patients with panic disorder. Am J Psychiatry, 1987, 144, 1080-1082.

GAFFNEY FA, FENTON BJ, LANE LD, LAKE CR. Hemodynamic, ventilatory, and biochemical responses of panic patients and normal controls with sodium lactate infusion and spontaneous panic attacks. Arch Gen Psychiatry, 1988, 45, 53-60.

GORMAN JM, FYER MR, LIEBOWITZ MR, KLEIN DF. Pharmacologic provocation of panic attacks. *In* Meltzer HY (ed.) Psychopharmacology: a third generation of progress, Raven press, New-York, 1987, 980-983.

GORMAN JM, LIEBOWITZ MR, FYER AJ, STEIN J. Neuroanatomical hypothesis for panic disorder. Am J Psychiatr, 1989a, 146, 148-161.

GORMAN JM, BATTISTA D, GOETZ RR et al. A comparison of sodium bicarbonate and sodium lactate infusion of panic attacks. Arch Gen Psychiatry 1989b, 46, 145-150.

GRIEZ EJ, LOUSBERG H, VAN DEN HOUT MA, VAN DER MOLEN GM. CO_2 vulnerability in panic disorder. Psychiatry Res, 1987, 20, 87-95.

GUTTMACHER LB, MURPHY DL, INSEL TR. Pharmacologic models of anxiety. Com Psychiatr, 1983, 24, 312-326.

KAHN RS, VAN PRAAG HM, WETZLER S, ASNIS GM, BARR G. Serotonin and anxiety revisited. Biol Psychiatry, 1988, 23, 189-208.

KLEIN DF, GORMAN JM. A model of panic and agoraphobic development. Acta Psychiatr Scand, 1987 (suppl), 335, 87-95.

KOSZYCKI D, BRADWEJN J, BOURIN M. Comparison of the effects of cholecystokinin and carbon dioxide in healthy volunteers. Eur Neuropharmacol, 1991, 1, 137-141.

LIEBOWITZ MR, FYER AJ, GORMAN JM et al. Specificity of lactate infusions in social phobia versus panic disorder. Am J Psychiatry, 1985, 142, 947-950.

MALINGE M. COLOMBEL MC, BOURIN M. Effects of CCK agonists and antagonists on morphine withdrawal in the mouse. Eur Neuropsychopharmacol, 1992, 2, 369-370.

MARGRAF J, EHLERS A, ROTH WT. Sodium lactate infusions and panic attacks: A review and critique, Psychosom Med, 1986, 48, 23-51.

Mc GRATH PJ, STEWART JW, LIEBOWITZ MR et al. Lactate provocation of panic attacks in depressed outpatients. Psychiatry Res, 1988, 25, 41-47.

POHL R, ETTEDGUI E, BRIDGES M et al. Plasma MHPG levels in lactate and isoproterenol anxiety states. Biol Psychiatr, 1987, 22, 1127-1136.

REDMOND DE Jr. Studies of the nucleus locus coeruleus in monkeys and hypothesis for neuropsychoparmacology. *In* Psychopharmacology : the third generation of progress (ed HY Meltzer) Raven Press, New-York, 1987.

REDMOND DE Jr, HUANG YH. Current concepts II: New evidence for a locus coeruleus norepinephrine connection with anxiety. Life Sci, 1979, 25, 2149-2162.

SANDERSON WC, RAPEE RM, BARLOW DH. The influence of an illusion of control on panic attacks induced via inhalation of 5.5% carbon dioxide enriched air. Arch. Gen Psychiatry, 1989, 46, 157-162.

SINGH L, LEWIS AS, FIELD MJ, HUGUES J, WOODRUFF GN. Evidence for an involvement of the brain cholecystokinin B receptor in anxiety. Proc Natl Acad Sci USA, 1991, 88, 1130-1133.

UHDE TW, BOULANGER JP, VITTONE B, JIMERSON DC, POST PM. Caffeine: Relationship to human anxiety plasma MHPG and cortisol. Psychopharmacol Bull, 1984, 20, 426-430.

UHDE TW. Caffeine: Practical facts for the psychiatrist. *In* Roy-Byrne PP (Ed) Anxiety: New research findings for the clinician, Washington DC American Psychiatric Press, 1988.

UHDE TW, STEIN MB, VITTONE BJ et al. Behavioral and physiologic effects of short-tem and long-term administration of clonidine in panic disorder. Arch Gen Psychiatry, 1989, 46, 170-177.

VASAR E, PEURANEN E, ÖÖPIK T, HARRO J, MÄNNISTÖ PT. Ondansetron, an antagonist of 5-HT3 receptors, antagonizes the anti-exploratory effect of caerulein, an agonist of CCK receptors, in the elevated plus-maze. Psychopharmacology, 1993, 110, 213-218.

WOODRUF GN, HUGUES J. Cholecystokinin antagonists. Ann Rev Pharmacol Toxicol, 1991, 31, 469-501.

YERAGANI VK, POHL R, BALON R, WEINBERG P, BERCHOU R, RAINEY J. Preinfusion anxiety predicts lactate-induced panic attacks in normal controls. Psychosom Med, 1987, 49, 383-389.

Résumé

L'utilisation d'agents inducteurs des attaques de panique a été très utile pour la compréhension du substratum biologique de ces troubles.. De nombreux agents tels que le lactate de sodium, le gaz carbonique (CO_2), la caféine, la yohimbine, l'isoproterénol et maintenant la cholecystokinine (CCK) sont utilisés comme agents panicogènes aussi bien chez des patients présentant un trouble panique que chez des volontaires sains. D'autre part, différents systèmes de neurotransmission ont été explorés afin de mieux comprendre l'étiologie des troubles paniques.

La plupart des agents inducteurs manquent de spécificité d'action et ne sont qu'un maillon pour comprendre le rôle biologique des neurotrasmetteurs impliqués dans les attaques de panique

Par ailleurs, la CCK semble apporter plusieurs avantages par rapport aux autres agents tels que le lactate, le CO_2 ou la caféine. En effet, la CCK est un neurotransmetteur du système nerveux central avec ses propres circuits neuronaux et ses propres récepteurs. Elle induit des attaques de panique dose dépendantes aussi bien chez le sujet sain que chez le patient présentant un trouble panique. Elle est désormais considérée comme un agent physiologique compatible avec des recherches chez l'homme, le blocage des récepteurs à la CCK peut conduire chez les patients présentant des attaques de panique à l'utilisation de médicaments efficaces.

Il reste cependant à élucider les relations existant entre la CCK, la noradrenaline et la sérotonine pour mieux comprendre la neurobiologie des attaques de panique.

Current behavioural models of anxiety in animals: how predictive are they for anxiolytic activity?

Marie-Hélène Thiébot

INSERM U.288, Faculté de Médecine Pitié-Salpêtrière, 91, boulevard de l'Hôpital, 75634 Paris Cedex 13, France

Summary. Current animal models for the study of anxiety and anxiolytic drugs are reviewed according to pharmacological and behavioural criteria: models based on conflict or conditioned fear and models using unconditioned behaviour. In comparison, one model not initially devoted to the study of anxiety, but in which a maladaptive behaviour is induced by an uncontrollable severe stress, is also considered. Their limits with regards to the various categories of human anxiety and their pharmacological validity are analysed.

Animal models of anxiety are developed with two essential aims: to predict the potency of compounds as clinically active anxiolytics, and to provide insights into the neurobiology of anxiety and the mechanisms whereby anxiolytic agents achieve their effects.

These objectives come up against various difficulties. The first one is the creation of an animal equivalent to human anxiety, expressed as an *observable behaviour*. The large variety of experimental situations used over the last decades present the common characteristic of inducing mild or severe "fear", broadly considered as an analogy to human anxiety. Almost all of these models have been pharmacologically validated by the prototypical anxiolytics, benzodiazepines (BZDs), and optimized for this class of compounds. In turn, the models have been considered as *predictive* for anxiolytic activity in humans.

However, behavioural pharmacologists are faced with a second difficulty, in that anxiety is not a unitary phenomenon (see Boulenger, this volume). The DSM-III-R diagnostic criteria allow the individualization of several forms of anxiety-related disorders, presenting various affective, cognitive, motivational, behavioural and autonomic aspects. Whereas the symptoms of generalized anxiety disorders (GAD) are usually alleviated by BZDs, the other forms of anxiety seem differentially sensitive to various psychotropic drugs, among which antidepressants frequently (re)appear whereas BZDs do not seem to be particularly potent against certain forms of anxiety such as phobias, obsessive compulsive disorders and even panic attacks. Furthermore, there are no clearcut boundaries between "normal" anxiety and maladaptive, "pathological" anxiety. Since the different categories of human anxiety are not yet precisely characterized, we are faced with the paradox of finding and using animal models which must be predictive of a therapeutic efficiency of drugs against human pathological states which are not clearly defined. Therefore, it is not surprising that face and construct validity of the animal models are not yet fully established.

In addition to the usual criteria of *feasibility* with pharmacological perspectives, *specificity* with a minimal number of false positive or false negative results and *reproducibility* with detection of dose-related effects, animal models are now required to predict an anxiolytic potential of newly developed agents. It is the case for BZD receptor partial agonists, drugs which interact with various serotonin (5-HT) receptor subtypes (more precisely 5-HT$_{1A}$ agonists, 5-HT$_{2/1C}$ and 5-HT$_3$ antagonists) or peptidergic compounds [cholecystokinin (CCK) or substance P receptor antagonists], whereas it is not yet known whether such substances will be active in the treatment of any anxiety disorder in humans (buspirone-like compounds and perhaps 5-HT$_2$ antagonists excepted). In addition, we also would like the situations to be able to detect possible anxiolytic-like effects of antidepressants or "anxiogenic" activities (Table 1).

Table 1 - Established and putative anxiolytic drugs.

Ligands for the GABA$_A$ receptor complex	Ligands for 5-HT receptors
Benzodiazepines (full and partial agonists)	5-HT$_{1A}$ (partial) agonists
Cyclopyrrolones	5-HT$_{2/1C}$ antagonists**
Imidazopyridines	5-HT$_3$ antagonists*
Triazolopyridazines	Other compounds
Barbiturates	Antidepressants
Carbamates	Neuroleptics
Alcohol	Antihistaminics
Neurosteroids*	β-adrenoceptor antagonists
Ligands for peptide receptors	α$_2$-adrenoceptor agonists
CCK$_B$ antagonists*	Opiates (morphine)
Substance P antagonists*	

* no available data as yet for anxiolytic action in man;
** no clear evidence for anxiolytic efficacy in man.

The aim of the present chapter is not to consider all the available models of anxiety. They have been reviewed and extensively discussed in several recent and very well documented papers (Treit, 1985,1991; Lister, 1990; Green & Hodges, 1991; Handley, 1991; Stephens & Andrews 1991). We will only consider the situations most frequently used (and whose pharmacological validity is therefore reasonably well established) and/or whose heuristic value could provide additional arguments for the analysis of anxiety-related behaviours.

Animal models of anxiety may be broadly divided into three classes: (i) Models based on conflict or conditioned fear in which secondary, well identified (often transitory) stimuli are patent or implicit signals which warn of a *known* aversive event. They do not necessitate a high level of interpretation since appropriate responses are already known. (ii) Models using unconditioned, continuous fear stimuli which are complex environmental signals of an *unknown* threat. They require a high level of processing and responses more likely vary according to arousal, previous experience, motor capacities, memory, cognitive ability. Some other procedures which were not initially devoted to the study of anxiety (e.g. the learned helplessness paradigm) may also provide data which deserve discussion with reference to anxiety. (iii) Models using "anxiety" reactions induced by patent aversive stimuli such as chemical compounds or electrical intracerebral stimulations, which have been reported to evoke intense anxiety in humans. These situations, such as drug discrimination paradigms or place conditioning, will not be considered here since they do not explore anxiety *per se*, but rather the overall stimulus effect they evoke.

Two main types of aversive stimuli are used: punishment (usually non noxious electric shocks) or conditioned signal of punishment, and novelty (uncertainty). A third kind of aversive event, frustative non-reward, is not used in current models. In most of the situations, these events induce a *reduction* or a *blockade* of ongoing (spontaneous or conditioned) behaviour. However, it must be pointed out that any paradigm using punishment cannot be considered as suitable for the study of anxiolytics. It is the case, for instance, for the conditioned emotional responses (CER) in which BZD-like agents exerted inconsistent effects. However, since only few other compounds have been studied in this procedure, it cannot be ascertained whether such emotional responses would be sensitive to atypical anxiolytics and/or to antidepressants (see refs. in Treit, 1985; Davis, 1990). In fact, the anti-punishment effect of drugs is closely dependent upon the relationships that exist between the animal and its surroundings, in particular on the patent consequences of responding or omission of responding. Therefore, any situation of punishment must be carefully characterized before being considered as a "model" suitable to approach the neurobiological bases of anxiety.

Some threatening situations *stimulate* the expression of ethologically-prepared behaviours such as burying, vocalizations or defensive responses (see Depaulis, this volume). Finally, it should be pointed out that none of the available situations are able to model one particular form of human anxiety in which the most distressful components are often anxious thoughts and not patent threatening stimuli.

1 - MODELS BASED ON CONFLICT OR CONDITIONED FEAR.

A number of experimental procedures used in this area involve mild electric shocks which induce blockade of behaviour, either exploration, drinking or lever pressing for food reward. The prototypical procedures are the conditioned conflict test (Geller & Seifter, 1960) and the acute punished drinking test (Vogel *et al.*, 1971), and their numerous variants, which have been shown to be reasonably reliable predictors of anxiolytic activity, or more precisely of BZD-like drug effects (see Table 2).

<u>Geller & Seifter-like conflict paradigms</u>

These paradigms typically consist in alternating punished and non-punished components of operant behaviour cued by different stimuli. During the *non-punished components*, lever presses result in food or water delivery. During the *punished components*, lever presses are both rewarded and punished by contingent footshocks. Well-trained animals stopped responding during punished periods and confine their responses to the non-punished periods. The suppression of the punished responses was reliably released by acute or chronic administration of BZD-like drugs. Responding during the non-punished periods was not notably modified, indicating that food consumption or motor capacities are probably not critically involved (Kilts *et al.*, 1981; Hodges & Green, 1987).

A large variety of non-BZD compounds, in particular $5-HT_{1A}$, $5-HT_{2/1C}$ and $5-HT_3$ receptor ligands, neuroleptics and antidepressants, almost completely failed to reduce (and more often further enhanced) the behavioural blockade, whatever the animal species. The pigeon, in which 5-HT$_{1A}$ agonists exert a potent release of punished behaviour, represents an exception which is still unexplained (see refs. in Gardner, 1986; Barrett & Gleeson, 1991).

Punished drinking test

In this paradigm, water drinking in thirsty rats is suppressed by the contingent delivery of shocks. BZD-related drugs released punished drinking. However, the results obtained with atypical anxiolytics such as buspirone and other 5-HT$_{1A}$ (partial) agonists are inconsistent both within and across studies. In fact, they have been found to be comparable to those observed with dopamine antagonists such as haloperidol or sulpiride (Merlo Pich & Samanin, 1986; and see refs. in Barrett & Gleeson, 1991). Conflict procedures also most often failed to detect a potential activity for compounds such as 5-HT$_{2/1C}$ or 5-HT$_3$ receptors antagonists and antidepressants (Gardner, 1986; Costall & Naylor, 1991).

With some modifications of the experimental parameters, in particular by manipulating the level of shock or habituation to the test chamber, the situation was also supposed to detect "anxiogenic"-like effects (i.e. a further reduction of punished drinking) such as those expected with drugs that may cause anxiety in humans, for example, BZD receptor inverse agonists or pentylenetetrazole (PTZ). In addition, the "proconflict" effect elicited by PTZ has been proposed as being suitable for detecting antipanic agents. This has been done on the basis of a dissociation of the doses of BZDs able to reduce conflict and proconflict drinking responses. However, several antidepressants used in the treatment of panic attacks only exhibited marginal efficacy (or may be "anxiogenic") even after chronic administration (Giusti et al., 1991). Thus, the proconflict procedure seems useful only to differentiate GABA$_A$/BZD receptor ligands.

Conditioned suppression of drinking

The procedure is a modification of the Geller & Seifter and Vogel conflict tests. It consists in non-punished drinking periods alternating with short signalled periods during which any contact with the drinking tube is punished by a shock. The conditioned suppression of drinking observed in well trained rats was released by BZD-like compounds, but not by either acute antidepressants or acute buspirone (Kilts et al., 1981; Ellis et al., 1990). In contrast, chronic administration of a variety of antidepressants resulted in a gradual increase in punished responding over the course of several weeks. In addition, a 1-2 week delayed offset was observed after drug discontinuation. These data might indicate that, under specific experimental conditions, some antidepressants exhibit an anxiolytic-like activity, an effect which is consistent with the reported efficacy of these drugs in anxiety disorders. On the basis of the active and inactive compounds, the conditioned suppression of drinking has been proposed as a "model" for panic disorders (Fontana et al., 1989; Commissaris et al., 1990). Face and construct validation of the situation remains to be established and a complete pharmacological study is necessary to substantiate this hypothesis.

In contrast to its marginal effect on acute injection, buspirone clearly increased punished drinking after several weeks of treatment. However, contrary to chronic antidepressants, buspirone exhibited this "anxiolytic"-like activity only if an acute pre-test challenge was superimposed to the chronic treatment (Schefke et al., 1989). Such delayed action is consistent with the reported efficacy of buspirone on anxiety states in humans only after 3-4 weeks. It would be interesting to further investigate whether, upon chronic administration, other 5-HT$_{1A}$ full or partial agonists and also specific 5-HT reuptake inhibitors —particularly active in several forms of anxiety disorders— would induce similar anxiolytic-like effects.

It should be pointed out that there are very few published reports on the effects of long chronic treatment with atypical anxiolytics in conflict procedures (but see Bodnoff et al., 1989). Therefore, it is not easy to ascertain if the conditioned suppression of drinking procedure presents some particular characteristics suitable for detecting an anxiolytic-like activity of non-BZD agents or if such activity has not been found in other tests because it has not been adequately studied.

Safety signal withdrawal conflict procedure (SSW)

In this procedure, a blockade of lever pressing for food is induced *not* by the presentation of a patent conditioned signal for punishment as in the Geller & Seifter test, but by the withdrawal of a conditioned signal for safety. This represents an unconditioned stimulus of an *unknown* threat to which animals have no readily prepared responses.

As in classical operant conflict paradigms, rats are trained under two alternating punished and non-punished components of a multiple schedule of food reinforcement, cued by two distinct light stimuli. On the test session, the safety signal was turned off at the end of the first non-punished period, but the punishment signal was not presented (presses were rewarded and no shocks were delivered). During the period associated with the safety signal withdrawal, control rats exhibited a marked, BZD-sensitive blockade of responding that lessened over time as shocks were omitted. The response suppression seemed not caused by intervening events such as novelty, temporal conditioning, schedule of food delivery or ambiguity of the signal presented. In addition, the procedure avoids the possible confounding effects of the drugs on shock perception, since shocks were omitted during the test sessions. As in other operant paradigms, responding during the non-punished components allows to control for nonspecific effects of drugs on motor and motivational capacities (Thiébot et al., 1991b).

In contrast to their lack of effect in classical operant conflict tests, a variety of 5-HT_{1A} agonists, upon acute administration, produced a robust and dose-related release in responding during the period associated with the safety signal withdrawal. Furthermore, the magnitude of the effect of MDL 73005EF, buspirone, gepirone and ipsapirone paralleled their partial agonist efficacy at post-synaptic 5-HT_{1A} receptors, whereas the full agonist 8-OH-DPAT was inactive. This suggests that, in addition to the reduction of 5-HT neuronal activity due to the stimulation of autoreceptors, a relative impairment of post-synaptic 5-HT_{1A} receptor function might be necessary for an "anxiolytic"-like effect of 5-HT_{1A} agents to be observed in the test. Acute administration of a small number of $5\text{-HT}_{2/1C}$ and 5-HT_3 antagonists, 5-HT uptake inhibitors and neuroleptics, failed to modify rats' behaviour during the period associated with the safety signal withdrawal (unpublished results).

Conversely, under identical procedural conditions, a number of compounds that may cause anxiety in humans (BZD inverse agonists, PTZ, amphetamine, picrotoxin) further enhanced the blockade of lever pressing induced by the safety signal withdrawal (Thiébot et al., 1991b).

Thus, this procedure seems sensitive to both "anxiolytic" and "anxiogenic" effects of drugs. Its ability to reproducibly detect acute effects of 5-HT_{1A} partial agonists (chronic treatments have not yet been studied) indicates that this paradigm might generate a kind of behavioural blockade (of anxiety?) different from that observed in the other conflict models. Whether this anxiety more closely resembles human anxiety generated by the disappearance of familiar cues (separation anxiety) than GAD remains to be established.

Table 2 - Effects of established and putative anxiolytics in some animal models of anxiety.

	BZP-R agon.		5-HT-R ligands			Anti-depressants		CCK$_B$ antag	Neuroleptics
	full	part.	1A agon		2antag	3antag				
	acute	acute	acute	chron	acute	acute	acute	chron	acute	acute
Geller & Seifter	+	+	0	[0]	0/[+]	0	-/0		[0(+)]	0
Vogel	+	+	0/(+)		0/(+)	0				0/[+]
CSD	+	+	(+)	[+]			0	+		
SSW	+	+	+		0	0				
CER	0/(+)		[+]							
Plus-maze	+	+	+/0/-	+/0/-	+/0/-	+/0/-	[+/0/-]	0	[+/0]	(0)
Light/dark box	+	+	+/[0]		+/0	+	0/-		[+/0]	+/0
Social interac.	+	+	+/[0/-]		0	+/0/-	0	0/-	[+]	0
LH	0		0		+	+	0	+		0
					(sub.ch)	(sub.ch)				

+ : anxiolytic-like effect; 0 : no effect; - : anxiogenic-like effect.
( ) : effects weak and not dose-related; [ ] : only few available data. See references in the text.

CSD : conditioned suppression of drinking; SSW : safety signal withdrawal conflict paradigm; CER : conditioned emotional response; LH : learned helplessness. BZP-R agon. full and part. : full and partial agonists at benzodiazepine receptors; 1A agon : 5-HT$_{1A}$ agonists; 2 antag : 5-HT$_{2/1C}$ antagonists; 3 antag : 5-HT$_3$ antagonists; sub.ch : subchronic administration.

2 - MODELS USING UNCONDITIONED BEHAVIOUR.

Recent models are based on novelty-induced variations in exploratory activity. They are thought to be naturalistic versions of conflict tests, wherein the natural tendency of rodents to explore novel surroundings is limited by the aversive characteristics of all or parts of the environment. They present the advantage of requiring no training and of avoiding confounding factors such as food-motivation or shocks. Conversely, exploratory behaviour most often varies in a non-monotonic manner and a low level of exploration may indicate either an increase or a decrease in fear drive. Thus, considerable caution must be exercised when interpreting pharmacological results in such situations. Furthermore, the effects of various manipulations of the experimental parameters such as size, familiarity, illumination, elevation, drug state, etc, are not always predictable. Finally, although claimed to be "naturalistic", these situations are not less artificial than conditioning procedures and, conversely, situations using shocks are usually easy to learn, indicating, as suggested by Green & Hodges (1991), that the brain mechanisms for evaluating and adapting to them are well developed.

Amongst the models most frequently used are the differential exploration of open and enclosed arms in the elevated plus-maze, of brightly lit and dark partition of a two-compartment box, and the social interactions in pairs of unfamiliar rats placed in a neutral area (see Table 2).

The elevated plus-maze

In this procedure, rats or mice are placed in a plus-shaped maze with two open and two enclosed arms, raised off the ground. They spend less time and make less entries onto the open than into the enclosed arms; a strategy which has been claimed to reflect rodents' aversion for open (and elevated) spaces (Pellow et al., 1985; Treit et al., 1993). Test-naive animals divide their activity more equally between the two types of arms when given BZD receptor agonists and partial agonists, but not neuroleptics or psychostimulants. The situation is also reported to be sensitive to agents such as PTZ, yohimbine and BZD receptor inverse agonists, as well as to withdrawal from chronic BZD, which further reduce the exploration of the open arms, suggesting an "anxiogenic"-like effect (Pellow et al., 1985; Lister, 1987; File, 1987). However, caution must be exercised in interpreting the real significance of the results, always expressed as percent, especially because of the frequent very low basal level of open arm activity. An additional problem occurs when the total number of arm entries is modified in the same way as open arm entries, although this value may also be related to the level of fear in the maze. More recently, measures of defensive behaviour or "risk assessment" (stretch attend postures, protected head-dipping, closed arm returns) have been proposed as additional indices of potential utility, especially for the detection of anxiogenic-like effects (Rodgers & Cole, 1993). Finally, it must be pointed out that numerous difficulties in establishing the plus-maze procedure have been signalled by several groups, mainly due to large inter-individual differences and poor reproducibility (see e.g. Green & Hodges, 1991; Stephens & Andrews, 1991).

As extensively reviewed (Chopin & Briley, 1987; Treit, 1991; Costall & Naylor, 1991), an impressive number of studies have been devoted to a variety of $5-HT_{1A}$ (partial) agonists and $5-HT_3$ antagonists in the plus-maze test. They failed to unequivocally give evidence of an anxiolytic-like effect of these compounds on acute administration, and sometimes an anxiogenic-like effect was reported. The few studies performed with $5-HT_{1A}$ agonists on chronic treatment were also inconsistent. The picture is no clearer for $5-HT_{2/1C}$ receptor ligands (see refs. in Handley & McBlane, 1993), nor is it for CCK-B and CCK-A receptor antagonists. However, preferential CCK-B agonists induced an anxiogenic-like reduction of open arm entries, consistent with the reported severe anxiety or panic attacks induced by CCK-4 in humans (see refs. in Bourin and in Daugé, this volume).

Contradictory results were reported with acute antidepressants which either increased, decreased or did not change open arm activity (see refs. in Chopin & Briley, 1987; Handley & McBlane, 1993). Chronic antidepressants also failed to enhance open arm activity or to reverse the anxiogenic-like effects of PTZ, yohimbine or FG 7142, a BZD receptors inverse agonist (File & Johnston, 1987, but see Cadogan et al., 1992).

The plus-maze test is one of the few situations which have been subjected to external (behavioural and physiological) validations. In particular, confinement to open arms resulted in more anxiety-related behaviours and greater plasma corticosterone levels than confinement to closed arms, giving some face validity to the test (Pellow et al., 1985). The situation also seems to be able to detect alterations in exploratory strategy induced by ecologically relevant stressful stimuli such as social defeat, scent of an aggressive conspecific or a predator (Rodgers & Cole, 1993). However, these behavioural manifestations have not yet been subjected to pharmacological validation.

It is possible that, in fact, incursions on the open arms did not reflect an approach behaviour (decreased anxiety ?) but rather attempts to escape the continual presence of mild aversive stimuli generated by the novelty of the situation. Indeed, repeated testing did not modify or even reinforce the avoidance of the open arms and habituation abolished the BZD-induced increase in exploration of open arms (Rodgers et al., 1992; File & Zangrossi, 1993; Treit et al., 1993). This might indicate that, as opposed to the fear generated by novelty, the fear of open spaces cannot habituate and perhaps models another category of anxiety which is not sensitive to BZD. The neurobiological bases for such a phenomenon (sensitization of fear ?) remain to be established.

Thus, despite its great popularity, if the plus-maze test really measures anxiety, its predictive value seems essentially specific to BZD-related drugs and restricted to the first trial. It would be interesting to determine whether the BZD-unresponsive avoidance of the open arms observed after repeated trials presents a specific pharmacological sensitivity.

The two-compartment test

The two-compartment test, or light / dark box, consists of one large, brightly lit (aversive) compartment and one smaller, dark (safe) compartment. Depending on the studies, drug effects are assessed (essentially in mice) by behavioural measures as different as the number of light-dark transitions, or the locomotor activity and the rearings in each compartment, the latency to first entry in the dark compartment, the time spent in each portion of the box. Increases in transitions or in the other activity parameters, without overall modification of locomotor activity, are viewed as indices of reduced anxiety. As expected, it was generally the case with BZD-related compounds (Crawley, 1981; Costall et al., 1989; Onaivi & Martin, 1989).

The situation has been extensively used for pharmacological studies, almost exclusively on acute administration. As reviewed elsewhere (Chopin & Briley, 1987; Costall & Naylor, 1991; Handley, 1991; Treit, 1991), there is generally good agreement that $5-HT_{1A}$ agonists enhance activity in the light section. Positive results were also found with $5-HT_{2/1C}$ and $5-HT_3$ antagonists. Antidepressants were globally inactive in the test and even enhanced the avoidance of the bright area (Costall et al., 1989; Onaivi & Martin, 1989). Some neuroleptics were also reported to enhance the preference of mice for the bright compartment and/or the number of light-dark transitions (Crawley, 1981; Merlo Pich & Samanin, 1986; Costall et al., 1987). A small number of studies devoted to CCK antagonists indicated a lengthening of the time spent in the light section (Singh et al., 1991).

The light / dark box has also been shown to detect behavioural modifications which would indicate an increase in anxiety. This was the case with several "anxiogenic" drugs (BZD receptor inverse agonists, PTZ) but, unexpectedly, also with morphine (Onaivi & Martin, 1989). In addition, an increase in preference for the dark section was also reported following a subchronic treatment with several compounds (BZD, alcohol, nicotine, cocaine), suggesting that the test is also able to detect behavioural changes (increased anxiety ?) associated with withdrawal from drugs of abuse (Costall et al., 1990).

The validity of the test was based upon two main facts. The avoidance of the bright compartment was a function of its level of illumination (Costall et al., 1989) and BZD did not modify the number of transitions when the two compartments were identical, either lighted or darkened (see Crawley, 1981). However, these data were challenged by the finding that corticosterone levels were *reduced* following the exposure of undrugged, naive mice to either the lighted or the darkened section (Onaivi & Martin, 1989). Furthermore, the aversion to the bright compartment was not modified by repeated exposure to the box. Thus, it cannot be excluded that, as for the plus-maze, the real drive for rodents to explore the bright section would reflect the animal's tendency to flee from the continual presence of threatening stimuli caused by the unknown environment, rather than an approach strategy. Whether or not anxiolytic compounds would be active in animals previously habituated in an undrugged state remains to be studied. A recent study indicated that a prior exposure to a plus-maze abolished the response to diazepam in the light / dark test (Rodgers & Shepherd, 1993). This suggests a possible cross habituation to the two experimental procedures.

The social interaction test in rats

The time spent on active social interactions by pairs of stranger male rats placed in a neutral arena has been proposed to reflect the stressful characteristics of the surroundings. Indeed, by manipulating both the light level and the familiarity with the chamber, social interactions vary. Undrugged rats spent less time interacting in high light / unfamiliar than in low light / familiar conditions and exhibited intermediate social behaviour in the other two conditions (File, 1980). The concomitant measure of locomotor activity may help to control for nonspecific effects of drugs (stimulation or sedation), but this measure is only valid so long as activity is not affected by changes in anxiety.

A number of BZDs and related compounds increased social interactions in the high light / unfamiliar condition, whereas in the low light / familiar arena (where the stanger conspecific is considered to be the only source of novelty), they were found to be either active or inactive (File, 1980; Guy & Gardner, 1985). Barbiturates enhanced interactions whatever the test condition, while neuroleptics did not specifically modify rats' behaviour. The situation also seemed to be able to give evidence of "anxiogenic"-like effects of a number of compounds such as BZD inverse agonists, PTZ and yohimbine, without substantial alteration of locomotor activity. However, amphetamine and caffeine were found to be either "anxiolytic" or "anxiogenic", depending on the test condition (Guy & Gardner, 1985; File, 1987)

Globally, acute $5\text{-}HT_{1A}$ agonists enhanced social interactions, although no effect or decreased interactions have also been reported with no clear relationship with the test condition. $5\text{-}HT_{2/1C}$ antagonists were inactive and $5\text{-}HT_3$ antagonists failed to induce consistent results whatever the test condition. (see refs. in Lister, 1990; Briley et al., 1991; Handley, 1991; Treit, 1991). Only a few studies have been devoted to antidepressant drugs. They did not enhance social behaviour upon acute or chronic administration, and in some cases, even caused a reduction in the interactions. They also failed to reverse the anxiogenic-like effect of FG 7142 and PTZ (Guy & Gardner, 1985; Pellow & File, 1987).

The variation in time spent on social interaction according to the experimental conditions represents a good internal validation of the test insofar as exploratory activity is controlled. However, it should be pointed out that in numerous studies, drugs were tested under only one condition, chosen according to the expected effect. This represents a serious procedural flaw. Plasma corticosterone levels were found to be higher under the high light than low light condition, but familiarization with the test arena does not seem to influence this parameter. File (1980) reported that the reduction in interaction was not due to changes inolfactory cues from the partner in the different test conditions. However, interpretation of the results in terms of anxiety is complex as the behaviour of one animal is critically dependent upon the behaviour of its partner. Thus, it cannot be ruled out that the drugs would affect the emission or the perception of social cues independently from anxiety levels.

The social interaction test is therefore essentially sensitive to BZD-like compounds and perhaps to 5-HT$_{1A}$ agonists, although numerous controversial results have been obtained with these agents.

3 - MODELS NOT INITIALLY DEVOTED TO THE STUDY OF ANXIETY.

As stressed above, it is now frequently required of animal models to be able to detect an anxiolytic-like activity of antidepressants. Although classically referring to depressive illness, the learned helplessness procedure can tentatively be considered in the scope of anxiety-related disorders. In this paradigm, experience with uncontrollable severe shocks in one situation has profound and *long-lasting* disruptive effects on the ability of the animals to learn to escape shocks in another situation such as the shuttle-box task. Animals also exhibit reduced locomotion, loss of appetite and weight and immunosuppression. Escape deficit has consistently been found to be reversed (and also prevented) by a large variety of established antidepressants, essentially upon chronic or subchronic administration (see refs. in Thiébot & Martin, 1991).

A main role of fear or anxiety during the induction phase is suggested by two sets of data. (i) BZD administered before the inescapable shocks *prevented* the development of the behavioural deficit. (ii) The BZD receptor inverse agonist, FG 7142, was reported to induce escape deficit in a shuttle-box task as was the case with uncontrollable shocks. Although we did not reproduce this result in a slightly different paradigm, we found FG 7142 able to potentiate the effects of otherwise ineffective shocks (unpublished results).

In contrast to antidepressants, BZD-related drugs were ineffective in *reversing* helpless behaviour when given after the induction phase, whereas several 5-HT$_{1A}$ agonists, 5-HT$_{2/1C}$ and 5-HT$_3$ antagonists, upon subchronic treatment, reduced escape deficit (see refs. in Thiébot & Martin, 1991).

In fact, the learned helplessnees procedure differs from all the others models in several aspects. An uncontrollable severe stress induces a long lasting, apparently maladaptive behaviour which develops over time, and is not limited to the experimental session. The lack of control over the aversive events seems to be the primary determinant for the induction of helpless behaviour, since the performance deficit is not seen in animals subjected to identical but controllable stressors, and previous experience with escapable shocks "immunized" against the disruptive effects of a subsequent uncontrollable stress (see refs. in Willner, 1986). On the contrary, the other situations include mild or low aversive events (usually controllable) which generate an adaptive behaviour. In this case, the behavioural alterations (adjustments ?) are limited to the test duration or even to small periods of the test sessions. They aim at (and generally succeed in) reducing the aversiveness of the situation. Therefore, the learned helplessness paradigm exemplifies the importance of the precipitating factors in the induction of anxiety-related behaviours and in their differential sensitivity to psychotropic drugs. One can wonder whether this situation models a different kind of anxiety which would be sensitive to antidepressants and 5-HT receptor ligands, but not to BZD-like anxiolytics. As a matter of fact, several recent studies indicated that antidepressants may be more effective than BZD for chronic GAD and anxiety linked to depression. Surprisingly no attempts have been made to study the behavioural strategy of such "helpless" animals in classical models of anxiety and the effects of the different classes of anxiolytics thereon (but see Van Dijken *et al.*, 1992).

To conclude, the general picture of the predictive value of animal models of anxiety is not fully satisfying. None of the current paradigms can claim to model one particular type of human anxiety. Since external validations are frequently missing, these paradigms come up against the problem of analogical reasoning. Furthermore, this reasoning often fails to take into account the fundamental difference which probably exists between reactions of fear and the expression of pathological anxiety. The definition of what would be an anti-anxiety effect is only given with regard to a clinical activity, but even this point is not always established by controlled studies. Moreover, the characteristics of the phenomena which are intented to be modelled are often not clearly defined. In particular, one can wonder whether reasoning in terms of general aspects of anxiety-related disorders is an adequate strategy. It would be more heuristic to dissect out the different categories of human anxiety into more elementary components, probably easier to model in animals, and to evaluate which of them constitute the core symptoms of anxiety and/or are shared with other psychiatric diseases. For instance, the anxiolytic-like effect of BZD and of some 5-HT$_{1A}$ ligands in conflict procedures has been linked to a reduced ability to withhold responding, that is a reduced impulse control (Thiébot et al., 1991a). Indeed, according to the theory of anxiety-related inhibition (Pull & Widlöcher, 1989), it could be proposed that a shift from passivity to activity, allowing momentary control over a situation, would contribute to a reduction in anxiety.

Therefore, it is probably by collating data from numerous drugs and a variety of situations referring to unitary components of anxiety disorders that a more precise picture of anxiety and its neurobiological substrates would emerge.

REFERENCES

Barrett, J.E. & Gleeson, S. (1991): Anxiolytic effects of 5-HT$_{1A}$ agonists, 5-HT$_3$ antagonists and benzodiazepines: Conflict and drug discrimination studies. In *5-HT$_{1A}$ agonists, 5-HT$_3$ antagonists and benzodiazepines. Their comparative behavioural pharmacology*, eds. R.J. Rodgers & S.J. Cooper, pp. 59-105, Chichester: Wiley.

Bodnoff, S.R., Suranyi-Cadotte, B., Quirion, R. & Meaney,M.J. (1989): A comparison of the effects of diazepam versus several typical and atypical antidepressant drugs in an animal model of anxiety. *Psychopharmacology*, 97: 277-279.

Briley, M., Chopin, P. & Moret, C. (1991): The role of serotonin in anxiety: Behavioural approaches. In *New concepts in anxiety*, eds. M. Briley & S. File, pp. 56-73, London: Macmillan Press.

Cadogan, A.K., Wright, I.K., Coombs, I., Marsden, C.A., Kendall, D.A., & Tulloch, I. (1992): Repeated paroxetine administration in the rat produces an anxiolytic profile in the elevated X-maze and a decreased ^{3}H-ketanserin binding. *Neurosci. Lett.*, 42(suppl): S8.

Chopin, P. & Briley, M. (1987): Animal models of anxiety: The effect of compounds that modify 5-HT neurotransmission. *Trends Pharmacol. Sci.*, 8:383-388.

Commissaris, R.L., Ellis, D.M., Hill, T.J., Schefke, D.M., Becker, C.A. & Fontana, D.J. (1990): Chronic antidepressant and clonidine treatment effects on conflict behavior in the rat. *Pharmacol. Biochem. Behav.*, 37: 167-176.

Corda, M.G. & Biggio, G. (1986): Proconflict effect of GABA receptor complex antagonists. *Neuropharmacology*, 25: 541-544.

Costall, B. & Naylor, R.J. (1991): Anxiolytic effects of 5-HT$_3$ antagonists in animals. In *5-HT$_{1A}$ agonists, 5-HT$_3$ antagonists and benzodiazepines. Their comparative behavioural pharmacology*, eds. R.J. Rodgers & S.J. Cooper, pp.133-157, Chichester: Wiley.

Costall, B., Hendrie, C.A., Kelly, M.E. & Naylor, R.J. (1987): Actions of sulpiride and tiapride in a simple model of anxiety in mice. *Neuropharmacology*, 26:195-200.

Costall, B., Jones, B.J., Kelly, M.E., Naylor, R.J. & Tomkins, D.M. (1989): Exploration of mice in a black and white test box: Validation as a model of anxiety. *Pharmacol. Biochem. Behav.*, 32:777-785.

Costall, B., Jones, B.J., Kelly, M.E., Naylor, R.J., Onaivi, E.S. & Tyers, M.B. (1990): Ondansetron inhibits a behavioural consequence of withdrawing from drugs of abuse. *Pharmacol. Biochem. Behav.*, 36:339-344.

Crawley, J.N. (1981): Neuropharmacologic specificity of a simple animal model for the behavioral actions of benzodiazepines. *Pharmacol. Biochem. Behav.*, 15:695-699.

Davis, M. (1990): Animal models of anxiety based on classical conditioning: The conditioned emotional response (CER) and the fear-potentiated startle effect. *Pharmacol.Ther.*, 47: 147-165.

Ellis, D.M., Fontana, D.J., McCloskey, T.M. & Commissaris, R.L. (1990): Chronic anxiolytic treatment effects on conflict behavior in the rat. *Pharmacol. Biochem. Behav.*, 37: 177-186.

File, S.E. (1980): The use of social interactions as a method for detecting anxiolytic activity of chlordiazepoxide-like drugs. *J. Neurosci. Meth.*, 2: 219-238.

File, S.E. (1987): The contribution of behavioural studies to the neuropharmacology of anxiety. *Neuropharmacology*, 26: 877-886.

File, S.E. & Johnston, A.L. (1987): Chronic treatment with imipramine does not reverse the effects of 3 anxiogenic compounds in a test of anxiety in the rat. *Neuropsychobiology*, 17: 187-192.

File, S.E. & Zangrossi, H. (1993): "One-trial tolerance" to the anxiolytic actions of benzodiazepines in the elevated plus-maze, or the development of a phobic state? *Psychopharmacology*, 110: 240-244.

Fontana, D.J., Carbary, T.J. & Commissaris, R.L. (1989): Effects of acute and chronic anti-panic drug administration on conflict behavior in the rat. *Psychopharmacology*, 98: 157-162.

Gardner, C.R. (1986): Recent developments of 5-HT-related pharmacology of animal models of anxiety. *Pharmacol. Biochem. Behav.*, 24: 1479-1485.

Geller, I. & Seifter, J. (1960): The effects of meprobamate, barbiturate d-amphetamine and promazine on experimentally-induced conflict in the rat. *Psychopharmacologia (Berlin)*, 1: 482-492.

Giusti, P., Guidetti, G., Costa, E. & Guidotti, A. (1991): The preferential antagonism of pentylenetetrazole proconflict responses differentiates a class of anxiolytic benzodiazepines with potential antipanic action. *J. Pharmacol. Exp. Ther.*, 257: 1062-1068.

Green, S. & Hodges, H. (1991): Animal models of anxiety. In *Behavioural models in psychopharmacology: Theoretical, industrial and clinical perspectives*, ed. P. Willner, pp. 21-49, Cambridge: Cambridge University Press.

Guy, A.P. & Gardner, C.R. (1985): Pharmacological characterisation of a modified social interaction model of anxiety in the rat. *Neuropsychobiology*, 13: 194-200.

Handley, S.L. (1991): Serotonin in animal models of anxiety: The importance of stimulus and response. In *Serotonin sleep and mental disorders*, eds. C. Idzikowski & P. Cowen, pp. 89-115, Petersfield: Wrightson Biomedical.

Handley, S.L. & McBlane, J.W. (1993): Serotonin mechanisms in animal models of anxiety. *Brazilian J. Med. Biol. Res.*, 26: 1-13.

Hodges, H. & Green, S. (1987): Are the effects of benzodiazepines on discrimination and punishment dissociable ? *Physiol. Behav.*, 41: 257-264.

Kilts, C.D., Commissaris, R.L. & Rech, R.H. (1981): Comparison of anti-conflict drug effects in three experimental animal models of anxiety. *Psychopharmacology*, 74: 290-296.

Lister, R.G. (1987): The use of a plus-maze to measure anxiety in the mouse. *Psychopharmacology*, 92: 180-185.

Lister, R.G. (1990): Ethologically-based animal models of anxiety disorders. *Pharmacol. Ther.*, 46: 321-340.

Merlo Pich, E. & Samanin, S. (1986): Disinhibitory effects of buspirone and low doses of sulpiride and haloperidol in two experimmental anxiety models in rats: Possible role for dopamine. *Psychopharmacology*, 89: 125-130.

Onaivi, E.S. & Martin, B.R. (1989): Neuropharmacological and physiological validation of a computer-controlled two-compartment black and white box for the assessment of anxiety. *Prog. Neuro-Psychopharmacol. & Biol. Psychiat.*, 13: 963-973.

Pellow, S. & File, S.E. (1987): Can anti-panic drugs antagonise the anxiety produced in the rat by drugs acting at the GABA-benzodiazepine receptor complex? *Neuropsychobiology*, 17: 60-65.

Pellow, S., Chopin, P., File, S.E. & Briley, M (1985): Validation of open:closed arm entries in an elevated plus-maze as a measure of anxiety in the rat. *J. Neurosci. Meth.*, 14: 149-167.

Pull, C.B. & Widlöcher, D. (1989): Anxiety-related inhibition. *Psychiatry Psychobiol.*, 4: 1-11.
Rodgers, R.J. & Cole, J.C. (1993): Anxiety enhancement in the murine elevated plus maze by immediate prior exposure to social defeat. *Physiol. Behav.*, 53: 383-388.
Rodgers, R.J. & Shepherd, J.K. (1993): Prior plus-maze experience abolishes anxiolytic response to diazepam in the murine light dark test. *Br. J. Pharmacol.*, 108: P50.
Rodgers, R.J., Lee, C. & Shepherd, J.K. (1992): Effects of diazepam on behavioural and antinociceptive responses to the elevated plus-maze in male mice depend upon treatment regimen and prior maze experience. *Psychopharmacology*, 106: 102-110.
Schefke, D.M., Fontana, D.J. & Commissaris, R.L. (1989): Anti-conflict efficacy of buspirone following acute versus chronic treatment. *Psychopharmacology*, 99: 427-429.
Singh, L., Field, M.J., Hughes, J., Menzies, R., Oles, R.J., Vass, C.A. & Woodruff, G.N. (1991): The behavioural properties of CI-988, a selective cholecystokinin$_B$ receptor antagonist. *Br. J. Pharmacol.*, 104: 239-245.
Stephens, D.N. & Andrews, J.S. (1991): Screening for anxiolytic drugs. In *Behavioural models in psychopharmacology: Theoretical, industrial and clinical perspectives*, ed. P. Willner, pp. 50-75, Cambridge: Cambridge University Press.
Thiébot, M.H. & Martin, P. (1991): Effects of benzodiazepines, 5-HT$_{1A}$ agonists and 5-HT$_3$ antagonists in animal models sensitive to antidepressant drugs. In *5-HT$_{1A}$ agonists, 5-HT$_3$ antagonists and benzodiazepines. Their comparative behavioural pharmacology*, eds. R.J. Rodgers & S.J. Cooper, pp. 159-194, Chichester: Wiley.
Thiébot, M.H., Bizot, J.C. & Soubrié, P. (1991a): Waiting capacity in animals: A behavioural component crossing nosologic boundaries of anxiety and depression? In *Animal models of psychiatric disorders, Vol 3: Anxiety, depression and mania*, ed P. Soubrié, pp. 48-67, Basel: Karger.
Thiébot, M.H., Dangoumau, L., Richard, G. & Puech A.J. (1991b): Safety signal withdrawal paradigm sensitive to both "anxiolytic" and "anxiogenic" drugs under identical experimental conditions. *Psychopharmacology*, 103: 415-424.
Treit, D (1985): Animal models for the study of anti-anxiety agents: A review. *Neurosci. Biobehav. Rev.*, 9: 203-222.
Treit, D (1991): Anxiolytic effects of benzodiazepines and 5-HT$_{1A}$ agonists: Animal models. In *5-HT$_{1A}$ agonists, 5-HT$_3$ antagonists and benzodiazepines. Their comparative behavioural pharmacology*, eds. R.J. Rodgers & S.J. Cooper, pp. 107-131, Chichester: Wiley.
Treit, D, Menard, J. & Royan, C. (1993): Anxiogenic stimuli in the elevated plus-maze. *Pharmacol. Biochem. Behav.*, 44: 463-469.
Van Dijken, H.H., Mos, J., Van Der Heyden, J.A.M. & Tilders, F.J.H. (1992): Characterization of stress-induced long-term behavioural changes in rats: Evidence in favor of anxiety. *Physiol. Behav.*, 52: 945-951.
Vogel, J.R., Beer, B. & Clody, D.E. (1971): A simple and reliable conflict procedure for testing antianxiety agents. *Psychopharmacologia (Berlin)*, 21: 1-7.
Willner, P. (1986): Validating criteria for animal models of human mental disorders: Learned helplessness as a paradigm case. *Prog. Neuro-Psychopharmacol. & Biol. Psychiat.*, 10: 677-690.

Résumé

Les situations expérimentales les plus fréquemment utilisées pour étudier l'anxiété et les anxiolytiques chez l'animal sont passées en revue, en fonction de critères comportementaux et pharmacologiques. Il s'agit de procédures de conflit ou de peur conditionnée et de situations exploitant des aversions non conditionnées. A titre de comparaison, une procédure non initialement destinée à l'étude de l'anxiété mais dans laquelle un comportement maladaptatif est induit par un stress incontrôlable, est aussi envisagée. Les limites de ces situations comme "modèles" des différentes catégories d'anxiété humaine et leur sensibilité relative aux diverses catégories d'anxiolytiques sont analysées.

Neurobiology of defensive reactions in animals as an approach to human anxiety

Antoine Depaulis

Laboratoire de Neurophysiologie et Biologie des Comportements, Centre de Neurochimie du CNRS, 5, rue Blaise Pascal 67084 Strasbourg Cedex, France

ABSTRACT

Defensive behavior is the main expression of fear in animals and shows several somatic and autonomic similarities with human reactions to danger (i.e., "normal anxiety"). Its study may thus constitute an interesting approach to human "pathological anxiety". Ethological observations suggest the existence of three main strategies used by animals to adapt to a natural threat (e.g., a predator, an aggressive conspecific): (i) flight; (ii) immobility and (iii) confrontation. Recent evidence suggests that these different strategies are coordinated by distinct neural circuits, especially within the periaqueductal gray matter. The data presented in this chapter suggest that the study of defensive behavior has increased our understanding of the neurobiology of fear and anxiety and that different mechanisms may underly different forms of anxiety.

INTRODUCTION

Parallel to studies which have used conditioned responses in animals to study the neurobiology of anxiety in humans and to test the anxiolytic effects of pharmacological compounds (see Thiébot, this volume), species-specific behavioral responses to a threat or a stress, so-called "defensive behavior", represent an alternative approach to the investigation of anxiety. Because it is the behavioral expression of fear in the animal it can easily be related to the "physiological" reaction of humans when confronted with an existing danger (e.g., aggression, war, disaster). The study of fear-promoted reactions in humans is certainly one of the most suitable way to study anxiety (i.e., fear without object) but is very difficult to achieve for obvious ethical reasons. Since defensive behavior can easily be observed spontaneously in wild as well as laboratory animals, its study may constitute an interesting approach of fear and anxiety in humans and several research groups have tried to better characterize this behavior and to unravel its neural substrate. The purpose of this paper is (i) to present recent ethological and neurobiological data which can provide some insights about the organization of defensive behavior and (ii) to address the possibility that defensive behavior in animals can model anxiety-mediated behavioral changes in humans.

Organization of defensive behavior

Different defensive strategies

Defensive behavior is a set of different species-specific behavioral reactions whose common aim is the protection of the individual. Because it is a critical response for the survival of all species, defensive behavior is very likely a "pre-programmed" behavior that appears quite early in the development of most species and is very rapidly "improved" by the animal's individual experience. Defensive behavior occurs in reaction to different kinds of threatening stimuli like the presence of a predator, an attacking conspecific, a dangerous situation or object (Blanchard & Blanchard, 1989). Furthermore, ethological studies in wild and laboratory animals have provided evidence that a wide variety of postures can be used by animals to reduce the probability of being injured or even killed. These postures vary across species and become more sophisticated in higher species. However, it is possible to categorize these reactions in mammals into three main defensive strategies: (i) *flight or escape* characterized by an animal trying to increase the distance, as rapidly as possible, between the source of threat and its own body; (ii) *immobility* characterized by a complete absence of motion in order to reduce the probability of detection and localization by the source of threat; (iii) *confrontation* characterized by the animal facing the source of threat and eventually trying to control it.

The choice of a defensive strategy depends on different factors such as (i) the characteristics of the source of threat (e.g., distance, size, species); (ii) the configuration of the environment (e.g., possibilities to escape, to hide); (iii) the animal's individual experience and also (iv) the animal's individual heritage. In addition, during a period of danger, an animal often needs to rapidly adapt its strategy according to the changes in the source of threat (e.g., a predator getting closer). For example, in the rhesus monkey, the presence of an experimenter showing his profile generally results in immobility and inhibition of calls in infant subjects, whereas a more active reaction associated with aggressive vocalization is elicited as soon as the experimenter turns his face towards the animal and stares at it (Kalin & Shelton, 1989). As well, a wild rat can rapidly switch from one strategy to another in reaction to an approaching predator (Blanchard & Blanchard, 1989). When the predator (e.g., an experimenter) is distant from the animal and when escape is not possible, immobility is the predominant response: the animal is motionless but remains oriented toward the predator and shows increased startle response to sonic or tactile stimuli. This posture corresponds to what is often called "freezing". If the predator approaches within a meter, defensive vocalizations and upright postures occur, eventually followed by jump attack at the predator. If escape is possible, the animal generally flees in a direction opposite to the predator. Although the intensity of their responses are reduced, laboratory rats show similar postures to a predator or to an aggressive conspecific. For example, an animal introduced into the home-cage of an aggressive conspecific or into a rat-colony will be attacked and will display mainly confrontational reactions (e.g., upright postures, backward movements) and eventually escape reactions (e.g., foward rapid locomotion, jumps). Different data suggest the existence of several forms of immobility. In particular the *freezing* reaction is characterized by the animal's orientation toward the source of threat along with signs of alertness and tension (hyperventilation, increased muscle tone; see Fanselow, 1991). This posture differs from the *quiescent* reaction characterized by an absence of orientation and muscle relaxation which is generally observed in defeated or injured animals (see Rodgers et al., 1983). This is further contrasted by the fact that tactile or sonic stimulation of a freezing animal leads to a more active defensive reaction (startle response) whereas quiescent animals remain hyporeactive. Whether this second form of immobility corresponds to a submissive posture or to a recuperative behavior remains to be examined.

Different autonomic concomitants

Autonomic changes are usually associated with the different behavioral defensive strategies. Hyperventilation is generally observed with most defensive reactions as well as an increase in arterial pressure (Adams et al., 1969; Viken et al., 1991). More specifically, in freely-moving cats, the approach of a dog or fire evokes a confrontational type of reaction (i.e., threat display) which is associated with an increase in cardiac ouput, hear rate and arterial blood pressure with vasoconstriction in renal and splanchnic beds but vasodilation in skeletal muscle beds (Mancia et al., 1972; 1974). As well, in rats attacked by a resident and showing mainly confrontational and immobility types of defensive reactions, increased heart rate with renal and mesenteric vasoconstriction and hindquarter vasodilation was observed (Viken et al., 1991). It has been suggested that the cardiovascular changes redistribute blood flow in favor of skeletal muscle in preparation for the defensive reaction (see Bandler, 1988). In addition, this redistribution of blood flow may be adapted to the defensive strategy used by the animal (e.g., increase of blood flow in head during confrontations versus increase of blood flow in limbs during flight). Data collected in the decerebrate animal following activation of specific groups of neurons tend to confirm this hypothesis (see below).

Strategies	Postures	Vocalizations	Autonomic changes	Situations
Flight	Running forward Hops Jumps		Hypertension Tachycardia Hyperventilation	Approaching predator Approaching aggressive conspecific
Immobility	Crouching	Ultrasonic (22-28 kHz)	Hypertension Tachycardia Hyperventilation	Distant predator Distant conspecific Dangerous place
Confrontation	Upright posture Boxing Backward motion,	Sonic Ultrasonic (22-28 kHz)	Hypertension Tachycardia Hyperventilation	Close predator Close aggressive conspecific

Table 1: Main characterics of the three defensive strategies in the rat

Vocalizations also often accompany defensive behavior in mammals. In the monkey, different qualities of calls have been described according to the type of defensive reactions. For instance, barking and cooing are generally observed during confrontational reactions in *Macaca mulatta* whereas the animals stop any vocalizations during immobility (Kalin & Shelton, 1989). In the cat, confrontational reactions are generally accompanied by hissing, howling and growling, whereas vocalizations are emitted less frequently during flight (Bandler, 1988). In the rat, different kinds of vocalizations are emitted along with defensive behavior. In addition to sonic vocalizations the rat, as most rodents, can emit and hear ultrasounds up to 80 kHz (Sales, 1972). In particular, long pulse (i.e., 1 to 3 s duration) vocalizations within the range of 22 to 28 kHz have been shown to be associated with defensive behavior in the rat (e.g., van der Poel & Miczeck, 1991; Blanchard et al., 1991; Portavella et al., 1993). These vocalizations do not simply result from painful or fearful stimuli and are generally emitted concomitantly with confrontational or immobile postures (van der Poel & Miczeck, 1991; Portavella et al., 1993). They have been suggested to have an alarm function since they are generally emitted in the presence of conspecifics and can eventually be relayed by others (Blanchard et al., 1991). Whether distinct kinds of call with different frequencies and/or modulations are associated in the rat with different defensive postures remains to be examined. However, the measurement of ultrasonic vocalization - which can be done via an ultrasound detector which transforms the ultrasonic tone into a sonic one - constitutes an objective variable to quantify defensive reactions in rodents and to help the interpretation of some defensive postures (i.e., immobility). The use of this variable in the isolated rat as a measurement of fear remains, however, quite questionable.

The critical role of the midbrain periaqueductal gray in the organization of defensive behavior

Recent data obtained in the cat and in the rat have confirmed the hypothesis that distinct neural circuits underly the different defensive strategies. This appears especially clear from the work that has been conducted during the last decade on the midbrain periaqueductal gray matter (PAG). That this brain region is one of the key structure in the organization of defensive behavior has become apparent from the many studies which have used electrical brain stimulations, lesions or even unitary recordings (for review see Bandler, 1988). Using intracerebral microinjections of excitatory amino acids in order to selectively activate cell bodies and their dendrites, and not fibers of passage (Goodchild et al., 1982), it is possible to evoke species-specific defensive reactions in the freely moving cat as well as in the rat (see Bandler, 1988; Bandler & Depaulis, 1991). For example, in the rat, PAG injection of low, non-toxic doses of kainic acid, evokes defensive reactions (e.g., uprights, backward motion or forward locomotion and jumps) in response to the non-aggressive investigations of a conspecific. These reactions are very similar to what is observed in natural conditions (e.g., after an attack by an offensive resident). Furthermore, these evoked-defensive reactions are clearly different according to the localization, whithin the PAG, of the site of injection. *Confrontational* defensive reactions, characterized by an animal facing its partner, are induced by activation of cell bodies in a region of the PAG which is *lateral* to the aqueduct and in the *intermediate* third of the midbrain (Figure 1; Depaulis et al., 1989; Bandler & Depaulis, 1991). By contrast, *flight reaction and escape* are evoked when the injections are made in the *caudal third of the lateral PAG* (Figure 1; Depaulis et al., 1992; Bandler & Depaulis, 1991). A totally different behavioral pattern characterized by *quiescence and hyporeactivity* of the animal is evoked when neurons located in the *ventrolateral quadrant of the caudal PAG* are activated (Zhang et al., 1990; Depaulis et al., 1993).

What also makes the PAG a most attractive structure for the study of the organization of defensive behavior is that evidence has been collected, mostly in the cat, suggesting that the above-mentioned regions of the PAG also integrate distinct cardiovascular modifications (see Bandler et al., 1991; Carrive, 1991). Activation of neurons located in the intermediate lateral PAG results in an increase of arterial pressure accompanied by vasodilation in the head region but vasoconstriction in limbs: a pattern quite adapted to a confrontational strategy. By contrast, activation of neurons in the caudal part of the lateral PAG results in an increase of arterial pressure accompanied by vasodilation in limbs and vasoconstriction in head and viscera: a pattern quite adapted to flight. Finally, activation of neurons in the ventrolateral part of the PAG results in hypotension (Carrive, 1991), an effect which has also been observed in the rat (Lovick, 1992) and which appears adapted with the quiescent and hyporeactive reaction observed in the animals after injection in this region. In addition to cardiovascular changes, neurons in the PAG appear to also coordinate defensive vocalizations. In both the cat and the rat, distinct types of vocalizations can be evoked according to the location of the neuronal population which is activated within the PAG (Davis & Zhang, 1991). In the rat, ultrasonic vocalizations in the 22-28 kHz range are evoked only after activation of neurons in the caudal lateral PAG, whereas no such vocalizations or only sonic ones are emitted by rats injected in the intermediate third of the lateral PAG or the ventrolateral quadrant of the caudal PAG (Depaulis et al., 1992).

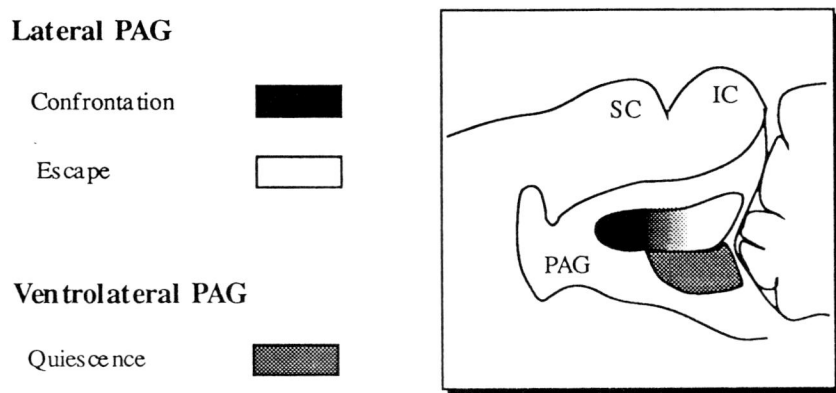

Figure 1: Schematic saggital representation of regions in the periaqueductal gray matter of the rat mediating confrontation, escape and quiescence. Abbreviations: IC: inferior colliculus; PAG: periaqueductal gray matter; SC: superior colliculus.

These data are thus in agreement with the existence of distinct neural circuits which coordinate the different defensive strategies and their physiological concomitants. The PAG is certainly not the only structure that organizes such adaptive response to threat. However, the fact that this structure receives quite direct projections from sensory systems (see Blomqvist & Craig, 1991) and sends projections to premotor neurons of the pons and medulla involved in the control of cardiovascular functions, locomotion and vocalization (see Carrive, 1991; Holstege, 1991) places the PAG as the core system in the organization of defensive behavior. This is confirmed by recent data showing that the different populations of neurons in the PAG described above are activated by different kinds of peripheral nociceptive stimuli (Keay & Bandler, 1993) and that such activation result in the corresponding defensive reaction (Keay et al., in preparation). If the neural circuitry within the PAG represents a basic and, perhaps even primitive system, which mediates and organizes the different defensive strategies, forebrain structures like the amygdala or the limbic cortices which project to specific areas of the PAG (see Shipley et al., 1991) can undoubtedly modulate the activity of this system.

An important feature of the data collected in the above-mentioned studies is that similar PAG regions appear to mediate similar defensive strategies in both the rat and the cat (Bandler & Depaulis, 1991). This suggests that a similar organization of defensive behavior in the PAG exists across mammals and may eventually have subsisted in humans. Indeed, it has been reported that electrical stimulation of the PAG in humans evokes intense feelings of fear and anxiety (see Bandler, 1988). The role of distinct PAG regions in mediating different basic patterns of human emotional expression remains, however, very speculative. A first question to address would be to determine if the human PAG has similar subdivisions as the functional/anatomical divisions suggested by the above mentioned studies in the cat and the rat. Using morphological approaches, (e.g., immunocytochemistry, receptor imaging) it should be possible in the future to verify this hypothesis.

Defensive behavior as a model of human anxiety

Although the neural system underlying defensive behavior is far from being understood, the different data presented in the first part of this chapter strongly suggest the existence of at least three different ways for an animal to cope with a threatening stimulation and that these responses imply different sets of neurons. These findings may thus provide an interesting conceptual framework to study fear and anxiety in humans. In the second part of this chapter, the possibility that defensive behavior models anxiety will be examined by addressing the different criteria (i.e., isomorphism, predictivity and homology) that are required for an experimental preparation to be considered as a valid model of a human pathology (Dantzer, 1986).

Defensive behavior in animals shares some components with human anxiety

Since defensive behavior is an essential behavioral feature along the evolution of the vertebrates, several of its basic characteristics in animals may have been preserved in humans. If one considers the three different defensive strategies described above, whether the behavioral reactions involved in each of these strategies are evocative of behavioral symptoms characterizing fear or anxiety in humans can be questioned. It is tempting to compare the immobility strategy in animals, and in particular the freezing response, to the behavioral inhibition showed by people facing a catastrophe or by most patients experiencing severe anxiety as it is the case during panic attack (Boulenger, 1987). Although, it is not always possible to distinguish this response from a "motoric" immobility, several studies have used freezing to measure fear in animals (e.g., Fanselow, 1991) and to model anxiety. The confrontational reactions are observed in invidualual protecting themselves from the aggression of another person and may correspond to the "reactive" symptoms of some forms of anxiety (i.e., hyperreactivity or paranoid symptoms). It is very likely that verbal communication in human plays an important role in this type of reaction and it is interesting to note that in animals, this strategy is associated with more vocalizations than the others (see Table 1). It is more difficult to find a human equivalence of the flight/escape strategy of an animal in response to a threat. It is interesting to note, however, that during a panic attack some patients try to leave the current situation (Boulenger, 1987).

The autonomic changes that accompany defensive behavior in animals provide further clues to eventually validate the isomorphic aspects of defensive behavior with fear and anxiety. The most evident similarities between animal defensive behavior and human anxiety relates to cardiovascular and respiratory changes. As in defensive behavior, fear and anxiety are generally associated with changes in arterial pressure, hear rate and ventilation (DSM-III-R classification, 1987). However, different kinds of cardiovascular changes can be observed in human experiencing fear and/or anxiety (e.g., hypertension and tachycardia or hypotension and bradycardia which can lead to syncope). Although it is very likely that local vascular changes differ with emotional reactions (e.g., blushing versus turning pale), there is no report of different modifications of regional blood flow according to the type of anxiety in human. As well, the changes in the tone of the voice which is reported in people during stage fright or in patients during panic attacks may also be compared with vocalizations accompanying defensive behavior in animals. That defensive behavior in animals shares both somatic and autonomic components with fear- and anxiety-mediated behavioral changes in humans appears supported by experimental and clinical data. However, whether the different defensive strategies are models of the different forms of anxiety (i.e., generalized anxiety, panic attack, phobia) in humans remains very speculative.

Anxiolytic and anxiogenic drugs differentially modify defensive behavior

During the last ten years, several experiments have been conducted in the animals (mainly rats and mice) using ethologically-based situations to examine the effects of either anxiolytic or anxiogenic treatments on the full repertoire of defensive behavior. It is not the purpose of the present section to provide a complete review of these data, but rather to show examples suggesting that the different defensive strategies can be differentially affected by treatments with know anxiolytic or anxiogenic effects in humans and what it might suggest for the mechanisms underlying anxiety.

Immobility appears to be generally decreased by *anxiolytic treatments* (Table 2). For examples, administration of diazepam, a benzodiazepine, reduces freezing and crouching postures induced, in the infant Rhesus monkey, by the presence of an experimenter (Kalin & Shelton, 1989). As well, immobile postures in response to the attacks of an offensive resident are reduced by a chronic treatment of diazepam or an acute injection of a partial agonist of the benzodiazepine receptor (Piret et al., 1991). Freezing responses in wild or laboratory rats are generally reduced in most situations either by benzodiazepines (Blanchard et al., 1990), $5HT_{1A}$ agonists (Blanchard et al., 1988) or ethanol (Blanchard et al., 1986). Conversely, administration of anxiogenic compounds like pentylenetetrazol or inverse agonists of the benzodiazepine receptor increases immobile freezing postures in rats confronted with an offensive resident (Piret et al., 1991; 1992). The fact that these compounds can induce non-convulsive seizures characterized by behavioral arrest (for discussion see Piret al., 1991) may, however, question the specificity of this effect. It is important to note that different results have been obtained after administration of yohimbine, another anxiogenic compound. In the laboratory mouse, this drug reduces immobile postures like crouching in reaction to the presence of a cat (Blanchard et al., 1993).

Treatments		Immobility	Flight	Confrontation
Anxiolytic	BZD agonist	decreased	no effect	increased/decreased
	$5\text{-}HT_{1A}$ agonist	decreased	increased?	decreased
	Ethanol	decreased	decreased	increased
Anxiogenic	BZD inverse agonist	increased		decreased
	pentylenetetrazol	increased		decreased
	Yohimbine	decreased	increased	

Table 2: Effects of systemic administration of anxiolytic and anxiogenic compounds on the different defensive strategies (summary from data in the literature).

Very likely because laboratory animals show very few *flight reactions* as compared to wild ones (Blanchard & Blanchard, 1989), there are less data on the effects of the various anxiolytic and anxiogenic compounds on this type of defensive strategy. Interestingly, this behavior appears quite resistant to most anxiolytic treatments, at least at doses without sedative/myorelaxant effects. In wild rats, flight and escape are unaffected or even enhanced by administration of buspirone or gepirone, two agonists of the 5-HT_{1A} receptor with anxiolytic effects (Blanchard et al., 1988). On the contrary, these reactions are reduced after administration of ethanol (Blanchard et al., 1986). Yohimbine, a drug with anxiogenic effects, has been reported to increase flight reaction in mice exposed to a cat (Blanchard et al., 1993).

Controversial data have been obtained concerning the effects of anxiolytic compounds on *confrontational reactions*. In wild rats, administration of buspirone or gepirone, significantly reduces confrontational reactions as observed in different test situations (Blanchard et al., 1988). Administration of diazepam reduced the amount of barking vocalizations induced in the infant Rhesus monkey by the presence of an experimenter (Kalin & Shelton, 1989) and decreased vocalizations in wild rat (Blanchard & Blanchard, 1989). However, benzodiazepine compounds and ethanol appear to have weaker effects on other component of this defensive reaction and to even increase some of them (Blanchard et al., 1986). In laboratory rats for instance, confrontational reactions like defensive upright postures and defensive sideways observed in response to the attack of an offensive resident were increased after a chonic treatment with a benzodiazepine full agonist or the acute injection of a partial agonist (Piret et al., 1991). Controversies in the effects of anxiolytic compounds on confrontational defensive reactions may come from the fact that this strategy involves postures which need to be constantly adjusted to the partner's or the predator's behavior. They are thus very sensitive to the sedative/myorelaxant effects of most of these compounds. Effects of chronic treatments - which reduce motor impairment - or of partial agonist may thus provide more reliable data. Anxiogenic treatments like benzodiazepine inverse agonist or pentylenetetrazol have been shown to decrease confrontational reactions in rats faced with an aggressive resident (Piret et al., 1991; 1992).

The data obtained after pharmacological treatments resulting in either known anxiolytic or anxiogenic effects in humans show that the different forms of defensive behavior are differentially affected by a given compound. This is in agreement with the existence of distinct neural mechanisms underlying the different defensive strategies. Furthermore, for a given test situation, different anxiolytics like benzodiazepines, 5-HT_{1A} agonists or ethanol have different profiles of action (see for instance Blanchard et al., 1988) on a given defensive strategy. This suggests that some compounds may act on the cognitive aspects of the stimulus (e.g., which is no longer perceived as dangerous) whereas other compounds act on the motor aspects of defensive reaction. Most of the anxiolytic compounds used in the studies (benzodiazepine, $5HT_{1A}$ agonists) are basically used in the clinic to treat generalized anxiety. Only immobility/freezing reaction appear to be consistently reduced by these treatments. This suggests that this strategy shows some predictivity for generalized anxiety which is in agreement with the general literature on models of behavioral inhibition (Thiébot, this volume). As for the other strategies, similar experiments with treatments used in the clinic for panic attacks and phobia will be of great interest. In particular, the effects of chronic treatments with antidepressants on flight/escape reactions will allow to further address the hypothesis that this strategy rather models panic attack forms of anxiety (see Graeff, 1991).

Defensive behavior: a fear-promoted adaptive behavior

All the defensive reactions described in the animals have been considered as "fear-promoted" behavior (Fanselow, 1991) and in this respect may certainly share some common mechanisms with fear-related behavior in humans. Whether each strategy is promoted by a different "quality" of fear is a very difficult question to address. Another aspect which needs also to be kept in mind is that defensive behavior is the *normal* reaction to threat and activation of this behavior in the appropriate context is certainly *adaptive*. As well, fear is the normal and adaptive reaction of a human being confronted with a dangerous situation. In contrast, what makes anxiety a pathology is (i) its maladaptive aspect: the symptoms may occur without any obvious reason (i.e., the fear without object) and/or the response is excessive to a threatening situation and (ii) its recurrent aspect (Hardy & Martinot, 1992). It may be thus argued that defensive behavior may model fear rather than "pathological" anxiety. However, there are instances where defensive behavior is maladaptive in animals: (i) when defensive reactions displayed are excessive or (ii) when the defensive strategy used is inappropriate. The lack of an adaptive response may reflect individual experience (e.g., non-aggressive exploration by a partner triggers defensive reactions in animals which have been previously defeated; van de Poll et al., 1982) - or a heritable trait in the coping strategy of the animals (e.g., Benus et al., 1991).

Conclusions

The data reported in the present paper demonstrate that different strategies are used by the animals to defend themselves. These strategies are mediated by distinct neural mechanisms and pharmacological anxiolytic and anxiogenic treatments differentially affect these strategies. This suggests that an individual have different ways to respond to fear and, although more speculative, that they may exist different qualities of fear. This is in favor of the very probable existence of different forms of anxiety with different brain mechanisms (see Dantzer, 1986, Thiébot, this volume). Whether each defensive strategy models one particular kind of anxiety is highly speculative and certainly more work is required both on the experimental and clinical aspects of fear and anxiety. A better understanding of the neural organization of defensive behavior and of the mechanisms that allow the animal to decide which strategy to use, will certainly provide important clues in the unravelling of human anxiety and the PAG appears one of the key structures. The fact that anxiolytic-like effects can be observed in the rat after injection of a benzodiazepine into this structure (Russo et al., 1993) further strengthens this idea.

References

Adams, D.B., Baccelli, G., Mancia, G. & Zanchetti, A. (1969): Cardiovascular changes during naturally elicited fighting behavior in the cat. *Am. J. Physiol.* 216, 1226-1235.
Bandler, R. (1988): Brain mechanisms of aggression as revealed by electrical and chemical stimulation: Suggestion of a central role for the midbrain periaqueductal grey region. In *Progress in Psychobiology and Physiological Psychology*, ed. A. Epstein & A. Morrison, vol. 13, pp. 67-154. New York: Academic Press.
Bandler, R., Carrive, P. & Zhang, S.P. (1991): Integration of somatic and autonomic reactions within the midbrain periaqueductal grey: Viscerotopic, somatotopic and functional organization. *Prog Brain Res.* 87, 269-305.
Bandler, R. & Depaulis, A. (1991): Midbrain periaqueductal gray control of defensive behavior in the cat and the rat. In: *The midbrain periaqueductal gray matter:*

functional, anatomical and neurochemical organization, ed. A. Depaulis & R. Bandler, pp. 175-198. New York, Plenum.

Benus, R.F., Bohus, B., Koolhass, J.M. & van Oortmerssen, G.A. (1991): Heritable variation for aggression as a reflection of individual coping strategies. *Experientia* 47, 1008-1019.

Blanchard, R.J., Blanchard, D.C., Flannelly, K.J. & Hori, K. (1986): Ethanol changes patterns of defensive behavior in wild rats. *Physiol. Behav.* 38, 645-650.

Blanchard, D.C., Rodgers, R.J., Hendrie, C.A. & Hori, K. (1988): "Taming" of wild rats (Rattus rattus) by $5HT_{1A}$ agonists buspirone and gepirone. *Pharmacol. Biochem. Behav.* 31, 269-278.

Blanchard, R.J. & Blanchard, D.C. (1989): Attack and defense in rodents as ethoexperimental models for the study of emotion. *Prog. Neuro-Psychopharmacol Biol. Psychiat.* 13, S3-S14.

Blanchard, D.C., Blanchard, R.J., Tom, P. & Rodgers, R.J. (1990): Diazepam changes risk assessment in an anxiety/defense test battery. *Psychopharmacology*, 101, 511-518.

Blanchard, R.J., Blanchard, D.C., Agullana, R. & Weiss, S.M. (1991): Twenty-two kHz alarm cries to presentation of a predator, by laboratory rats living in visible burrow systems. *Physiol. Behav.* 50, 967-972.

Blanchard, R.J., Taukulis, H.K., Rodgers, R.J., Magee, L.K. & Blanchard D.C. (1993): Yohimbine potentiates active defensive responses to threatening stimuli in swiss-webster mice. *Pharmacol. Biochem. Behav.* 44, 673-681.

Blomqvist, A. & Craig, A.D. (1991): Organization of spinal and trigeminal input to the PAG. In: *The midbrain periaqueductal gray matter: functional, anatomical and neurochemical organization,* ed. A. Depaulis & R. Bandler, pp. 345-364. New York, Plenum.

Boulenger, J.P. (1987): Troubles anxieux paroxystiques (troubles panique) et agoraphobie. In *L'attaque de panique: un nouveau concept?* ed. J.P. Boulenger, pp. 79-118. Paris, Editions Jean-Pierre Goureau.

Carrive, P. (1991): Functional organization of PAG neurons controlling regional vascular beds. In: *The midbrain periaqueductal gray matter: functional, anatomical and neurochemical organization,* ed. A. Depaulis & R. Bandler, pp. 67-100. New York, Plenum.

Dantzer, R. (1986): Les modèles animaux: différents types d'anxiété? *Suppl. Act. Méd. Int.-Psychiatrie* 3, 4-10.

Davis, P.J. & Zhang, S.P. (1991): What is the role of the midbrain periaqueductal gray in respiration and vocalization? In: *The midbrain periaqueductal gray matter: functional, anatomical and neurochemical organization,* ed. A. Depaulis & R. Bandler, pp. 57-66. New York, Plenum.

Depaulis, A., Bandler, R. & Vergnes, M. (1989): Characterization of pretentorial periaqueductal gray neurons mediating intraspecific defensive behaviors in the rat by microinjections of kainic acid. *Brain Res.* 486, 121-132.

Depaulis, A., Keay, K.A. & Bandler, R. (1992): Longitudinal neuronal organization of defensive reactions in the midbrain periaqueductal gray region of the rat. *Exp. Brain Res.* 90, 307-318.

Depaulis, A., Keay, K.A. & Bandler, R. (1993): Quiescence and hyporeactivity evoked by activation of cell bodies in the ventrolateral midbrain periaqueductal gray of the rat. *Exp. Brain Res.*, in press.

Fanselow, M. (1991): The midbrain periaqueductal gray as a coordinator of action in response to fear and anxiety. In: *The midbrain periaqueductal gray matter: functional, anatomical and neurochemical organization,* ed. A. Depaulis & R. Bandler, pp. 151-174. New York, Plenum.

Goodchild, A.K., Dampney, R.A.L., Bandler, R. (1982): A method for evoking physiological responses by stimulation of cell bodies, but not axons of passage, within localized regions of the central nervous system. *J. Neurosci. Meth.* 6, 351-363.

Graeff, F.G. (1991): Neurotransmitters in the dorsal periaqueductal grey and animal models of panic anxiety. In *New concepts in anxiety*, ed. M. Briley & S.E. File, pp. 288-312. London: The Macmillan Press.

Hardy, P. & Martinot, J.L. (1992): Les états anxieux. In *Les états névrotiques*, ed. J. Ades & F. Rouillon, pp. 61-106. Paris, Editions Jean-Pierre Goureau.

Holstege, G. (1991): Descending pathways from the periaqueductal gray and adjacent areas. In: *The midbrain periaqueductal gray matter: functional, anatomical and neurochemical organization,* ed. A. Depaulis & R. Bandler, pp. 239-266. New York, Plenum.

Kalin, N.H. & Shelton, S.E. (1989): Defensive behaviors in infant rhesus monkeys: environmental cues and neurochemical regulation. *Science* 243, 1718-1721.

Keay, K.A., Li, Q.F., Depaulis, A. & Bandler, R. (1993): Deep and superficial pain have a different representation in the midbrain periaqueductal gray and upper cervical spinal cord of the rat., submitted for publication.

Keay, K.A. & Bandler, R. (1993): Deep and superficial noxious stimulation increases foslike immunoreactivity in different regions of the midbrain periaqueductal gray. *Neurosci Lett..* 154, 23-26.

Lovick, T.A. (1992): Inhibitory modulation of the cardiovascular defence response by the ventrolateral periaqueductal grey matter in rats. *Exp. Brain Res.* 89, 133-139.

Mancia, G., Baccelli, G. & Zanchetti, A. (1972): Hemodynamic responses to different emotional stimuli in the cat: patterns and mechanisms. *Am. J. Physiol.* 223, 925-933.

Mancia, G., Baccelli, G. & Zanchetti, A. (1974): Regulation of renal circulation during behavioral changes in the cat. *Am. J. Physiol.* 227, 536-542.

Piret, B., Depaulis, A. & Vergnes, M. (1991): Opposite effects of agonist and inverse agonist ligands of benzodiazepine receptor on self-defensive and submissive postures in the rat. *Psychopharmacology.* 103, 56-61.

Piret, B., Depaulis, A. & Vergnes, M. (1992): Opposite effects of pentylenetetrazol on selfdefensive and submissive postures in the rat. *Psychopharmacology.* 107, 457-460.

Portavella, M., Depaulis A. & Vergnes, M. (1993): 22-28 kHz ultrasonic vocalizations associated with defensive reactions in male rats do not result from fear or aversion. *Psychopharmacol.ogy* 111, 190-194.

Rodgers, R.J., Hendrie, C.A. & Waters, A.J. (1983): Naloxone partially antagonizes postencounter analgesia and enhances defensive responding in male rats exposed to attack from lactating conspecifics. *Physiol. Behav.* 30, 781-786.

Russo, A.S., Guimaraes, F.S., De Aguiar, J.C. & Graeff, F.G. (1993): Role of benzodiazepine receptors located in the dorsal periaqueductal grey of rats in anxiety. *Psychopharmacology* 110, 198-202.

Sales, G.D. (1972): Ultrasound and aggressive behaviour in rats and other small mammals. *Anim. Behav.* 20, 88-100.

Shipley, M.T., Ennis, M., Rizvi, T.A. & Behbehani, M.M. (1991): Topographical specificity of forebrain inputs to the midbrain periaqueductal gray: evidence for discrete longitudinally organized input columns. In: *The midbrain periaqueductal gray matter: functional, anatomical and neurochemical organization,* ed. A. Depaulis & R. Bandler, pp. 417-448. New York, Plenum.

Van der Poel, A.M. & Miczeck, K.A. (1991): Long ultrasonic calls in male rats following mating, defeat and aversive stimulation - frequency modulation and bout structure. *Behaviour* 119, 127-142.

Van de Poll, N.E., de Jonge, F., van Oyen, H.G. & van Pelt, J. (1982): Aggressive behaviour in rats: effects of winning or losing on subsequent aggressive interactions. *Behav. Proc.* 7, 143-155.

Viken, R.J., Johnson, A.K. & Knutson, J.F. (1991): Blood pressure, heart rate, and regional resistance in behavioral defense. *Physiol. Behav.* 50, 1097-1101.

Zhang, S.P., Bandler, R. & Carrive, P. (1990): Flight and immobility evoked by excitatory amino acid microinjection within distinct parts of the subtentorial midbrain periaqueductal grey of the cat. *Brain Res.* 520, 73-82.

Résumé

Les comportements de défense sont, chez l'animal, la principale expression de la peur et présentent plusieurs similitudes comportementales et physiologiques avec les réactions humaines face à un danger ("anxiété normale"). L'étude de ces comportements constituent ainsi une approche intéressante de la "pathologie anxieuse" chez l'être humain. Les observations éthologiques suggèrent l'existence de trois principales stratégies utilisées par l'animal pour s'adapter à une menace naturelle (un prédateur, un congénère agressif): (1) la fuite; (2) l'immobilité et (3) la confrontation. Des données récentes suggèrent que ces différentes stratégies sont coordonnées par des circuits nerveux différents, en particulier au niveau de la substance grise periaqueducale du mésencéphale. Les données présentées dans ce chapitre montrent que l'étude des comportements de défense a permis d'accroître notre connaissance de la neurobiologie de la peur et de l'anxiété et que différents mécanismes sont susceptibles de sous-tendre différentes formes d'anxiété.

II. Biological aspects of stress and anxiety

II. *Aspects biologiques du stress et de l'anxiété*

Stress and GABAergic transmission in the rat brain: the effect of carbon dioxide inhalation

Giovanni Biggio, Tonino Cuccheddu, Stefania Floris, Enrico Sanna, Maria Luisa Barbaccia*, Gianna Roscetti*, Mariangela Serra and Alessandra Concas

*Department of Experimental Biology, University of Cagliari, Italy and * Department of Experimental Medicine, University of Rome «Tor Vergata», Italy*

Summary

Several experimental data suggest that the $GABA_A$ receptor complex plays a major role in the pharmacology neurochemistry and physiopathology of stress and anxiety. This idea has received further support by the finding that stress, like anxiogenic drugs, reduces the function of $GABA_A$ receptor complex, an effect mimicked by the in vivo administration of different inhibitors of GABAergic transmission and opposite to the effect of anxiolytics.

More recently, we found that a brief exposure to CO_2 inhalation, a treatment known to induce anxiety and panic attack in man, produces on $GABA_A$ receptor function an effect similar to that elicited by stress and anxiogenic drugs. Accordingly, this treatment shares with stress and anxiogenic drugs the capability to induce proconflict behaviour in rats and to reduce the capability of GABA to stimulate $^{36}Cl^-$ uptake in the brain of these rodents. Moreover, like stress CO_2 inhalation enhances the brain content of different steroid derivatives.

Taken together, these data further indicate that anxiety and $GABA_A$ receptor function are interdependent. In fact, changes in the emotional state of the animals elicited by different stressful stimuli is paralleled by a rapid plastic changes of central GABAergic synapses.

A crucial finding to understand the neurochemical mechanisms involved in the neurobiology and pharmacology of stress and anxiety has been the discovery that several anxiolytic and anxiogenic drugs have specific recognition sites at the level of $GABA_A$ receptor complex. Accordingly, these studies suggested that the central GABAergic transmission is directly or indirectly involved not only in the pharmacology of those anxiogenic and anxiolytic drugs but also in the neurochemistry and physiopathology of a variety of neurologic and psychiatric diseases mainly related to alterations of the emotional state, sleep and neuronal excitability (see for review Biggio and Costa, 1986; Biggio et al., 1990).

The idea that the emotional states, fear and GABAergic transmission are interdependent has received a further support by our finding showing that a stressful condition alters the function of $GABA_A$ receptors in the rat brain (see for review Biggio et al., 1990). In agreement with the latter finding, several papers have more recently shown that different environmental stimuli known to change the emotional state of the animals alter the biochemical parameters usually used to evaluate the functional state of the GABA-gated chloride channel (Biggio, 1983; Havoundjian et al., 1986; Concas et al., 1987, 1988; Serra et al., 1989a, Drugan et al., 1989) and modify the sensitivity of the animals to the effect of anxiolytic and anxiogenic drugs (Corda and Biggio, 1986; Boix et al., 1989; Mennini et al., 1988; File et al., 1990, 1992; Andrews et al., 1992).

Altogether these experimental data strongly suggest that in the mammalian brain the GABAergic synapses play a key role in the physiological and pharmacological modulation of the behaviour and neuropsychiatric diseases related to stress and anxiety.

Stress, emotional state and GABAergic function

The evidence that in rats a rapid change in the emotional state may result in a parallel change in the function of central GABAergic synapses was obtained in our laboratory using the handling-habituated rats (see for review Biggio, 1983). The animals habituated to the manipulations that precede killing were considered an "unstressed animal model" while the acute handling of the naive rats before sacrifice constituted the emotional stimulus responsible for the changes in GABAergic transmission. Consistent with this idea foot-shock delivered just before sacrifice to both naive and handling-habituated rats markedly modified $GABA_A$ receptor function only in the brain of handling-habituated "unstressed" rats and failed to change significantly $GABA_A$ receptors in the same tissue preparation from naive ones (Biggio et al., 1980; 1981).

All together the above data indicated that handling-habituated rats represent a relatively nonstressed condition while the acute handling of the naive rats or foot-shock constitutes a stressful condition which modifies both the emotional state of the animals and the function of the GABA-coupled chloride channel. In fact, those stressful stimuli markedly reduced ^3H-GABA binding and chloride fluxes and increased ^{35}S-TBPS binding in the brain of handling-habituated rats (Concas et al., 1987, 1988; Serra et al., 1989b).

Anxiogenic drugs, stress and GABAergic function

A major contribution to understand the functional meaning of the changes in the GABAergic biochemical parameters elicited by stress was clearly provided by the finding that inhibitors of $GABA_A$ receptor function and negative allosteric modulators (anxiogenic ß-carbolines) of the GABAergic transmission mimicked in vitro the effect of stress on those parameters. In fact, bicuculline, isoniazid, FG 7142 and other drugs known to reduce the function of GABAergic transmission and to induce proconflict effect in rats and experimental anxiety in primates, man included (Ninan et al., 1982; Corda et al., 1983a; Dorow et al., 1983) shared with stress the capability to enhance ^{35}S-TBPS binding and to reduce the function of the GABA coupled chloride channel (Biggio et al., 1984; Concas et al., 1987; 1988; Serra et al., 1989b; 1991).

The evidence that anxiogenic drugs, which decrease the activity of the GABA associated chloride channel, shared with stress the capability to induce the same modification of ^{35}S-TBPS binding, chloride fluxes and ^3H-GABA binding in the rat brain, suggested that stress might decrease the function of the GABA-coupled chloride channel.

To further verify the above conclusion and to better understand the functional significance of the changes in ^{35}S-TBPS binding produced by the in vitro addition of anxiolytic and anxiogenic drugs, we measured ^{35}S-TBPS binding "ex vivo" following the in vivo administration of GABAergic drugs. As expected, we found that the in vivo administration of anxiolytic benzodiazepines or anxiogenic ß-carbolines, modulates ^{35}S-TBPS binding in the "ex vivo" preparation from rat cerebral cortex as they do in vitro. Thus, the intraperitoneal administration of benzodiazepines induced a marked decrease in ^{35}S-TBPS binding in the "ex vivo" membrane preparation from rat cerebral cortex and other brain areas (Serra et al., 1989b, 1991; Sanna et al., 1989b, 1990). Vice versa, the intravenous injection of anxiogenic ß-carbolines increased ^{35}S-TBPS binding (Sanna et al., 1989a). The effect of both ß-carbolines and benzodiazepines was completely antagonized by the previous administration to rats of the specific benzodiazepine receptor antagonist, flumazenil.

Altogether these results demonstrated that the "ex vivo" measurement of ^{35}S-TBPS binding allows the detection of changes in the activity of the GABA-dependent chloride channel induced by the

administration of positive and negative modulators of GABAergic transmission. This conclusion was confirmed by our recent finding (Serra et al., 1989b) that isoniazid, a drug which fails to affect ^{35}S-TBPS binding in vitro modifies it after in vivo administration. In fact, isoniazid increased in a dose-related manner ^{35}S-TBPS binding in the rat cerebral cortex.
Since isoniazid inhibits the GABAergic transmission by reducing the GABA synthesis and consequently the amount of GABA present at the presynaptic level (Horton et al., 1979), our results suggested that the in vivo decrease in the availability of GABA at the receptor site may cause a conformational modification of the postsynaptic molecular components (α-ß-γ subunits) of the GABA$_A$ receptor complex (Barnard and Seeburg, 1988; Pritchett et al., 1989; Shivers et al., 1989), that persists in vitro in the membrane preparations.
The evidence that the in vitro addition or in vivo administration of anxiolytic drugs, which enhance GABAergic transmission and modulate ^{35}S-TBPS binding, ^{3}H-GABA binding and ^{36}Cl$^-$ uptake in a manner opposite to that of anxiogenic ß-carbolines, completely abolished the effect elicited by acute handling and foot-shock in handling-habituated rats further suggested that stress might have an inhibitory action on the function of central GABAergic synapses. This conclusion was also supported by the finding that foot-shock potentiated the convulsant activity of isoniazid (Serra et al., 1991) while the latter drug markedly enhanced the proconflict action induced by FG 7142 in rats (Corda et al., 1983b).

Carbon-dioxide inhalation and anxiety
Several clinical studies suggest that carbon dioxide inhalation produces anxiety both in healthy subjects and in anxious patients. These studies have clearly shown that patients with panic disorder react to carbon dioxide with greater anxiety and more panic attacks than normal controls (Griez et al., 1990; Woods et al., 1986; Gorman et al., 1987).
The finding that the inhalation of carbon dioxide is panicogenic in patients with an hystory of spontaneous panic attack but much less in normal subjects has allowed to suggest the hypothesis that carbon dioxide hypersensitivity plays a major role in the physiopathology of panic disorder. Accordingly, it has been suggested that patients with panic disorder have an altered sensitivity of carbon dioxide receptors both in periphery and in the central nervous system (Gorman et al., 1987). However, the neuronal mechanisms whereby carbon dioxide inhalation produces anxiety and panic attack are still unknown.
Experimental studies have only suggested that in laboratory animals carbon dioxide inhalation enhances the function of noradrenergic neurons in the locus coeruleus and increases the plasma level of catecholamines (Stone, 1993). This finding is consistent with several lines of evidence suggesting that an enhancement of brain noradrenergic pathways is intimately related to the neurobiology and physiopathology of anxiety disorders (Charney and Redmond, 1983).
As reported in the previous paragraphes, several experimental evidences have shown that the central GABA$_A$ receptor and their coupled modulatory recognition sites play a major role in the neurobiology and pharmacology of stress, emotional states and fear. Accordingly, benzodiazepines, drugs known to enhance the function of the central GABA$_A$ receptors are the most efficacious drugs used in the treatment of different anxiety disorders. On the contrary, drugs known to reduce the function of the GABA$_A$ receptors such as the inverse agonists of the benzodiazepine recognition site, tetrazol and other negative modulators elicit a proconflict behaviour in rat, experimental anxiety in monkeys and severe anxiety attack in man. Finally, environmental stress and changes of the emotional states reduce the function of the GABA-coupled chloride channel in the rat brain and modifies the sensitivity of the animals to the effects of anxiolytic drugs.
On the basis of these studies we decided to evaluate the effect of the exposure to carbon dioxide on the function of the GABA-ionophore receptor complex in the rat brain. This study may improve the knowledge of the neurochemical events involved in the anxiogenic and panicogenic effects elicited by carbon dioxide inhalation as well as in the physiopathology of stress and anxiety.

CO_2 inhalation reduces $GABA_A$ receptor function

Male-Sprague Dawley rats (Charles River, Como, Italy) weighing 200-250 g were used. Animals were housed under 12 h light-dark cycles at a constant temperature of 22 ± 2 °C with water and standar laboratory food ad libitum. In order to avoid the stress associated with sacrifice (Biggio et al., 1990) rats were habituated to the new environment (hermetically closed box) and to the handling manouvers that precede killing. Thus, they were picked up from the cages, held for 1 min in a hermetically closed box followed by a forced introduction of the animal head through the blades of a guillotine for animal sacrifice and then put back in the former cages. This procedure were repeated 3 times a day for 1 week.

The day of the experiment the animals were exposed for 1 min to the gas mixture (35% CO_2, 65% O_2) in an hermetically closed box with a capacity of 35 l and killed by decapitation 10 min later unless otherwise specified. The control animals were kept in the same cage but not exposed to the gas. In order to evaluate the $GABA_A$ receptor function animals were sacrificed and $^{36}Cl^-$ uptake and ^{35}S-TBPS binding measured in membranes of different brain areas.

As shown in Fig 1, $^{36}Cl^-$ uptake into membrane vesicles from cerebellum of the control group was stimulated by GABA (50-100 μM) in a concentration-dependent manner. The exposure of rats to the following concentrations of CO_2 (35% - 1 min) significantly reduced the enhancement of $^{36}Cl^-$ uptake elicited by 50-100 μM GABA. In fact, CO_2 treatment reduced by about 50% the capability of GABA to stimulate $^{36}Cl^-$ uptake. Similar results were obtained measuring $^{36}Cl^-$ uptake into membrane vesicles from cerebral cortex and hippocampus. On the contrary, basal $^{36}Cl^-$ uptake was not modified by this treatment.

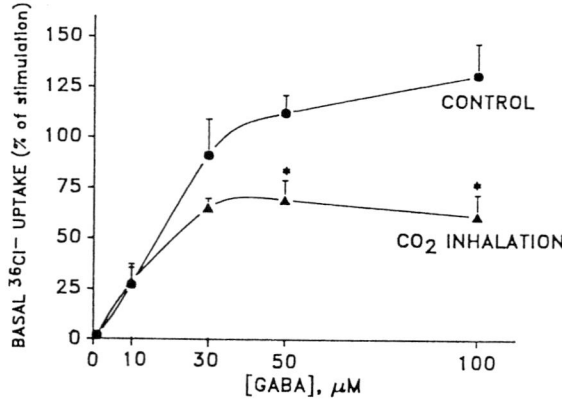

Fig. 1. CO_2 inhalation reduces GABA-stimulated $^{36}Cl^-$ uptake into membrane vesicles from rat cerebellum. The animals were exposed for 1 min to the gas mixture (35% CO_2, 65% O_2) and killed 10 min later. Pooled tissue from two rats from each group was used in each experiment. Data are mean ± S.E. of five separate experiments. Similar results were obtained using membrane vesicles from cerebral cortex and hippocampus.
*$p < 0.05$ versus control.

To evaluate further the action of CO_2 inhalation on the function of the chloride channel coupled to $GABA_A$ receptor we investigated whether this treatment was able to modify the binding of ^{35}S-TBPS to recognition sites coupled to the GABA gated chloride channel.

As shown in Fig. 2, the inhalation of a gas mixture (35% CO_2, 65% O_2) increased ^{35}S-TBPS binding in the cerebral cortex, cerebellum and hippocampus. The time course of the CO_2 inhalation-induced increase of ^{35}S-TBPS binding showed that the effect of this treatment was already significant (+

34%) in rats sacrificed immediately after 1 min inhalation, reached a peak (+ 55%) at 10 min and returned to control value in about 2 hr (Fig. 3). The action of CO_2 inhalation on the function of the $GABA_A$ receptor complex was similar to that induced by the anxiogenic and proconvulsant ß-carboline derivatives ßCCE and FG 7142. In fact, as already shown (Sanna et al., 1989a; Biggio et al., 1990) these inverse agonists for benzodiazepine receptors, produced a marked and dose-dependent (0.2 - 1 mg/kg i.v.) increase of ^{35}S-TBPS binding in the rat brain (Fig. 3).

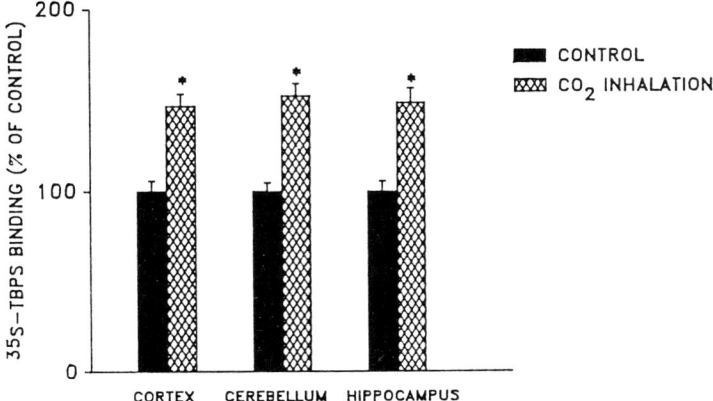

Fig. 2. CO_2 inhalation enhances ^{35}S-TBPS binding in different areas of the rat brain. Rats were killed 10 min after 1 min exposure to CO_2. Pooled tissue from two rats from each group was used in each experiment. Data are the means ± S.E. of 5 separate experiments.
*$p < 0.01$ versus the respective control group.

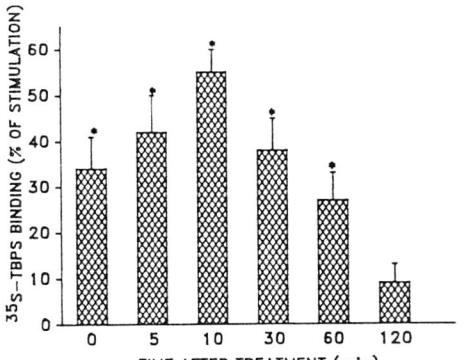
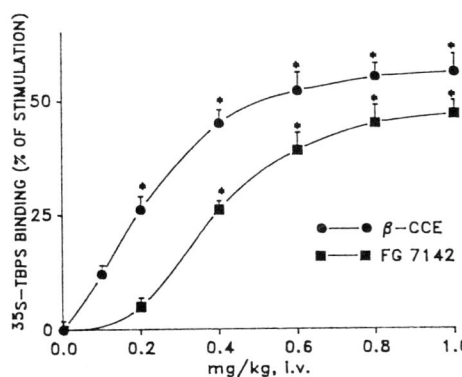

Fig. 3. Increase of ^{35}S-TBPS binding by CO_2 inhalation and anxiogenic ß-carbolines in the rat cerebellum. Rats were killed at different times after exposure for 1 min to the gas mixture (time 0). FG 7142 and ßCCE were administered intravenously as a saline suspension containing 1 drop of Tween 80 per 3 ml 15 min before killing. Data are the means ± S.E. of three to five separate experiments.
*$p < 0.05$ versus the respective control group.

Anxiolytic drugs and CO_2 inhalation
The finding that CO_2 inhalation reduces the function of $GABA_A$ receptor prompted us to investigate whether different benzodiazepine recognition site ligands which prevent the action of stressful stimuli

on GABAergic transmission were able to antagonize the action of CO_2 on ^{35}S-TBPS binding.
As reported in Fig. 4 the previous administration of different benzodiazepine receptor ligands classified as partial (imidazenil, bretazenil), full agonists (alprazolam, diazepam) and a selective ligand (abecarnil) prevented the reduction in $GABA_A$ receptor function exerted by CO_2 inhalation. On the contrary, the anxiogenic ß-carboline derivatives FG 7142 and ßCCE, like CO_2 inhalation, markedly enhanced ^{35}S-TBPS binding in the same brain areas (Fig. 3). The latter finding shows that CO_2 inhalation shares with anxiogenic ligands and foot-shock stress (Concas et al., 1988) the capability to reduce the function of GABA gated chloride channel, an effect opposite to that elicited by different anxiolytic benzodiazepine receptor ligands.

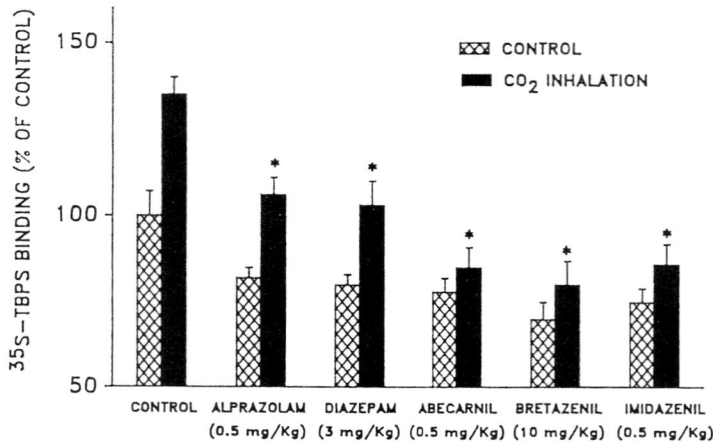

Fig. 4. Different anxiolytic drugs antagonize the action of CO_2 inhalation on ^{35}S-TBPS binding in the rat cerebellum. Rats were killed 10 min after 1 min exposure to CO_2 inhalation. Drugs were administered intraperitoneally 30 min before CO_2 inhalation.
*$p < 0.05$ versus CO_2 treated animals.

CO_2 inhalation and brain steroids

Steroids may reach their site of action in brain via the blood stream or may be produced in situ and for this they have been called neurosteroids (Le Goascogne et al., 1987). It is known, in fact, that glial cell cultures, which express the cytochrome P450 side chain cleavage enzyme (Le Goascogne et al., 1987), can synthesize pregnenolone (the major precursor of all steroids) from cholesterol (Hu et al., 1987) via activation of the mitochondrial DBI receptor (MDR). This is an oligomeric receptor complex located on the outer mitochondrial membrane (Anholt et al., 1986) that binds with high affinity the peptide Diazepam Binding Inhibitor (DBI) and a series of so-called "peripheral benzodiazepine receptor" ligands (Mukhin et al., 1989; Papadopoulos et al., 1992; Romeo et al. 1992). Moreover, like in adrenal, also in brain cortical minces from adult male rats, the process of steroidogenesis can be stimulated by a short term exposure to dibutyryl-cyclic AMP or forskolin (Barbaccia et al., 1992).

Steroids interact with at least two types of receptors in brain: 1) a nuclear/cytosolic type, directly participating in gene transcription regulation and 2) a membrane receptor located in the transmembrane domain of the $GABA_A$ and possibly other ligand-gated ionotropic receptors. The evidence for the latter site of steroid action comes from several lines of independent investigation showing that a series of ring-A reduced derivatives of pregnenolone and progesterone 19 modulate the GABA-operated chloride current trough either native or recombinant $GABA_A$ receptors (Lambert et al., 1987; Majewska et al., 1986; Puia et al., 1990) and 2) interacts with several ligand binding sites on the $GABA_A$ receptor complex: they have been reported to increase the affinity of GABA for its receptor, to decrease the binding of ^{35}S-TBPS and to modulate the binding of various benzodiazepine receptor ligands to their site on the $GABA_A$/chloride channel receptor complex (Gee et al, 1988; Majewska et al., 1986; Morrow et al., 1990). In line with these electrophysiological and biochemical data, the ring-A reduced derivatives of pregnenolone (PRE), progesterone (PRO) and desoxycorticosterone (DOC), such as 5alpha-pregnan-3alpha-ol-20 one and tetrahydrodesoxycorticosterone, have been shown to possess anticonvulsant (Romeo et al., 1992), antineophobic (Romeo et al., 1992) and sedative (Holzbauer, 1975) properties, further pointing towards a positive interaction with the $GABA_A$ receptors also in vivo. On the other hand, some pregnenolone derivatives (pregnenolone-sulphate and dehydroepiandrosterone-sulphate) have been reported to negatively modulate the $GABA_A$ receptor function (Majewska and Schwartz, 1987). On this ground we asked whether the decreased $GABA_A$ receptor function, elicited by CO_2 inhalation, could be paralleled by an alteration of the brain content of neuroactive steroids.

The concentrations of PRE, PRO and DOC (the direct precursors of the $GABA_A$ receptor active steroids) were measured in ethylacetate extracts of brain cerebral cortex taken from adult male rats, either control or CO_2-exposed, previously habituated to the experimental procedure. The rats were sacrificed by focussed microwave irradiation (5-6 seconds) to the head, in order to instantaneously fix the brain tissue, thus minimizing the post mortem steroid metabolism. Trace amounts (6-8000 cpm) of each ^3H-steroid were added to the homogenate in order to monitor their recovery throughout the entire extraction and purification procedure. After extraction, the steroids were purified by HPLC on a Silica-diol column (Merck), developed with a gradient of 2-propanol (from 0 to 30%) in hexane. PRE, PRO and DOC were then quantified in the respective HPLC fractions by radioimmunoassay run with specific antibodies.

As shown in Table 1, in the brain cortex of rats killed 10 minutes after the CO_2 inhalation there was a robust increase in the levels of PRE, PRO and DOC (3, 27 and 14 folds, respectively); while in the brain cortex of rats killed right after the CO_2 exposure only DOC was significantly increased (86%). It is interesting to note that this time dependence in the effect of CO_2 inhalation on brain steroid levels is reminiscent of the time dependence of the CO_2 effect on the ^{35}S-TBPS binding and on the GABA-stimulated $^{36}Cl^-$ uptake. We are now investigating whether the increase of brain steroid content after CO_2 could be functionally related to the observed changes in $GABA_A$ receptor function and whether is due to the activation of peripheral (adrenal and/or gonadal) or central steroidogenesis, as it has been previously shown that both pathways may be activated following stressful stimuli (Purdy et al., 1991).

TABLE 1

CO_2 INHALATION ENHANCES THE CONTENT OF STEROIDS IN THE RAT BRAIN

	PRE	PRO	DOC
	(ng/g protein)		
CONTROL	46 ± 2.8	1.7 ± 0.34	6.6 ± 1.2
CO_2 time 0	50 ± 5.4	2.4 ± 0.46	$12.3 \pm 1.7^*$
CO_2 time 10	$130 \pm 8.0^{**}$	$47.0 \pm 8.4^{**}$	$95.0 \pm 7.5^{**}$

$^*p < 0.01$, $^{**}p < 0.001$ when compared to the respective control values

CO_2 inhalation and conflict behaviour

Conflict test is one of the most used animal models to study the neurochemical mechanisms underlying anxiety. Accordingly, using the Vogel's punished drinking test it has been clearly shown that in rats, drugs (ß-carbolines, $GABA_A$ receptor antagonists and inhibitors cf GABAergic transmission) known to reduce the function of $GABA_A$ receptors elicited a proconflict responce enhancing the shock induced suppression of drinking in thirsty rats (Corda et al., 1983a,b).

On the basis of this evidence we evaluate the capability of CO_2 inhalation in suppressing punished behaviour in rats. This study should allow to better understand whether the biochemical modifications of the GABAergic function elicited by CO_2 inhalation had a functional significance. As shown in Table 2 a proconflict response similar to that induced by the anxiogenic benzodiazepine receptor ligand, FG 7142, was elicited also by the CO_2 inhalation. Accordingly, rats tested 10 min after CO_2 exposure (35% CO_2 - 65% O_2) resulted much more sensitive to the low intensity (0.4 mA) electric stimulus than control animals. In fact, the number of licking periods in CO_2 treated rats was markedly reduced in comparison with not treated animals. Moreover, pretreatment with imidazenil (0.5 mg/kg) or alprazolam (0.5 mg/kg) prevented the proconflict effect elicited by CO_2 inhalation.

TABLE 2

CO_2 INHALATION ENHANCES SHOCK-INDUCED SUPPRESSION OF DRINKING IN RATS

	SHOCKS/3 MIN
Control	26 ± 2.1
CO_2 inhalation	19 ± 1.8*
Imidazenil + CO_2	32 ± 2.4
Alprazolam + CO_2	29 ± 2.2

The test was performed 10 min after 1 min exposure to CO_2. Imidazenil (0.5 mg/kg i.p.) or alprazolam (0.5 mg/kg i.p.) were injected 30 min before CO_2 inhalation. Licking periods were measured during the punished session at 0.4 mA current. Each value is the mean ± S.E. of 1-5 rats per group. *$p < 0.05$ versus the control group.

CONCLUSIONS

The results presented here show that a brief exposure to CO_2 inhalation shares with stress due to handling and foot shock and anxiogenic drugs the capability to reduce the $GABA_A$ receptor function and to enhance punishment-suppressed behaviour in rats.

This conclusion is supported by the reduction of the number of licking periods elicited by CO_2 inhalation as well as by the reduced capability of GABA to stimulate $^{36}Cl^-$ uptake and by the higher content of ^{35}S-TBPS binding found in the brain of CO_2 treated rats. Since inhalation of carbon dioxide induces anxiety in healthy subjects and panic attack in patient with panic disorder (Woods et al., 1986) our biochemical and behavioural findings are in line with several reports showing that a reduced GABAergic transmission is a major neurochemical event involved in the pharmacology and physiopathology of different anxiety disorders.

In the brain of CO_2 treated rats the levels of PRE, PRO and DOC were markedly increased with respect to control animals. Thus, CO_2 inhalation exerted on brain content of steroid derivatives an effect similar to that elicited by swim stress (Purdy et al., 1991). This finding further suggests a role of these compounds as endogenous modulators of $GABA_A$ receptor complex during stress.

In conclusion, all the present results further indicate that anxiety may result from a decrease in the GABAergic transmission following the inhibition of the GABA-coupled chloride channel. Thus, the present data are consistent with previous results showing a functional correlation between the emotional state of the animals and the degree of function of central $GABA_A$ receptors.

ACKNOWLEDGMENT

This study was in part supported by grant 92.00022.PF41 from the National Research Council (CNR) [target project "Prevention and Control Disease Factor"] Subproject "Stress".

REFERENCES

Andrews, N., Zharkovsky, A., and File, S.E. (1992): Acute handling stress downregulates benzodiazepines receptors: reversal by diazepam. Eur. J. Pharmacol. 210: 247-251.

Anholt, R.R.H., Pedersen, P.L., De Souza, E.B., and Snyder, S.H. (1986): The peripheral type benzodiazepine receptor. Localization to the mitochondrial outer membrane. J. Biol. Chem. 261: 576-583.

Barbaccia, M.L., Roscetti, G., Trabucchi, M., Ambrosio, C. and Massotti, M. (1992): Cyclic AMP-dependent increase of steroidogenesis in brain cortical minces. European J. Pharmacology 219: 485-486.

Barnard, E.A., and Seeburg, P.H. (1988): Structural basis of the GABA-activated chloride channels: molecular biology and molecular electrophysiology. In Chloride Channels and Their Modulation by Neurotransmitters and Drugs, eds. G. Biggio and E. Costa, pp. 1-18. New York: Raven Press.

Biggio, G., Corda, M.G., Demontis, G., Concas, A., and Gessa, G.L. (1980): Sudden decrease in cerebellar GABA binding induced by stress. Pharmac. Res. Comm. 12: 489-493.

Biggio, G., Corda, M.G., Concas, A., Demontis, G., Rossetti, Z., and Gessa, G.L. (1981): Rapid changes in GABA binding induced by stress in different areas of the rat brain. Brain Res. 229: 363-369.

Biggio, G. (1983): The action of stress, ß-carbolines, diazepam and Ro 15-1788 on GABA receptors in the rat brain. In Benzodiazepine Recognition Site Ligands: Biochemistry and Pharmacology, eds. G. Biggio and E. Costa, pp. 105-117. New York: Raven Press.

Biggio, G., Concas, A., Serra, M., Salis, M., Corda, M.G., Nurchi, V., Crisponi, C., and Gessa, G.L. (1984): Stress and ß-carbolines decrease the density of low affinity GABA binding sites: an effect reversed by diazepam. Brain Res. 305: 13-18.

Biggio, G., and Costa, E. eds (1986): GABAergic Transmission and Anxiety. Advances in Biochemical Psychopharmacology, Vol. 41. New York. Raven Press.

Biggio, G., Concas, A., Corda, M.G., Giorgi, O., Sanna, E., and Serra, M. (1990) GABAergic and dopaminergic transmission in the rat cerebral cortex: effect of stress, anxiolytic and anxiogenic drugs. Pharmac. Ther. 48: 121-142.

Boix, F., Fernandez Teruel, A., and Tobena, A. (1989): The anxiolytic action of benzodiazepines is not present in handling-habituated rats. Pharmacol. Biochem. & Behav. 31: 541-546.

Charney, D.S., and Redmond, D.E., Jr. (1983): Neurobiological mechanism in human anxiety. Evidence supporting central noradrenergic hyperactivity. Neuropharmacol. 22: 1531-1536.

Concas, A., Mele, S., and Biggio, G. (1987): Foot-shock stress decreases chloride efflux from rat brain synaptoneurosomes. Eur. J. Pharmac. 135: 423-427.

Concas, A., Serra, M., Atsoggiu, T., and Biggio, G. (1988): Foot-shock stress and anxiogenic ß-carbolines increase t-[^{35}S]butylbicyclophosphorothionate binding in the rat cerebral cortex, an effect opposite to anxiolytics and γ-aminobutyric acid mimetics. J. Neurochem. 51: 1868-1876.

Corda, M.G., Blaker, W.D., Mendelson, W.B., Guidotti, A., and Costa, E. (1983a): ß-carbolines enhance shock-induced suppression of drinking in rats. Proc. Natn. Acad. Sci. U.S.A. 80: 2072-2076.

Corda, M.G., and Biggio, G. (1986) Stress and GABAergic transmission: biochemical and behavioural studies. In GABAergic Transmission and Anxiety, eds G. Biggio and E. Costa, pp. 121-136. New York: Raven Press.

Corda, M.G., Costa, E., and Guidotti, A. (1983b): Involvement of GABA in the facilitation of punishment suppressed behaviour induced by ß-carbolines in rats. In Benzodiazepine Recognition Site Ligands: Biochemistry and Pharmacology, eds. G. Biggio and E. Costa, pp. 121-128. New York: Raven Press.

Dorow, R., Horowski, R., Paschelke, G., Amin, M., and Braestrup, C. (1983): SEvere anxiety induced by FG 7142, a ß-carboline ligand for benzodiazepine receptors. Lancet II: 98-99.

Drugan, R.C., Morrow, A.L., Weizman, R., Weizman, A., Deutsch, S.I., Crawley, J.N., and Paul, S.M. (1989): Stress-induced behavioural depression in the rat is associated with a decrease in GABA receptor-mediated chloride ion flux and brain benzodiazepine receptor occupancy. Brain Res. 487: 45-51.

File, S.E., Andrews, N., and Zharkovsky, A. (1990): Handling habituation and chlordiazepoxide have different effects on GABA and 5-HT function in the frontal cortex and hippocampus. Eur. J. Pharm. 190: 229.

File, S.E., Andrews, N., Wu, P.Y., Zharkovsky, A., and Zangrossi, H., Jnr (1992): Modification of chloridazepoxide's behavioural and neurochemical effects by handling and plus-maze experience. Eur. J. Pharmacol. 218: 9-14.

Gee, K.W., Bolger, M.B., Brinton, R.E., Coirini, H. and McEwen, B. (1988): Steroid modulation of the chloride ionophore in rat brain: structure-activity requirements, regional dependence and mechanism of action. J. Pharmacol. Exper. Ther. 246(2): 803-812.

Gorman, J.M., Fyer, M.R., Liebowitz, M.R., and Klein, D.F. (1987): Pharmacologic provocation of panic attacks. In Psychopharmacology: The Third Generation of Progress, ed. Meltzer H.Y., pp. 985-993. New York: Raven Press.

Griez, E., Zandbergen, J., Pols, H., and de Loof, C. (1990): Response to 35% CO_2 as a marker of panic in severe anxiety. Am. J. Psychiatry 147: 796-797.

Havoundjian, H., Paul, S.M., and Skolnick, P. (1986): Acute, stress-induced changes in the benzodiazepine/γ-aminobutyric acid receptor complex are confined to the chloride ionophore. J. Pharmac. Exp. Ther. 237: 787-793.

Holzbauer, M. (1975): Physiological variations in the ovarian production of 5-pregnane derivatives with sedative properties in the rat. J. Steroid Biochem. 6: 1307-1310.

Horton, W.R., Chapman, A.G., and Meldrum, B.S. (1979): Isoniazid, as a glutamic acid decarboxylase inhibitor. J. Neurochem. 33: 745-750.

Hu, Z.Y., Bourreau, E., Jung-Testas, I., Robel, P., and Baulieu, E.-E. (1987): Neurosteroids: oligodendrocyte mitochondria convert cholesterol to pregnenolone. Proc. Natl. Acad. Sci. U.S.A. 84: 8215-8219.

Lambert, J.J., Peters, J.A., and Cottrell, G.A. (1987): Actions of synthetic and endogenous steroids on the $GABA_A$ receptor. Trends Pharmacol. Sci. 8: 224-227.

Le Goascogne, C., Robel, P., Gouezou, M., Sananes, N., Baulieu, E.-E., and Waterman, M. (1987): Neurosteroids: cytochrome P450 scc in rat brain. Science 237: 1212-1215.

Majewska, M.D., Harrison, N.L., Schwartz, R.D., Barker, J.L., and Paul, S.M. (1986): Steroid hormone metabolites are barbiturate-like modulators of the GABA receptors. Science (Wash., D.C.) 232: 1004-1007.

Majewska, M.D., and Schwartz, R.D. (1987): Pregnenolone-sulfate: an endogenous antagonist of the γ-aminobutyric acid receptor complex in brain? Brain Res. 404: 355-360.

Mennini, T., Gobbi, M., Perin, L., and Salmona, M. (1988): Rapid internalization of benzodiazepine receptors in the rat cortex induced by handling. In Chloride Channels and their Modulation by Neurotransmitters and Drugs, Eds G. Biggio and E. Costa, p. 263. New York: Raven Press.

Morrow, L.A., Pace, J.R., Purdy, R.H., and Paul, S.M. (1990): Characterization of steroid interactions with γ-aminobutyric acid receptor-gated chloride ion channels: evidence for multiple steroid recognition sites. Mol. Pharmacol. 37: 263-270.

Mukhin, A.G., Papadopoulos, V., Costa, E., and Krueger, K.E. (1989): Mitochondrial benzodiazepine receptors regulate steroid biosynthesis. Proc. Natl. Acad. Sci. U.S.A. 86: 9813-9816.

Ninan, P.T., Insel, T.M., Cohen, R.M., Cook, J.M., Skolnick, P., and Paul, S.M. (1982): Benzodiazepine receptor-mediated experimental "anxiety" in primates. Science 218: 1332-1334.

Papadopoulus, V., Guarneri, P., Krueger, K.E., Guidotti, A. and Costa, E. (1992): Pregnenolone biosynthesis in C6-2B clioma cell mitochondria: regulation by a mitochondrial diazepam binding inhibitor receptor. Proc. Natl. Acad. Sci. U.S.A. 89: 5113-5117.

Pritchett, D.B., Sonthelmer, H., Shivers, B.D., Ymer, S., Kettnmann, H., Schofield, P.R. and Seeburg, P.H. (1989): Importance of a novel $GABA_A$ receptor subunit for benzodiazepine pharmacology. Nature 338: 582-585.

Puia, G., Santi, M., Vicini, S., Pritchett, D.B., Purdy, R.H., Paul, S.M., Seeburg, P.H., and Costa, E. (1990): Neurosteroids act on recombinant human $GABA_A$ receptors. Neuron 4: 759-765.

Purdy, R.H., Morrow, A.L., Moore, P.H., Jr., and Paul, S.M. (1991): Stress-induced elevations of γ-aminobutyric acid type A receptor-active steroids in the rat brain. Proc. Natl. Acad. Sci. U.S.A. 88: 4553-4557.

Romeo, E., Auta, J., Kozikowski, A.P., Papadopoulos, V., Puia, G., Costa, E., and Guidotti, A. (1992): 2-aryl-3-indoleacetamides (FGIN- 1): a new class of potent and specific ligands for the mitochondrial DBI receptor (MDR). J. Pharmacol. Exper. Ther. 262(3): 971-978.

Sanna, E., Concas, A., Serra, M., and Biggio, G. (1989a): "In vivo" administration of anxiogenic ß-carbolines enhances ^{35}S-TBPS binding in the rat cerebral cortex. Eur. J. of Neurosci. Suppl. 2: 287.

Sanna, E., Serra, M., Pepitoni, S., and Biggio G. (1989b): Dramatic increase in nigral t-[^{35}S]butylbicyclophosphorothionate binding sites elicited by the degeneration of the striato-nigral GABAergic pathway: reversal by diazepam. Brain Res. 501: 144-149.

Sanna, E., Concas, A., Serra, M., and Biggio, G. (1990): In vivo administration of ethanol enhances the function of the GABA-dependent chloride channel in the rat cerebral cortex. J. Neurochem. 54: 696-698.

Serra, M., Concas, A., Atsoggiu, T., and Biggio, G. (1989a): Stress like bicuculline and DMCM reduces the basal ^{36}Cl⁻ uptake in the rat cortical membrane vesicles: an effect reversed by GABA. Neurosci. Res. Commun. 4: 41-50.

Serra, M., Sanna, E., and Biggio, G. (1989b): Isoniazid, an inhibitor of GABAergic transmission enhances ^{35}S-TBPS binding in the rat cerebral cortex. Eur. J. Pharmacol. 164: 385-388.

Serra, M., Sanna, E., Concas, A., Foddi, C., and Biggio, G. (1991): Foot-shock stress enhances the increase of ^{35}S-TBPS binding in the rat cerebral cortex and the convulsions induced by isoniazid. Neurochem. Res. 16: 17-22.

Shivers, B.D., Killisch, I., Sprengel, R., Sontheimer, H., Kohler, M., Schofield, P.R., and Seeburg, P.H. (1989): Two novel $GABA_A$ receptor subunits exists in distinct neuronal subpopulations. Neuron 3: 327-337.

Stone, E. (1983): Rapid adaptation of the stimulatory effect of CO_2 on brain norepinephrine metabolism. Naunyn-Schmiedeberg's Arch. Pharmacol. 324: 313-315.

Woods, S.W., Charney, D.S., Loke, J., Goodman, W.K., Redmond, D.E., and Heninger, G.R. (1986): Carbon dioxide sensitivity in panic anxiety. Arch. Gen. Psychiatry 43: 900-909.

Résumé

De nombreuses données expérimentales suggèrent que le complexe-récepteur $GABA_A$ joue un rôle majeur dans la pharmacologie, la neurochimie et la physiopathologie du stress et de l'anxiété. En particulier, le stress, comme les agents anxiogènes, diminue la fonction de ce récepteur, et cet effet peut être reproduit par des traitements avec des inhibiteurs de la transmission GABAergique. Au contraire, les anxiolytiques augmentent l'activité du récepteur $GABA_A$.

Récemment, nous avons observé qu'une inhalation brève de CO_2 (qui peut déclencher une crise d'angoisse et une attaque de panique chez l'homme) provoque des altérations fonctionnelles du récepteur $GABA_A$ tout à fait semblables à celles induites par le stress ou les agents anxiogènes. En particulier, chez le rat, tous ces traitements renforcent l'inhibition comportementale dans des situations aversives appropriées et diminuent l'effet stimulant du GABA sur l'influx neuronal de $^{36}Cl^-$ dans le cerveau. Enfin, comme le stress, l'inhalation de CO_2 entraine une élévation de la concentration cérébrale de différents stéroïdes.

Ces données confirment l'existence d'un lien étroit entre l'état fonctionnel du récepteur $GABA_A$ et l'anxiété. D'ailleurs, les changements dans l'état émotionnel des animaux soumis à différents stress interviennent parallèlement à des adaptations rapides de la transmission GABAergique centrale.

Stress and catecholamines: similarities and differences between NA and DA systems

Jean-Pol Tassin

Chaire de Neuropharmacologie, Collège de France, INSERM U.114, 11, place Marcelin Berthelot, 75231 Paris Cedex 05, France

SUMMARY

Numerous studies have shown that stressful situations induce increased brain noradrenaline (NA) turnover. Different methodologies, including electrophysiology, biochemical determination of neurotransmitter tissue contents and brain dialysis have given concordant results. Since most of the NA innervation of the forebrain originates from the locus coeruleus, this nucleus is considered as playing a major role in stress response. Ascending mesencephalic dopaminergic (DA) neurons are also activated by stressful situations but the amplitude of the effects decreases from the mesocortical to the mesolimbic and nigro-striatal DA neurons, the latter group being only slightly or not affected. Minor tranquillizers, such as benzodiazepines, can prevent the stress-induced activations of both NA and DA neurons. Neuronal corticotropin-releasing factor may be a primary factor responsible for the stress-induced NA activations, whereas pituitary-hypophysial corticosterone may induce a sensitization of DA neurons. Finally, it is proposed that the differences observed between the reactivities to stress of NA and DA neurons are due to their respective functional roles, in particular as regards the importance of mesocortical DA neurons in cognitive representational processes.

INTRODUCTION

The concept of stress arose as a result of Hans Selye's observations that a large number of damaging or potentially damaging stimuli led to similar physiological reactions. It is well known, for example, that sympathoadrenal activation is an essential component of the physiological response to stress (Cannon, 1914; Mason et al., 1961; Levi, 1967). Various stimuli, aversive or considered as a challenge to the organism, increase heart rate and plasma adrenaline, NA and 17-hydroxycorticosteroid levels.

In the central nervous system, the activation of NA neurons following stress has become increasingly documented (Maynert & Levi, 1964; Thierry et al., 1968; Korf et al., 1973; Stone, 1975). The locus coeruleus, which contains as many as half of all the brain NA cell bodies (Chu & Bloom, 1974; Jones & Moore, 1974), has therefore been hypothesized to play an important role in stress response (Korf et al., 1973; Cassens et al., 1980; Glavin, 1985). Locus coeruleus has even been proposed as a central analog of peripheral sympathetic ganglia (Amaral & Sinnamon, 1977; Aghajanian & VanderMaelen, 1982; Elam et al., 1986; Reiner, 1986).

Like locus coeruleus cells, DA neurons connect the brain stem reticular formation (ventral tegmental area (VTA) and substantia nigra) to the forebrain. However, unlike the locus coeruleus projections which present most diffuse projections (Swanson & Hartman, 1975; Moore & Bloom, 1979), mesencephalic DA neurons seem to innervate only selected brain regions, and much of that innervation is topographically organized (Björklund & Lindvall, 1978; Moore & Bloom, 1978). This may thereby provide an anatomical basis for the ascending DA neurons to influence phasic extrapyramidal motor activities as well as emotive and cognitive functions. In agreement with this proposition, we will see that DA neurons are, like NA cells, activated by stressful situations but that the amplitudes of these activations are dependent on the DA subgroup taken into account, i.e. mesocortical, mesolimbic or nigro-striatal (Lavielle et al., 1979).

Different techniques are available to study modifications of activity of catecholaminergic neurons. These methods include electrophysiology, cup technique, push-pull cannula, biochemical estimations of metabolites and neurotransmitters, voltammetry and, more recently, brain dialysis. As far as stressful situations are concerned, only those methods which allow the utilization of awake animals seem to be adapted. Fortunately, among the numerous papers published on this subject, data obtained with different methodologies do not exhibit important discrepancies. It should be kept in mind, however, that the estimation of catecholamine release *in vivo* is not sufficient to fully describe neurotransmission in the behaving animal for at least two reasons. First, it cannot be expected that modifications of neuronal activities may be determined biochemically for stressful situations shorter than few minutes. Clearly, this limitation does not stand for electrophysiological methods. Second, it cannot be excluded that changes in the sensitivities of post-synaptic receptors occur during stress and thus modify the integrated function of catecholamine synapses in such a way that the neurotransmission could be temporarily blocked.

Finally, if most authors agree that stress increases brain NA turnover, some controversies exist about the relationship between stress and DA neurons (Antelman et al., 1988). More precisely, Antelman and his colleagues note that a stressor which induces a ninefold increase in plasma corticosterone fails to affect the mesocortical DA neurons, a DA subgroup generally accepted as being the most sensitive to stressful situations (Thierry et al., 1976; Fadda et al., 1978; Lavielle et al., 1979; Herman et al., 1982; Abercrombie et al., 1989). This observation emphasizes that the link between stress and DA neurons is obviously not as tight as it is with NA neurons. Such discrepancies may be due to differences in the functional roles of each catecholamine and this will be tentatively discussed at the end of this short review.

STRESS AND NORADRENALINE

As mentioned previously, most of the NA innervation of the forebrain originates from one sole nucleus, the locus coeruleus. The electrophysiological activity of these neurons is highly responsive to stressful stimulation (Abercrombie et al., 1987) and this can explain that sufficiently intense stressors can reduce the NA content of brain (see review Stone, 1975). In addition, whatever the stressor, footshock, cold, restraint, heat, treadmill, aggregation, burns, limb ischemia etc.., acute or chronic, an increase of NA turnover has been observed (Corrodi et al., 1967; Bliss et al., 1968; Thierry et al., 1968; Korf et al., 1973; Stone, 1975; Tsuda et al., 1982).

More recently, the development of *in vivo* microdialysis brought a confirmation of these data by measuring the release of NA in brain areas of freely moving rats. A 30 minutes restraint stress or tailshocks increase the release of NA in the hippocampus by more than 200 % (Abercrombie et al., 1988). Similarly, Rossetti et al. (1990) have reported an increase in NA release in the frontal cortex after tailshock in rats, and Yokoo et al. (1990a,b) have also found increased NA release in the hypothalamus following either inescapable footshock or immobilization stress. It is interesting to note that diazepam, a minor tranquillizer, is able to prevent the increased NA release in the frontal cortex induced by stressful situations (Rossetti et al., 1990).

Corticotropin-releasing factor (CRF) is presumed to play a crucial role in eliciting the coordinated set of endocrine, autonomic and behavioural events which constitute the stress response. This peptide has been reported to be principally localized to cell bodies located in the hypothalamus and the median eminence (Olschowka et al., 1982). Some of the fibers arising from these cell bodies travel caudally in the braistem, and the locus coeruleus appears to be one of the nuclei receiving such an innervation (Swanson et al., 1983). Valentino et al. (1983) have found that CRF administered intraventricularly increases the discharge rates of locus coeruleus neurons of anesthetized rats. Very recently, in an *in vivo* microdialysis study, Lavicky and Dunn (1993) found that an intracerebroventricular administration of CRF dose-dependently increased release of NA in the medial hypothalamus and medial prefrontal cortex. In addition, there is some evidence that NA can be stimulatory on CRF release (Plotsky, 1987) which suggests that CRF can both activate and be activated by NA systems. It must be noted, however, that the activation of NA systems occurs at relatively high doses of CRF and Dunn and Berridge (1990) have proposed to divide behavioral and physiological responses to CRF into high-dose and low-dose effects. Decreased feeding and sexual behavior, decreased locomotor activity in a novel environment, increased locomotor activity in a familiar environment and exacerbated acoustic startle response would correspond to the high-dose (aversive doses > 0.5 µg i.c.v.) effects, whereas enhancement of locomotor behaviour in a novel environment, decreased social interaction, increased feeding and shock-induced fighting are observed at lower doses (0.005-0.1 µg i.c.v.). Dunn and Berridge (1990) propose that the low-dose effects correspond to mild or moderate activations of NA systems associated with arousal and mild anxiety whereas the higher doses of CRF may directly activate locus coeruleus NA neurons and perhaps also DA systems.

The problem of the differentiation between stressful stimuli and behaviorally activating but nonstressful stimuli has been adressed by Abercrombie and Jacobs (1987) in a very elegant electrophysiological study. Simultaneous recordings of the electrophysiological activity of locus coeruleus cells and measurements of plasma NA levels and heart rate have allowed these authors to show that behavioral activation *per se* is not sufficient to evoke a tonic activation of NA neurons. Their study demonstrates that the locus coeruleus is involved in the CNS response to stress and confirms that the activity of these neurons increases in association with sympathoadrenal activation.

STRESS AND DOPAMINE

The cell bodies of ascending DA pathways are located in the mesencephalon and innervate cortical (prefrontal, cingular, entorhinal), limbic (nucleus accumbens, septum, amygdala, hippocampus) and striatal structures (Björklund and Lindvall, 1978). Since 1976, numerous studies have reported that stressful stimuli activate the mesocortical DA neurons (Thierry et al., 1976; Fadda et al., 1978; Lavielle et al., 1979; Hervé et al., 1979; Tassin et al., 1980; Blanc et al., 1980; Herman et al., 1982; Reinhard et al., 1982; Bannon et al., 1983; Dantzer et al., 1984; Deutch et al., 1985; Claustre et al., 1986; D'Angio et al., 1988; Abercrombie et al., 1989; Kaneyuki et al., 1991). Although some specificity has been claimed for the sensitivity of the mesocortical DA neurons to stress, analysis of the literature clearly indicates that DA meso-nucleus accumbens neurons are also activated by stress. It appears, however, that the mesocortical DA neurons are the most reactive whereas the DA nigro-striatal pathway is only very slightly or not affected (Lavielle et al., 1979; Herman et al. 1982; Abercrombie et al., 1989). Most authors have also noted that the activation of DA mesocortical neurons can be blocked by a pretreatment with minor tranquillizers such as benzodiazepines (Fadda et al., 1978; Lavielle et al., 1979; Reinhard et al., 1982; Claustre et al., 1986; Kaneyuki et al., 1991). Interestingly, it seems that the effects of anxiolytics is exerted at brain sites other than the VTA and the prefrontal cortex (Claustre et al., 1986). Since benzodiazepines can also prevent the stress-induced NA release, it can be suggested that the blockade occurs upstream to DA and NA neurons, at the level of CRF release, as it has been proposed by Vargas et al. (1992).

Experiments have also been performed on rats which did not receive shocks but were submitted to environmental stimuli associated with shocks (Herman et al., 1982; Kaneyuki et al., 1991). Although these situations are clearly stressful since plasma corticosterone levels are increased, the DA activation in these experimental conditions is confined to the mesoprefrontocortical neurons. These effects could therefore be related to the implication of mesocortical DA neurons in cognitive representational processes (Brozoski et al., 1979; Simon et al., 1980; Sawaguchi & Goldman-Rakic, 1991).

The role of the DA mesocortical neurons in the control of emotional behaviour has also been analyzed on two strains of mice, BALB/C and C57/BL6, presenting high and low emotionality, respectively. When submitted to electric footshocks, the increase in turnover of mesocortical DA neurons was higher for the BALB/C than for C57/BL6 mice (Hervé et al., 1979). When both strains were submitted to a two-minute open field session, the mesocortical DA neurons of BALB/C mice were the only ones affected (Tassin et al., 1980).

The general agreement which arises from the different studies analyzing the reactivity of DA neurons to stress should not, however, hide the presence of some discrepancies.

First, many authors have noted an absence of correlation between the amplitude of the changes in plasma corticosterone levels and the reactivity of mesocortical DA neurons (Herman et al, 1982; Antelman et al., 1988; Kaneyuki et al., 1991).

Second, when the voltammetric determination of extracellular DOPAC was used, immobilization as well as tail-pinch induced a much higher increase of DOPAC in the nucleus accumbens than in the prefrontal cortex (Bertolucci-D'Angio et al., 1990). It cannot be excluded that differences in the rates of elimination of extracellular DOPAC and DA in the nucleus accumbens and in the prefrontal cortex are responsible for these discrepancies. This would explain why a technology measuring DOPAC with a short time constant (voltammetry) gives different results than microdialysis which estimates DA with a larger time constant. In any case, these data suggest that the reactivity to stress of mesolimbic DA pathway is probably very similar to that of the mesocortical DA system.
Same authors (D'Angio et al., 1988) have compared two genetically selected lines of rats (Roman high (RHA/Verh) and low (RLA/Verh) avoidance), the former presenting a much lower level of emotionality than the latter. As expected, all of the stressful situations investigated (mild tail pinch, high intensity loud noise, or immobilization) induced a greater augmentation of heart rate in RLA/Verh than RHA/Verh rats. However, increases of extracellular DOPAC levels in the anteromedial cortex occurred only in RHA/Verh animals, i.e. those presenting the lower level of emotionality.

Third, a long-term isolation, which may represent a stressful stimulus, <u>decreases</u> the turnover of DA in the prefrontal cortex (Blanc et al., 1980). Interestingly, isolated animals exposed to footshocks exhibit ampler behavioural responses as well as a higher reactivity of the mesocortical DA system, when compared to grouped animals. In other words, chronic isolation induces a sensitization to stress, although it decreases the basal turnover of DA in the prefrontal cortex.

DIFFERENCES BETWEEN NA AND DA SYSTEMS

As mentioned previously, CRF seems particularly important in situations where an organism must mobilize not only the pituitary-adrenal system but also the CNS in response to environmental challenge. Acute as well as chronic stress have been shown to double the levels of CRF-like immunoreactivity in the locus coeruleus, suggesting that it may mediate stress-induced modifications of NA turnover (Chappell et al., 1986). On the other hand, increases in corticosterone secretion, which is one of the final consequence of a pituitary-adrenal axis activation, induce a sensitization of DA systems to amphetamine psychomotor effects (Deroche et al., 1992). Moreover, there is some evidence that high doses of CRF induce aversion (Heinrichs et al., 1991), whereas corticosterone increases the reinforcing properties of addictive drugs (Piazza et al., 1991). It is thus tempting to propose the existence of a link between CRF, NA and aversion and corticosterone, DA and reward.

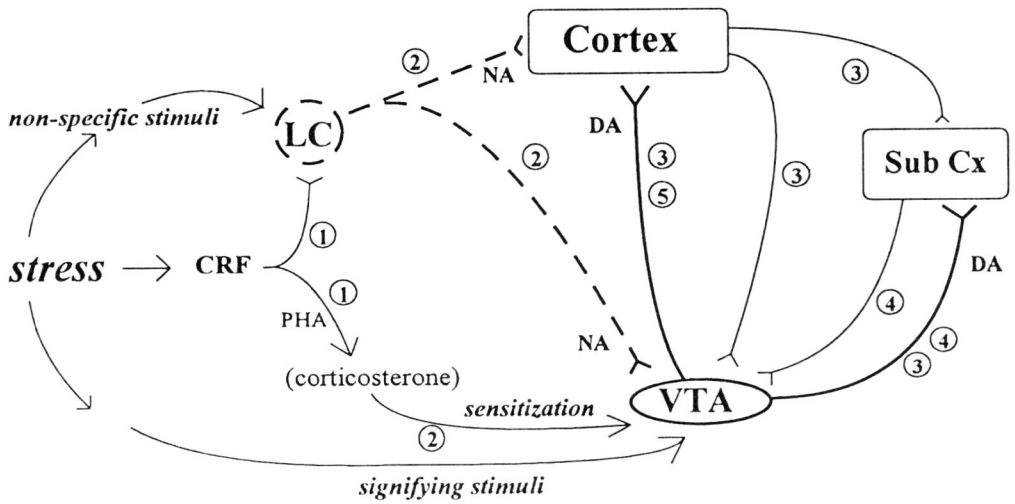

Fig.1: Schematic diagram of sequential events ending up to an activation of NA and DA systems by stress.
Non-specific stimuli and neuronal CRF activate NA locus coeruleus cells. Mesocortical and mesolimbic DA ascending pathways, previously sensitized by corticosterone, are activated by signifying stimuli and, among others, by NA neurons. Other activating neurons, such as habenulo-interpeduncular substancePergic ones (Lisoprawski et al. 1981; Bannon et al., 1983), have not been represented. Numbers in circles correspond to putative sequential events. Abbreviations: CRF: corticotropin-releasing factor; DA: dopamine; LC: Locus coeruleus; NA: noradrenaline; PHA: pituitary-hypophysial axis; Sub Cx: subcortical structures; VTA: ventral tegmental area. See text for details.

In freely moving animals, NA cells of the locus coeruleus respond to a variety of stimuli, including auditory, visual and tactile, with an excitation-inhibition pattern (Aston-Jones & Bloom, 1981). The most effective and reliable stimuli for eliciting locus coeruleus responses are those that disrupt behaviour and evoke orienting responses. In contrast, modifications of activity of DA neurons seem to be related to motivational arousal elicited by stimuli with appetitive properties (Steinfels et al., 1983; Romo & Schultz, 1990).
We have previously shown that locus coeruleus cells tonically activate mesocortical DA neurons (Hervé et al., 1982). More recently, we have obtained data suggesting the existence of multiple levels of interaction between NA and DA systems in the prefrontal cortex (see review Tassin, 1992). Moreover, we have shown that the stimulation by NA of cortical α1-adrenergic receptors is necessary for the expression of subcortical DA function (Blanc et al, 1993).

Taking all these observations into account, a summary of the different effects of stress on NA and DA systems is tentatively proposed on Fig. 1:

- The CRF released by a stressful situation acts simultaneously through a neuronal pathway which activates locus coeruleus NA cells and *via* the pituitary-hypophysial axis which increases corticosterone levels (1).
- An increased release of NA will then occur in the cerebral cortex and the VTA, while corticosterone will sensitize DA neurons located in the VTA (2).
- The NA released in the VTA is then able to activate mesocortical DA neurons. In addition, the NA released in the prefrontal cortex will, through cortico-subcortical and cortico-VTA pathways, allow the processing of information in subcortical structures, partly *via* an activation of DA mesolimbic pathways (3).

- Depending on the result of this processing and on the nature of the initial stimuli, subcortico-VTA pathways will induce an increased activity of DA mesolimbic (4) or mesocortical (5) systems.

CONCLUSION

There is a general agreement to consider that stressful situations activate both NA and DA pathways in the CNS. However, experimental data suggest that activations of NA systems are more directly linked to any type of situation which can be considered as a challenge to the organism than DA cells. Indeed, it seems that an increased release of hypothalamic CRF can parallely activate locus coeruleus cells activity through a neuronal pathway and augment corticosterone levels *via* the pituitary-adrenal axis. In contrast, although DA cells also respond to stressful situations, they are sensitive to more complex stimuli. Two factors at least suggest that the responses of DA neurons are linked to the animal's experienced past. First, the reactivity of DA neurons depends upon previous levels of corticosterone which have sensitized or not VTA-DA neurons. Second, DA neurons are responsive to stimuli whose signification has been previously encoded. Finally, it cannot be excluded that part of the activation of mesocortical DA neurons is due to a representational process triggered by the necessity of coping with the situation.

REFERENCES

Abercrombie, E.D., & Jacobs, B.L. (1987): Single-unit response of noradrenergic neurons in the locus coeruleus of freely moving cats. I. Acutely presented stressful and nonstressful stimuli. *J. of Neurosci.* 7, 2837-2843.

Abercrombie, E.D., Keller, R.W., & Zigmond, M.J. (1988): Characterization of hippocampal norepinephrine release as measured by microdialysis perfusion: Pharmacological and behavioral studies. *Neuroscience* 27, 897-904.

Abercrombie, E.D., Keefe, K.A., DiFrischia, D.S., & Zigmond, M.J. (1989) Differential effect of stress on *in vivo* dopamine release in striatum, nucleus accumbens, and medial frontal cortex. *J. Neurochem.* 52, 1655-1658.

Aghajanian, G.K., & VanderMaelen, C.P. (1982): α2-Adrenoreceptor-mediated hyperpolarization of locus coeruleus neurons: Intracellular studies in vivo. *Science* 215, 1394-1396.

Amaral, D.G. & Sinnamon, H.M. (1977): The locus coeruleus: Neurobiology of a central noradrenergic nucleus. *Prog. Neurobiol.* 9, 147-196.

Antelman, S.M., Knopf, S., Caggiula, A.R., Kocan, D., Lysle, D.T., & Edwards D.J. (1988): Stress and enhanced dopamine utilization in the frontal cortex: The Myth and the Reality. In *The mesocorticolimbic dopamine system*, eds P.W. Kalivas and C.B. Nemeroff, Vol. 537, pp. 262-272, Ann. N. Y. Acad. Sci., New York.

Aston-Jones, G., & Bloom, F.E. (1981): NE-containing locus coeruleus neurons in behaving rats exhibit pronounced responses to non-noxious environmental stimuli. *J. Neurosci.* 1, 887-900.

Bannon, M.J., Elliot, P.J., Alpert, J.E., Goedert, M., & Iversen, S.D. (1983): Selective activation of mesocortical dopamine neurons by stress: The role of substance P afferents demonstrated using *in vivo* application of substance P monoclonal antibody. *Nature* 306, 791-792.

Bertolucci-D'Angio, M., Serrano, A., & Scatton, B. (1990): Differential effects of forced locomotion, tail-pinch, immobilization and methyl-β-carboline carboxylate on extracellular DOPAC levels in the rat striatum, nucleus accumbens and prefrontal cortex : *in vivo* voltammetric study. *J. Neurochem.* 55, 1208-1215.

Björklund, A., & Lindvall, O. (1978): The meso-telencephalic dopamine neuron system: a review of its anatomy. In *Limbic mechanisms*. eds K.E. Livingstone and O. Hornykiewicz, Plenum Press, New York.

Blanc, G., Hervé, D., Simon, H., Lisoprawski, A., Glowinski, J., & Tassin, J.P. (1980): Response to stress of mesocortico-frontal dopaminergic neurones in rats after long-term isolation. *Nature* 284, 265-267.

Blanc, G., Trovero, F., Vézina, P., Godeheu, A-M., Glowinski, J., & Tassin, J.P. (1993): Blockade of prefronto-cortical α1-adrenergic receptors prevents locomotor hyperactivity induced by subcortical D-amphetamine injection (submitted).

Bliss, E.L., Ailion, J, & Zwanziger, J. (1968): Metabolism of norepinephrine, serotonin and dopamine in rat brain with stress. *J. Pharmacol. Exp. Ther.* 164, 122-131.

Brozoski, T.J., McBrown, R., Rosvold, H.E., & Goldman, P.S. (1979): Cognitive deficit caused by regional depletion of dopamine in prefrontal cortex of rhesus monkey. *Science* 205, 929-932.

Cannon, W.B. (1914): The emergency function of the adrenal medulla in pain and in the major emotions. *Am. J. Physiol.* 33, 356-360.

Cassens, G., Roffman, M., Kuruc, A., Orsulak, P.J., & Schildkraut, J.J. (1980): Alterations in brain norepinephrine metabolism induced by environmental stimuli previously paired with inescapable shock. *Science* 209, 1138-1140.

Chappell, P.B., Smith, M.A., Kilts, C.D., Bissette, G., Ritchie, J., Anderson, C., & Nemeroff, C.B. (1986): Alterations in corticotropin-releasing factor-like immunoreactivity in discrete rat brain regions after acute and chronic stress. *J. of Neurosci.* 6, 2908-2914.

Chu, N. & Bloom, F.E. (1974): The catecholamine-containing neurons in the cat dorsolateral pontine tegmentum: Distribution of the cell bodies and some axonal projections. *Brain Research* 66, 1-21.

Claustre, Y., Rivy, J.P., Dennis, T., & Scatton, B. (1986): Pharmacological studies on stress-induced increase in frontal cortical dopamine metabolism in the rat. *J. Pharmacol. Exp. Ther.* 238, 693-700.

Corrodi, H., Fuxe, K., & Hökfelt, T. (1967): A possible role played by central monoamine neurons in thermoregulation. *Acta Physiol. Scand.* 71, 224-231.

Dantzer, R., Guilloneau, D., Mormède, P., Herman, J.P., & Le Moal, M. (1984): Influence of shock-induced fighting and social factors on dopamine turnover in cortical and limbic areas of the rat. *Pharmacol. Biochem. Behav.* 20, 331-335.

D'Angio, M., Serrano, A., Driscoll, P., & Scatton, B. (1988): Stressful environmental stimuli increase extracellular DOPAC levels in the prefrontal cortex of hypoemotional (Roman high-avoidance) but not hyperemotional (Roman low-avoidance) rats. An *in vivo* voltammetric study. *Brain Research* 451, 237-247.

Deroche, V., Piazza, P.V., Casolini, P., Maccari, S., Le Moal, M., & Simon, H. (1992): Stress-induced sensitization to amphetamine and morphine psychomotor effects depend on stress-induced corticosterone secretion. *Brain Research* 598, 343-348.

Deutch, A.Y., Tam, S-Y., & Roth, R.H. (1985): Footshock and conditioned stress increase 3,4-dihydroxyphenylacetic acid (DOPAC) in the ventral tegmental area but not substantia nigra. *Brain Research* 333, 143-146.

Dunn, A.J., & Berridge, C.W. (1990): Physiological and behavioral responses to corticotropin-releasing factor administration: is CRF a mediator of anxiety or stress responses? *Brain Research Reviews* 15, 71-100.

Elam, M., Yao, T., Svensson, T.H., & Thoren, P. (1984): Regulation of locus coeruleus neurons and splanchnic, sympathetic nerves by cardiovascular afferents. *Brain Research* 290, 281-287.

Fadda, F., Argiolas, A., Melis, M.R., Tissari, A.H., Onali, P.L., & Gessa, G.L. (1978): Stress-induced induced increase in 3,4-dihydroxy-phenylacetic acid (DOPAC) levels in the cerebral cortex and in N. accumbens: reversal by diazepam. *Life Sci.* 23, 2219-2224.

Glavin, G.B. (1985): Stress and brain noradrenaline: A review. *Neurosci. Biobehav. rev.* 9, 233-243.

Heinrichs, S.C., Britton, K.T., & Koob, G.F. (1991): Both conditioned taste preference and aversion induced by corticotropin-releasing factor. *Pharmacol. Biochem. & Behav.* 40, 717-721.

Herman, J.P., Guillonneau, D., Dantzer, R., Scatton, B., Semerdjian-Rouquier, L., & Le Moal, M. (1982): Differential effects of inescapable footshocks and of stimuli previously paired with inescapable footshocks on dopamine turnover in cortical and limbic areas of the rat. *Life Sci.* 30, 2207-2214.

Hervé, D., Tassin, J.P., Barthelemy, C., Blanc, G., Lavielle, S., & Glowinski, J. (1979): Difference in the reactivity of the mesocortical dopaminergic neurons to stress in the BALB/C and C57 BL/6 mice. *Life Sci.* 25, 1659 1664.

Hervé, D., Blanc, G., Glowinski, J., & Tassin, J.P. (1982): Reduction in dopamine utilization in the prefrontal cortex but not in the nucleus accumbens after selective destruction of noradrenergic fibers innervating the ventral tegmental area in the rat. *Brain Research* 237, 510-516.

Jones, B.E. & Moore, R.Y. (1974): Catecholamine-containing neurons of the nucleus locus coeruleus in the cat. *J. Comp. Neurol.* 157, 43-51.

Kaneyuki, H., Yokoo, H., Tsuda, A., Yoshida, M., Mizuki, Y., Yamada, M., & Tanaka, M. (1991): Psychological stress increases dopamine turnover selectively in mesoprefrontal dopamine neurons of rats: reversal by diazepam. *Brain Research* 557, 154-161.

Korf, J., Aghajanian, G.K., & Roth, R.H. (1973): Increased turnover of norepinephrine in the rat cerebral cortex during stress: Role of the locus coeruleus. *Neuropharmacology* 12, 933-938.

Lavicky, J., & Dunn, A. (1993): Corticotropin-releasing factor stimulates catecholamine release in hypothalamus and prefrontal cortex in freely moving rats as assessed by microdialysis. *J. Neurochem.* 60, 602-612.

Lavielle, S., Tassin, J.P., Thierry, A-M., Blanc, G., Hervé, D., Barthélémy, C., & Glowinski, J. (1979) Blockade by benzodiazepines of the selective high increase in DA turnover induced by stress in mesocortical DA neurons in the rat. *Brain Research* 168, 585-594.

Levi, L. (1967): Stressors, stress tolerance, emotions and performance in relation to catecholamine excretion. In *Emotional Stress*, ed L. Levi, pp. 192-200, Elsevier, New York.

Lisoprawski, A., Blanc, G., & Glowinski, J. (1981): Activation by stress of the habenulo-interpeduncular substance P neurons in the rat. *Neurosci. Lett.* 25, 47-51.

Mason, J.W., Mangan Jr, G., Brady, J.V., Conrad, D. & McK. Rioch, D. (1961): Concurrent plasma epinephrine, norepinephrine and 17-hydroxycorticosteroid levels during conditioned emotional disturbance in monkeys. *Psychosom. Med.* 23, 344-353.

Maynert, E.W. & Levi, R. (1964): Stress induced release of brain norepinephrine and its inhibition by drugs. *J. Pharmacol. Exp. Ther.* 143, 90-95.

Moore, R.Y., & Bloom, F.E. (1978) Central catecholamine neuron systems: Anatomy and physiology of the dopamine systems. *Ann. Rev. Neurosci.* 1, 129-169.

Moore, R.Y., & Bloom, F.E. (1979) Central catecholamine neuron systems: Anatomy and physiology of the norepinephrine and epinephrine systems. *Ann. Rev. Neurosci.* 2, 113-168.

Olschowka, J.A., O'Donohue, T.L., Mueller, G.P., & Jacobowitz, D.M. (1982): Hypothalamic and extrahypothalamic distribution of CRF-like immunoreactive neurons in the rat brain. *Neuroendocrinology* 35, 305-308.

Piazza, P.V., Maccari, S., Deminière, J.M., Le Moal, M., Mormède, P., & Simon, H. (1991): Corticosterone levels determine individual vulnerability to amphetamine self-administration. *Proc. Natl. Acad. Sci. USA* 88, 2088-2092.

Plotsky, P.M. (1987): Facilitation of immunoreactive corticotropin-releasing factor secretion in the hypophysial-portal circulation after activation of catecholaminergic pathways or central norepinephrine injection. *Endocrinology* 121, 924-930.

Reiner, P.B. (1986): Correlational analysis of central noradrenergic neuronal activity and sympathetic tone in behaving cats. *Brain Research* 378, 86-96.

Reinhard, J.F., Bannon, M.J., & Roth, R.H. (1982): Acceleration by stress of dopamine synthesis and metabolism in prefrontal cortex: antagonism by diazepam. *Naunyn-Schmiedeberg's Arch. Pharmacol.* 318, 374-377.

Romo, R., & Schultz, W. (1990): Dopamine neurons of the monkey midbrain: contingencies of responses to active touch during self-initiated arm movements. *J. Neurophys.* 63, 592-606.

Rossetti, Z.L., Portas, C., Pani, L., Carboni, S., & Gessa, G. (1990): Stress increases noradrenaline release in the rat frontal cortex: prevention by diazepam. *Eur. J. Pharmacol.* 176, 229-231.

Sawaguchi, T., & Goldman-Rakic, P.S. (1991): D1 dopamine receptors in prefrontal cortex: Involvement in working memory. *Science* 251, 947-950.

Simon, H., Scatton, B., & Le Moal, M. (1980): Dopaminergic neurons are involved in cognitive functions. *Nature* 286, 150-151.

Steinfels, G.F., Heym, J., Strecker, R.E., & Jacobs, B.L. (1983): Behavioural correlates of dopaminergic unit activity in freely moving cats. *Brain Research* 258, 217-228.

Stone, E.A. (1975): Stress and Catecholamines. In *Catecholamines and Behavior*, ed. A.J. Friedhoff, Vol. 2, pp.31-72, Plenum, New York.

Swanson, L.W., & Hartman, B.K. (1975): The central adrenergic system. An immunofluorescence study of the location of cell bodies and their efferent connections in the rat utilizing DA-β-hydroxylase as a marker. *J. Comp. Neurol.* 163, 467-506.

Swanson, L.W., Sawchenko, P.E., Rivier, J., & Vale, W. (1983): The organization of ovine corticotropin releasing factor (CRF)-immunoreactive cells and fibers in the rat brain: an immunohistochemical study. *Neuroendocrinology* 36, 165-186.

Tassin, J.P. (1992): NE/DA interactions in prefrontal cortex and their possible roles as neuromodulators in schizophrenia. *J. Neural Transm.* 36, 135-162.

Tassin, J.P., Hervé, D., Blanc, G., & Glowinski, J. (1980): Differential effects of a two-minute open-field session on dopamine utilization in the frontal cortices of BALB/C and C57 BL/6 mice. *Neurosci. Lett.* 17, 67-71.

Thierry, A-M., Javoy, F., Glowinski, J. & Kety, S.S. (1968): Effects of stress on the metabolism of norepinephrine, dopamine and serotonin in the central nervous system of the rat. I. Modifications of norepinephrine turnover. *J. Pharmacol. Exp. Ther.* 163, 163-171.

Thierry, A-M., Tassin, J.P., Blanc, G., & Glowinski, J. (1976): Selective activation of the DA mesocortical system by stress. *Nature* 263, 242-244.

Tsuda, A., Tanaka, M., Kohno, Y., Nishikawa, T., Iimori, K., Nakagawa, R., Hoaki, Y., Ida, Y., & Nagasaki, N. (1982): Marked enhancement of noradrenaline turnover in extensive brain regions after activity-stress in rats. *Physiol. Behav.* 29, 337-341.

Vargas, M.A., Bissette, G., Owens, M.J., Ehlers, C.L., & Nemeroff, C.B. (1992): Effects of chronic ethanol and benzodiazepine treatment and withdrawal on corticotropin-releasing factor neural systems. In *The neurobiology of drug and alcohol addiction*, eds P.W. Kalivas and H.H. Samson, Vol. 654, pp. 145-152. Annals N. Y. Acad. Sci., New-York.

Yokoo, H., Tanaka, M., Yoshida, M., Tsuda, A., Tanaka, T., & Mizoguchi, K. (1990a): Direct evidence of conditioned fear-elicited enhancement of noradrenaline release in the rat hypothalamus assessed by intracranial microdialysis. *Brain Research* 536, 305-308.

Yokoo, H., Tanaka, M., Tanaka, T., & Tsuda, A. (1990b): Stress-induced increase in noradrenaline release in the rat hypothalamus assessed by intracranial microdialysis. *Experientia* 46, 290-292.

Résumé

Un grand nombre d'études ont montré que les situations anxiogènes entrainent une augmentation de l'utilisation de la NA cérébrale. Différentes méthodes, parmi lesquelles on peut citer l'électrophysiologie, la mesure des taux de neurotranmetteur tissulaire et la dialyse cérébrale, ont donné des résultats concordants. La majeure partie de l'innervation NA du cerveau antérieur provenant du locus coeruleus, ce noyau est considéré comme jouant un rôle fondamental dans la réponse au stress. Les neurones DA ascendants mésencéphaliques sont aussi activés par les situations anxiogènes mais l'amplitude des effets décroît selon qu'il s'agit des neurones DA mésocorticaux, mésolimbiques ou nigro-striataux, ce dernier groupe n'étant que peu ou pas affecté. Les tranquillisants mineurs, tels que les benzodiazépines, bloquent les activations des neurones NA et DA induites par le stress. C'est la libération neuronale au cours du stress du peptide responsable de la libération de l'hormone corticotrope qui semble être un des premiers éléments entrainant l'activation des neurones NA. D'autrepart, la corticostérone libérée à l'occasion de l'activation de l'axe hypothalamo-hypophysaire sensibiliserait les neurones DA. Enfin, nous proposons que les réactivités différentes des neurones NA et DA vis-à-vis du stress soient dûes à leurs rôles fonctionnels respectifs, en particulier en ce qui concerne l'importance des neurones DA mésocorticaux dans les processus cognitifs.

Serotonergic mechanisms and animal models of anxiety

Charles A. Marsden, Michael Bickerdike, Anna-Karina Cadogan, Ian Wright, Andre Rex* and Heidrun Fink*

*Department of Physiology and Pharmacology, Nottingham University Medical School, Queen's Medical Centre, Nottingham NG7 2UH, England and * Institute of Pharmacology and Toxicology, Humboldt University, PF140, 1040 Berlin, Germany*

SUMMARY

Two animal models of state anxiety, elevated plus maze and social interaction test, were used in combination with microdialysis measurement of hippocampal 5-hydroxytryptamine (5-HT) in the freely moving rat and guinea pig. Extracellular 5-HT increased on exposure to the elevated plus maze in both the rat and guinea pig and this effect was prevented by pretreatment with diazepam (1 mg/kg i.p.). A similar rise in extracellular 5HT was seen in the rat during the social interaction test and there was an associated increase in extracellular c-AMP. Both these changes were reduced by pretreatment with diazepam. These findings support the hypothesis that one of the actions of diazepam is to reduce an increase in 5-HT release caused by anxiety. Rats reared in social isolation from weaning show an anxiogenic profile on the elevated plus maze and marked supersensitivity of post-synaptic 5-HT receptors. Interestingly these rats have reduced pre-synaptic 5-HT function and fail to show an increase in 5-HT release on exposure to the elevated plus maze compared to group reared controls. Social isolation may correspond to trait anxiety and the results indicate that under these conditions there is not a simple relationship between 5-HT release and aversion.

INTRODUCTION

Animal models of mental diseases have two major uses; firstly as predictors of clinical potency and efficacy for new drugs. Their second role is a means of understanding the psychological, neural and biochemical events that may underlie specific human mental diseases. The models used to investigate potential anxiolytic drugs are either based on conditioned conflict tests, such as the Geller-Seifter conflict procedure, or social situations involving aversion. The tests in the latter group include the elevated plus maze and the social interaction between pairs of rats in either high or low light conditions. Anxiety, however, is not just a state condition but could also involve a trait situation. The development of animal models to look at trait conditions is a relatively new but important development in the study of the neurobiology of disease. One such model that may be of relevance to anxiety is rearing rats from weaning in social isolation.

The development of techniques for monitoring extracellular transmitter levels offers the possibility of investigating changes in neurotransmitters of possible relevance to anxiety during behaviour associated with the models. More recently it has been suggested that changes in extracellular cyclic AMP (cAMP) might also be used to monitor changes in post-synaptic receptor activation (Egawa et al, 1988, Sibjesma et al, 1991). The present study has investigated the changes in extracellular 5-hydroxytryptamine (5-HT) and cAMP during behaviour on the elevated plus maze (Handley and Mithani, 1984), during social interaction (Rile, 1987) and in rats reared from weaning in social isolation (Jones et al, 1992). The aim was to determine whether aversive situations are commonly associated with increased 5-HT release with subsequent post-synaptic 5-HT receptor activation.

EXPOSURE TO THE ELEVATED PLUS MAZE INCREASES EXTRACELLULAR 5-HT IN THE RAT AND GUINEA PIG

Male Lister hooded rats had microdialysis probes implanted into the ventral hippocampus (Wright et al, 1992b). The following day 5-HT and its metabolite 5-hydroxyindole acetic acid (5-HIAA) were measured using HPLC with electrochemical detection in 20 min dialysis samples collected for 80 mins in the home cage after which the rat was placed on the elevated plus maze for 20 mins and a sample collected at the end of this period. The rat was then returned to the home cage and 20 min samples collected for a further 140 mins.

Exposure of the rat to the elevated plus maze caused an increase in extracellular 5-HT but no change in 5-HIAA and the levels returned to the pre-exposure value on return to the home cage. This result indicates that the aversive conditions of the elevated plus maze results in increased 5-HT release. When the experiment was repeated but half the rats were given diazepam (2.5 mg/kg i.p.), the increase in extracellular 5-HT was only observed in saline pretreated rats, while those given diazepam showed no increase in 5-HT on exposure to the elevated plus maze, a significant decrease in 5-HT on their return to the home cage and a significant increase in the number of open arm entries (Fig. 1). This result indicates that the increase in extracellular 5-HT is associated with aversion and that drugs such as diazepam, which reduce aversion, prevent the rise in 5-HT (Wright et al, 1992b).

The increase in 5-HT on exposure to the elevated plus maze is not only observed in the rat but also in the guinea pig. The guinea pig (Leeds coloured) needs to be handled daily from birth for it to show measurable behaviour on the maze (Rex et al, 1993). Unhandled guinea pigs placed on the maze simply freeze on the centre square; however, handled guinea pigs explore the maze spending a limited time in the open arms but this is increased by pretreatment with diazepam (1.0 mg/kg i.p.), an effect reversed by the benzodiazepine receptor antagonist flumazenil (10.0 mg/kg i.p.) In a similar manner to the rat exposure of the handled guinea pig results in an increase (+ 161 ± 13%, n = 6) in frontal cortical extracellular 5-HT, an effect reduced but not fully blocked by pretreatment with diazepam. Again flumazenil prevented this effect of diazepam. Interestingly and unexpectedly flumazenil alone, like diazepam, markedly reduced the rise in 5-HT observed on the elevated plus maze but had no effect on behaviour. Previous studies have suggested that flumazenil may demonstrate a partial agonist action and/or could have different pharmacological actions at subtypes of the benzodiazepine/GABA receptor complex (Robertson and Riives, 1983, Dantzer and Perio, 1982, Massotti et al, 1991). An explanation for the present findings could be that flumazenil acts as an antagonist at benzodiazepine receptors with regard to the behaviour but a partial agonist with respect to its effects on 5-HT release under normal but not aversive situations (Rex et al, 1993).

Further evidence of a relationship between the increase in 5-HT and behaviour comes from the finding that in the guinea pig the 5-HT_{1A} agonist (8-OHDPAT, 0.3 m/kg s.c.) has an anxiolytic action in the elevated plus maze and completely prevents the rise in 5-HT, both effects being prevented by pretreatment with the non-selective 5-HT_1 antagonist methiothepin (10.0 mg/kg) which had no effect on its own on the behaviour. In contrast 5-carboxamidotryptamine (5-CT, 0.1 mg/kg i.p.) prevented in the rise in 5-HT but had no anxiolytic effect.

In summary the results with the elevated plus maze demonstrate that aversion is associated with increased 5-HT release but that inhibition of this increase is not necessarily associated with an anxiolytic response. This indicates that there is not a simple relationship between inhibition of 5-HT release and behaviour indicative of anxiolytic drug action. Further experiments were designed to investigate whether increased 5-HT release occurred in other aversive situations and whether such an increase in release was accompanied by activation of post-synaptic 5-HT_{1A} receptors. One explanation for the lack of effect with drugs acting at 5-HT_{1A} receptors may relate to the presence of these receptors at pre- (somatodendritic autoreceptors) and post-synaptic sites and a balance of agonist action at these two sites might determine the end behavioural state of the animal under the test conditions.

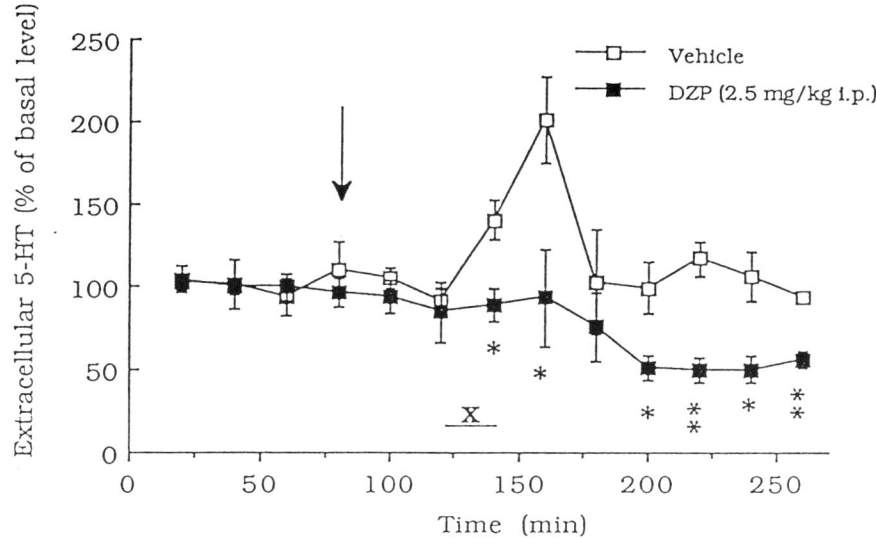
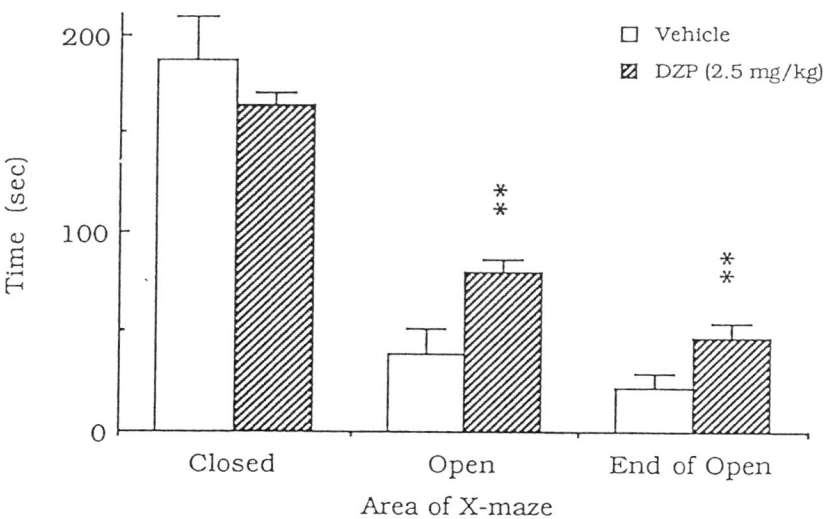

Fig. 1. Effect of diazepam (2.5 mg/kg^{-1} i.p.) on the increase in extracellular 5-HT observed when rats are placed on the elevated plus maze (X) and behaviour on the maze. Note that diazepam prevents the rise in 5-HT (top graph) and increases open arm entries (bottom histogram). (Data from Wright et al, 1992b). Values are the mean of 6 animals/group.

SOCIAL INTERACTION BETWEEN PAIRS OF RATS IN HIGH LIGHT CONDITIONS RESULTS IN INCREASED HIPPOCAMPAL 5-HT RELEASE AND ACTIVATION OF POST-SYNAPTIC 5-HT$_{1A}$ RECEPTORS

Cyclic AMP functions as an intracellular second messenger by activating cAMP-dependent protein kinase in response to activation of a number of neurotransmitter receptors. There is also evidence that there is an egress of cAMP out of cells into the extracellular space. The rate of egress of cAMP has been found to be proportional to its intracellular concentration over a wide range of values in both cultured cells and tissue slices (Stoof and Kebabian, 1981; Barber and Butcher, 1983; Lazareno et al, 1985). This relationship has been used by some investigators as an index of changes in the intracellular cAMP levels and hence of the function of some adenylyl cyclase-coupled receptors. More recently, *in vivo* studies utilising the technique of microdialysis, have shown increases in extracellular cAMP in rat frontal cortex, striatum and hippocampus following activation with noradrenergic (Egawa et al, 1988; Stone and John, 1990; Stone et al, 1989), dopaminergic (Hutson and Suman-Chauhan, 1990) and serotonergic (Sibjesma et al, 1991) agonists.

In vivo microdialysis was initially used to examine the efflux of cAMP and effect of 5-HT$_{1A}$ receptor activation into the extracellular fluid of the ventral hippocampus in the freely-moving rat. The changes in extracellular cAMP concentration were monitored in response to forskolin and the 5-HT$_{1A}$ receptor agonist, 8-OH-DPAT. The basal level of hippocampal extracellular cAMP was 2.3 ± 0.2 pmol/ml (n = 6), after a 3 hour post-surgery stabilisation period. Perfusion of forskolin (100 µM) through the probe for 30 mins significantly increased the efflux of cAMP, which returned to baseline levels within 90 mins. 8-OH-DPAT (0.3 mg/kg s.c.) also significantly increased cAMP efflux, whereas a similar volume of saline had no effect. Desensitisation of the 8-OH-DPAT-induced increased in cAMP efflux was observed following a second administration of 8-OH-DPAT after a 4 hour interval. Administration of 8-OH-DPAT did not alter the efflux of cAMP when forskolin was perfused through the probe. Pretreatment with WAY100135 [N-tert-butyl 3- 4-(2-methoxyphenyl) piperazine-l-yl-2-phenylpropanamide dihydrochloride] (5 mg/kg s.c.) a specific 5-HT$_{1A}$ receptor antagonist, prevented the 8-OH-DPAT-induced increase in cAMP efflux. The data from these preliminary studies indicate that the 8-OH-DPAT-induced increase in cAMP efflux *in vivo* is mediated by a 5-HT$_{1A}$ receptor.

Microdialysis probes were then implanted in male Wistar rats into the ventral hippocampus 24 hours before the start of the experiments using the social interaction test (File, 1987). The probes were perfused with artificial cerebrospinal fluid at 1µl/min with sample collection every 30 minutes. Three control samples were taken before the rats underwent a 10 minute period of social interaction, followed by 30 minute samples for a further 3 hours. The social interaction test involved monitoring the behaviour of a pair of unfamiliar rats in an equally unfamiliar, high light environment. One of the pair of rats had been implanted 24 hours previously and kept isolated, while the other rat came from an established group of five rats. Levels of 5-HT were measured by HPLC with electrochemical detection as before, while levels of cAMP were evaluated using a radio-receptor assay.

A 10 minute period of social interaction significantly increased extracellular levels of 5-HT and cAMP, as compared to basal levels (Fig. 2). Pretreatment with diazepam (1 mg/kg i.p.) significantly increased the total time spent in social contact, while causing a significant reduction in the aversion-induced increases in 5-HT and cAMP. These findings indicate that increased 5-HT release in the ventral hippocampus of the rat produced by aversive conditions was associated with increased cAMP efflux probably mediated by a post-synaptic receptor linked to adenylyl cyclase, the most likely candidate being the 5-HT$_{1A}$ receptor. These findings also support the hypothesis that one of the actions of diazepam is through a reduction in the anxiety-induced increase in 5-HT in the hippocampus of the rat and that this action of diazepam could be related to its anxiolytic properties.

ISOLATION REARING AND EFFECTS ON 5-HT FUNCTION

Both the behavioural models discussed so far are concerned with a state of anxiety. In the human anxiety will also be a trait condition and in future animal models should be more directed towards the investigation of the neurochemical events associated with trait anxiety. We have investigated the involvement of 5-HT neuronal function in rats reared in social

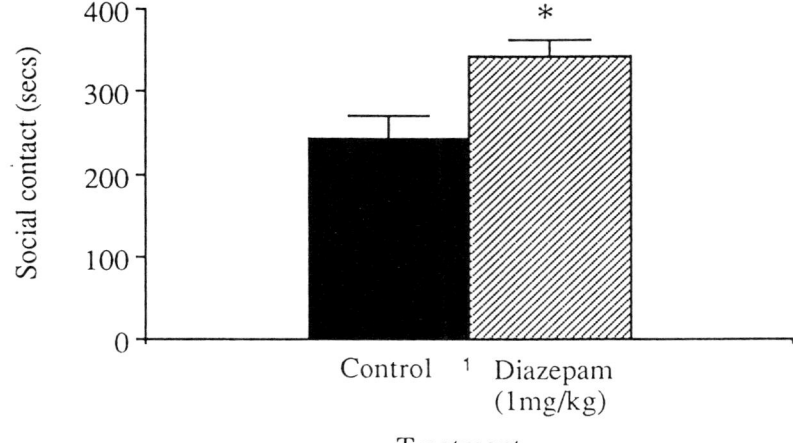
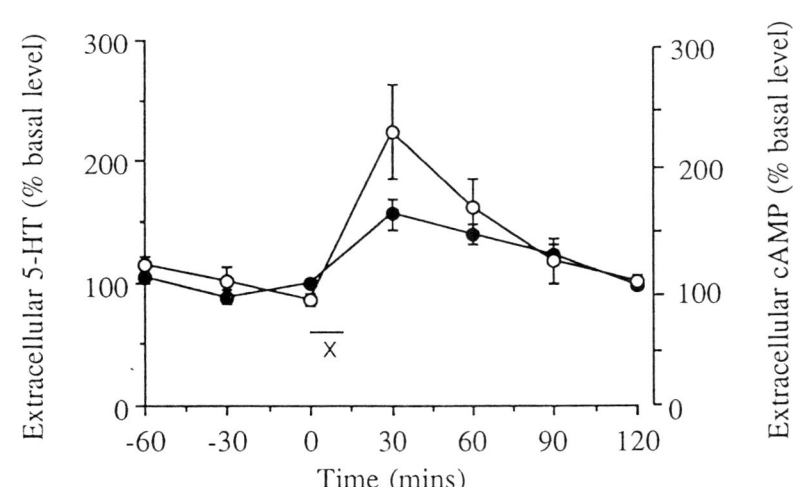

Fig. 2 Effects of diazepam in the social interaction test in rats (A) and effects of the aversive conditions, produced by the social interaction test, on extracellular levels of 5-HT and cAMP measured by *in vivo* microdialysis in the rat hippocampus.
A. Mean time spent in active social interaction by pairs of rats, treated with either saline (■) or diazepam (1mg/kg, i.p.) (▨) in a high light, unfamiliar environment. Values represent the mean ± sem of 10 pairs. *$P < 0.05$ (2-tailed Mann Whitney U-test).
B. Effect of a 10 minute period of social interaction, marked by X, on extracellular levels of 5-HT (●) and cAMP (○) in the hippocampus of the rat. Samples were collected every 30 minutes. Levels of both 5-HT and cAMP in dialysate samples are expressed as a percentage of the average amount of the substance collected in the two 30 minute samples directly before the social interaction period. Values represent the mean ± sem of 6 rats.

isolation from weaning as these animals show anxiogenic behaviour on the elevated plus maze when compared with group (5/group) reared controls (Wright et al, 1992a).

Rats reared in social isolation in the weeks post-weaning show many behavioural disturbances in comparison with socially-reared control rats. Krech et al (1962) first showed that rats raised in "impoverished" environments demonstrated learning deficits compared with rats raised in "enriched" environments. Further disturbances in behaviour produced by isolation rearing have been revealed in many other studies. These include a hyperactive response to a novel environment (Sahakian et al, 1975), maze-learning deficits (Greenough et al, 1972), impaired spatial memory (Juraska et al, 1984) and an anxious profile on the elevated x-maze (Parker and Morinan, 1986). It has been shown that resocialization of previously isolated rats does not reverse the anxious behaviour revealed by the elevated x-maze model.(Wright et al, 1992a). This suggests that isolation rearing induced a permanent development change in the rats" response to the maze. Persistent changes in an ethological response to a cue would appear to require a corresponding alteration in forebrain neurochemistry to account for the changes observed. The investigation of the developmental changes in rat brain neurochemistry that occur during isolation rearing has predominantly centred on the dopaminergic system: for example, isolated rats show an enhanced release of dopamine in response to d-amphetamine stimulation (Jones et al, 1992). There has, however, been a more limited interest in the effects of isolation rearing on the central 5-hydroxytryptamine (5-HT) system. Studies of *post-mortem* monoamine tissue levels have shown decreased 5-HT in nucleus accumbens but not in caudate putamen or frontal cortex of isolated rats (Jones et al, 1992). A study of the behavioural effects of 5-HT receptor agonists has revealed that isolated rats show an enhanced responsiveness to these agonists (Wright et al, 1991). Wright and co-workers demonstrated that 8-OH-DPAT, the selective 5-HT$_{1A}$ agonist and 1-(2,5-dimethoxy-4-iodophenyl)-2-aminopropane (DOI), a 5-HT$_{2/1C}$ agonist, produced enhanced 5-HT syndrome and back-muscle contractions, respectively, in the isolated rats. These data suggest that isolated rats may have supersensitive post-synaptic 5-HT receptors. Receptor supersensitivity, as indicated by this study, could develop from a reduced endogenous synaptic release of the neurotransmitter.

We have recently looked at the increase in extracellular 5-HT induced by K^+ (100 mM perfused the probe) in group and isolation reared rats and found a reduced response in the isolation reared animals indicative of reduced pre-synaptic 5-HT function. In a further study we have shown that exposure of the group reared rats to the elevated plus maze increases extracellular 5-HT by 86% as previously demonstrated but there was no increase in the isolation reared rats (Bickerdike e al, 1993) (Table 1). Thus isolation rearing results in a loss of the increase in 5-HT release normally observed with aversive stimuli but a marked post-synaptic 5-HT supersensitivity. The pre-synaptic change is not associated with altered sensitivity of the 5HT$_{1A}$ somatodendritic autoreceptor (measured using 8-OHDPAT induced inhibition of firing) and so may reflect a long-term, change in 5-HT neuronal state produced by the environmental conditions of post-weaning rearing, together with changes in other neurotransmitter systems sensitive to the environmental state.

CONCLUSIONS

Animal models of acute anxiety are associated with increased release of 5-HT in the hippocampus (rat) and frontal cortex (guinea pig) but drug studies show that there is not a simple relationship between inhibition of this increase and anxiolytic effects. Anxiogenic behaviour produced by rearing rats in social isolation from weaning is associated with marked post-synaptic 5-HT receptor supersensitivity but reduced pre-synaptic 5-HT function. These animals also show marked changes in other neurotransmitter systems, including enhanced dopaminergic function, and a greater understanding of the neurobiology of anxiety may come from careful analysis of neurotransmitter interactions using models such as the isolation reared rat.

Table 1

Effect of isolation rearing on extracellular 5-HT in rat ventral hippocampus during exposure to the elevated plus maze.

	Group reared	Isolation reared
	5-HT (fmol/10µl)	
Basal	18.3 ± 4.1 (7)	14.7 ± 3.4 (7)
X-maze	37.4 ± 6.6 (7)	20.3 ± 4.5 (7)
	+ 104%	+ 38%
	$p < 0.05$	NS

Male Hooded Lister rats were either kept in groups of 5 or in social isolation from weaning at 21 days. 4-6 weeks later microdialysis measurements of 5-HT were made before (basal) and during exposure to the X-maze. Results are the mean values ± SEM. Basal values are the mean of the three 20 min samples collected before the rats went on the X-maze and the X-maze value is the mean of the sample collected immediately after a 20 min exposure to the maze.

ACKNOWLEDGEMENTS

This work was financially supported by the MRC, SERC, British Council, SmithKline Beecham and Wyeth (UK) Ltd.

REFERENCES

Barber, R. & Butcher, R.W. (1983): The egress and cyclic AMP from metazoan cells. *Adv.Cycle Nucleotide Res.* 15, 119-138.

Bickerdike, M.J., Wright, I.K. & Marsden, C.A. (1993): Social isolation attenuates rat forebrain 5-HT release induced by KCL stimulation and exposure to a novel environment. *Behavioural Pharmacology* (in press).

Dantzer, R, Perio, A. (1982): Behavioural evidence for partial agonist properties of Ro 15-1788, a benzodiazepine receptor antagonist. *Eur.J.Pharmacol.* 81, 655-658.

Egawa, M., Hoebel, B.G. & Stone, E.A. (1988): Use of microdialysis to measure brain noradrenergic function *in vivo*. *Brain Res.* 458, 303-308.

File, S.E. (1987): The contribution of behavioural studies to the neuropharmacology of anxiety. *Neuropharmacology* 26, 877-886.

Handley, S.L. & Mithani, S. (1984): Effects of alpha-adrenoceptor agonists and antagonists in a maze-exploration model of 'fear'-motivated behaviour. *Naunyn Schmeidebergs Archives of Pharmacology* 327, 1-5.

Hutson, P.H. & Suman-Chauhan, N. (1990): Activation of postsynaptic striatal dopamine receptors, monitored by efflux of cAMP *in vivo*. *Neuropharmacology* 29, 1011-1016.

Jones, G.H., Hernandez, T.D., Kendall, D.A., Marsden, C.A. & Robbins, T.W. (1992): Dopaminergic and serotonergic function following isolation rearing in rats: study of behavioral responses and postmortem and *in vivo* neurochemistr. *Pharmacology, Biochemistry and Behavior* 43, 17-35.

Juraska, J.M., Henderson, C. & Muller, J. (1984): Differential rearing experience, gender and radial maze performance. *Developmental Psychobiology* 17, 209-215.

Krech, D. Rosenzweig, M.R. & Bennett, E.L. (1962): Relations between brain chemistry and problem-solving among rats raised in enriched and impoverished environments. *Journal of Comparative Physiology and Psychology*, 55, 801-807.

Lazareno, S., Marriott, D.B. & Nahorski, S.R. (1985): Differential effects of selective and non-selective neuroleptics on intracellular and extracellular cyclic AMP accumulation in rat striatal slices. *Brain Res.* 361, 91-98.

Massotti, M., Schlichting, J.L., Antonacci, M.D., Giusti, P., Memo, M., Costa, E., Guidotti, A. (1991): Gamma-aminobutyric acid A receptor heterogeneity in rat central nervous system: studies with clonazepam and other benzodiazepine ligands. *J.Pharmacol.Exp.Ther.* 256, 1154-1160.

Parker, V. & Morinan, A. (1986): The socially-isolated rat as a model for anxiety. *Neuropharmacology* 25, 663-664.

Rex, A., Marsden, C.A. & Fink, H. (1993): Effect of diazepam on cortical 5-HT release and behaviour in the guinea pig on exposure to the elevated plus maze. *Psychopharmacology* 110, 490-496.

Robertson, H.A., Riives, M.L. (1983): A benzodiazepine antagonist is an anticonvulsant in an animal model for limbic epilepsy. *Brain Res.* 270, 380-382.

Sahakian, B.J., Robbins, T.W., Morgan, M.J. & Iversen, S.D. (1975): The effects of psychomotor stimulants on stereotype and locomotor activity in socially-deprived and control rats. *Brain Res.* 84, 195-205.

Sijbesma, H., Schipper, J., Molewijk, H.E., Boson, A.I., & De Kloet, E.R. (1991): 8-hydroxy-2-(di-N-propylamino)tetralin increases the activity of adenylate cyclase in the hippocampus of freely moving rats. *Neuropharmacology* 30, 967-975.

Stone, E.A. & John, S.M. (1992): Stress-induced increase of extracellular levels of cylic AMP in rat cortex. *Brain Res.*. 597, 144-147.

Stone, E.A., Egawa, M. & Colbjornsen, C.M. (1989): Catecholamine-induced desensitization of brain beta adrenoceptors *in vivo* and reversal by corticosterone. *Life Sci.* 44, 209-213.

Stoof, J.C. & Kebabian, J.W. (1981): Opposing roles for D-1 and D-2 dopaminereceptors in efflux of cAMP from rat neostriatum. *Nature* 294, 366-368.

Wright, I.K., Ismail, H., Upton, N. & Marsden, C.A. (1991): Effect of isolation-rearing on 5-HT agonist-induced responses in the rat. *Psychopharmacology* 105, 259-263.

Wright, I.K., Upton, N. & Marsden, C.A. (1992a): Resocialisation of isolation-reared rats does not alter their anxiogenic profile on the elevated x-maze model of anxiety. *Physiology and Behaviour* 50, 1129-1132.

Wright, I.K., Upton, N. & Marsden, C.A. (1992b): Effect of established and putative anxiolytics on extracellular 5-HT and 5-HIAA in the ventral hippocampus of rats during behaviour on the elevated X-maze. *Psychopharmacology* 109, 338-346.

Résumé

La libération de sérotonine a été mesurée par microdialyse dans l'hippocampe de rats et de cobayes libres de leurs mouvements, et placés dans deux situations anxiogènes modèles: le labyrinthe en croix surélevé et le test d'intéraction sociale. La libération de l'amine augmente aussi bien chez le rat que chez le cobaye placés dans le labyrinthe en croix surélevé, et cet effet peut être supprimé par un prétraitement avec du diazépam (1 mg/kg i.p.). Une augmentation de la libération de 5-HT est également observée chez le rat au cours du test d'intéraction sociale. De plus, cet effet est associé à une élévation de la concentration extracellulaire d'AMP cyclique dans l'hippocampe. Un prétraitement avec le diazépam supprime les deux effets. Ces données s'accordent avec l'hypothèse selon laquelle l'une des actions du diazépam est de s'opposer à l'augmentation de la libération de 5-HT normalement induite par une situation anxiogène. Des rats maintenus isolés depuis le sevrage présentent un comportement de type anxieux dans le labyrinthe en croix surélevé. On note aussi chez ces animaux une hypoactivité sérotoninergique en présynaptique et une hypersensibilité des récepteurs postsynaptiques. Enfin, la libération de 5-HT au niveau de l'hippocampe n'augmente pas lors du test du labyrinthe en croix surélevé appliqué à ces rats qui ont été élevés séparément. L'isolement social induisant probablement un état anxieux, ces résultats suggèrent qu'il n'existe pas de relation claire entre la libération centrale de 5-HT et un comportement aversif.

Stress and neuroendocrine systems

Francis Héry, Anne-Marie François-Bellan, Michel Grino, Micheline Héry and Charles Oliver

Laboratoire de Neuro-Endocrinologie Expérimentale, INSERM U.297, Faculté de Médecine secteur Nord, boulevard Pierre-Dramard, 13916 Marseille Cedex 20, France

SUMMARY

Among other biological adaptative reactions (neurovegetative and behavioural), stress exposure induces neuroendocrine changes i.e. stimulation of ACTH, Prolactine; inhibition of gonadotropins; stimulation or inhibition of GH and TSH depending upon type of stress and species. Central neurotransmitters and especially serotonin are involved in neuroendocrine changes as well as in the other biological reactions of the organism to stress. Modifications of brain serotoninergic activity (during development or after drug administration) can induce short and long term alterations in hormonal response to stress.

INTRODUCTION

Exposure to various stress situations induces biological changes which have been separated in behavioral, neurovegetative and endocrine changes. The influence of stress on endocrine function has been recognized in the early works of Cannon (1919) and Selye (1936). Sympathetic and adrenal medulla activation and glucocorticoid release have been described by these authors during stress. Changes in pituitary hormones secretion have been observed during stress. In this report, we will report shortly neuroendocrine changes during stress and analyze their potentiel relationships with serotoninergic systems. First, we will briefly report some informations on the functional anatomy of the hypothalamus.

FUNCTIONAL ANATOMY OF THE HYPOTHALAMUS AND ITS POTENTIAL RELATIONSHIP WITH NEUROENDOCRINE RESPONSE TO STRESS

Hypothalamic nuclei

Stress exposure is followed by changes in the secretion of various pituitary hormones. The hypothalamus controls the regulation of pituitary hormones. This control is mediated by several neurohormones which are synthetized in several hypothalamic nuclei, then released into portal capillaries at the level of median eminence and secreted into the hypophysial portal blood (HPB) to the pituitary cells. These hypothalamic nuclei are located in the hypothalamic periventricular area : the arcuate nucleus (ACN) synthetizes LHRH, dopamine, GH-RH; the paraventricular nucleus (PVN) synthetizes CRH, TRH; the periventricular nucleus synthetizes SRIH; the preoptic nuclei contains more or less LHRH synthetizing cells according to the species studies. These hypothalamic nuclei send their projections to the median eminence where neurohormones are released into HPB; but also to brain stem; medulla and other parts of the brain giving support for an action of hypothalamic neurons on behavior and autonomous system. They receive several projections from extrahypothalamic brain structures (hippocampus, amygdala, brain stem, medulla, thalamus etc...) which may carry informations related to stress. Besides, intra-hypothalamic connections between these nuclei have been described (see Swanson, 1987, for review).

The pathways responsible for the activation of the hypothalamic structures following stress exposure are unknown. The informations carried out by other brain structures may influence one or several hypothalamic nuclei and induce an hormonal response. Alternatively, the information may be treated at the level of a single nucleus i.e. the PVN. This hypothalamic structure is a central feature since it receives a dense innervation from other parts of the brain. Furthermore, it contains CRH neurons which, upon activation, stimulate ACTH release and autonomous neuronal system activity. Besides, it has clearly been shown that activation of CRH neurons may generate behavioral, neurovegetative and endocrine changes. Indeed, hyperactivity of CRH neurons can induce a stimulation of the pituitary-adrenal system and other hormonal changes. Indeed, intrahypothalamic connections between PVN and other hypothalamic nuclei such as the arcuate and the periventricular nuclei have been demonstrated supporting an action of CRH upon LHRH and SRIH synthetizing cells i.e. upon the gonadotropic and somatotropic functions. Central CRH increases sympathetic tone and may be responsible for vegetative reactions of stress. Besides, it has also been shown to induce behavioural reaction i.e. anxiety, similar to that observed during stress (Dunn & Berridge, 1990). Moreover, several line of evidence indicate that other endocrine systems can also be influenced by physical and/or psychological variables. These include mammotropic and thyrotropic axis (Van de Kar et al.1991 for review).

Serotoninergic innervation of the hypothalamus

Although all hypothalamic nuclei receive serotoninergic fibers, the density of this innervation differs markedly from one nucleus to another (Steinbusch and Nieuwenhuys 1981). A large serotoninergic innervation has been particularly found in the suprachiasmatic (SCN), mammilary, ventromedialis (VMN) and arcuate (ACN) nuclei. A moderate serotoninergic innervation has been described in the paraventricular (PVN), supraoptic (SON) and dorsomedialis (DMN) nuclei. Moreover, the distribution of the serotoninergic innervation is heterogeneous inside some nuclei. Serotoninergic terminals are more abundant in the ventral part of the SCN (Bosler and Beaudet 1985), in the parvocellular area of the PVN (Liposits et al. 1987) and in the ventral part of the DMN. All the hypothalamic nuclei receive their serotoninergic innervation from both the dorsal and the medial raphe nuclei, excepted the median eminence and the dorso- and ventromedialis nuclei, in which 5-HT nerve terminals originate exclusively from the dorsal raphe nucleus (DRN) (Sawchenko et al. 1983). Moreover, some 5-HT nerve cell bodies have been observed in the ventral part of the DMN (Beaudet and Descarries 1979). More recently, we have reported that 5-HT was synthetized from tryptophan in hypothalamic primary cell cultures, indicating the presence of serotoninergic nerve cell bodies in the hypothalamus (Becquet et al. 1990b). These 5-HT neurons may innervate some hypothalamic nuclei and the pituitary gland.

Although hypothalamic serotoninergic innervation has been extensively studied, only few reports are devoted on 5-HT receptors distribution in various hypothalamic nuclei. Studies reporting the general distribution of 5-HT receptors in entire CNS indicate that the density of $5-HT_1$ and $5-HT_2$ receptors are low in the hypothalamus (Pazos and Palacios, 1985; Pazos et al. 1985). Recently, the distribution of $5-HT_{1A}$ and $5-HT_{1B}$ binding sites labeled respectively with ^3H-8-OH-DPAT and ^{125}I-S-CM-GTNH$_2$ (Boulenguez et al. 1992) was investigated by quantitative autoradiography in the rat hypothalamus. The density of $5-HT_{1A}$ (Manrique, personnal communication) and $5-HT_{1B}$ (Manrique et al. 1993) binding sites is moderate in the hypothalamic nuclei as compared with extrahypothalamic structures. The highest density of $5-HT_{1A}$ binding sites was observed in the ventromedial nucleus whereas the paraventricular and suprachiasmatic nuclei exhibited the lowest density. The hypothalamus showed a moderate density of $5-HT_{1B}$ binding sites, especially when compared with extrapyramidal structures. However, some individual nuclei appeared consistently labeled. The anterior and dorsomedial nuclei had the greatest densities of labeling. A weaker, but still consistent density was observed in the PVN and the VMN. The medial preoptic area, the suprachiasmatic and arcuate nuclei exhibited only weak labeling (Manrique et al. 1993).

Neuroanatomical studies have shown that 5-HT fibers contact peptidergic or dopaminergic hypophysiotropic neurons. Synaptic contacts were observed 1) on somatodendritic elements of VIP neurons in the ventral part of the SCN (Bosler and Beaudet 1985) 2) on dendrites of LHRH neurons in the preoptic nucleus (Kiss and Halasz 1985a) 3) on dopaminergic neurons in the arcuate nucleus (Kiss and Halasz 1985b) 4) on CRH neurons in the parvocellular part of the PVN (Liposits et al. 1987). In the median eminence, 5-HT nerve terminals projected onto catecholaminergic, LHRH and TRH nerve endings. This anatomical organization suggests that 5-HT can modulate neuropeptide release by an action both on nerve cell bodies and nerve terminals of neuropeptide secreting neurons (Van de Kar, 1991 for review)).

STRESS AND NEUROENDOCRINE FUNCTIONS

Stress and corticotropic function

The stimulation of ACTH and glucocorticoids secretion during exposure to various stress situations is known since several years. Physiological control of ACTH release is multifactorial although the main role is devoted to two neuropeptides : CRH and Arginine Vasopressin (AVP). CRH stimulates both synthesis and release of ACTH after binding to membrane specific receptors and stimulation of adenyl cyclase activity. AVP action is limited to the release of ACTH (Antoni, 1986). Both peptides are synthetized in the PVN which is divided into two main portions. The magnocellular area contains AVP neurons which project mostly to the posterior lobe and the parvocellular portion contains CRH neurons. Under basal conditions, a various percentage (5-50% depending upon the studies) of CRH neurons expresses AVP. These cells are designated CRH^+/AVP^+. The percentage of CRH^+/AVP^+ neurons increases strikingly after adrenalectomy or chronic stress exposure. The rest of the cells does not express AVP and is designated CRH^+/AVP^- (Whitnall, 1993). Extensive studies on the respective role of CRH and AVP in ACTH regulation in the rat have been performed in several laboratories . In most experiments, both CRH and AVP appears to be involved in the stimulation of ACTH secretion during stress exposure. In our laboratory, another animal model has been used, the sheep, for a direct investigation of CRH and AVP release into HPB . Indeed, it is possible to collect HPB in conscious sheep. Under moderate conditions of stress, CRH and AVP release into HPB increase. When the situation of stress become more intense, the increase of AVP secretion predominates, as compared with that of CRH. The source of AVP (magno- or parvocellular portion of the PVN) responsible for the corticotropic response to stress is yet undetermined . Further experiments in sheep using active immunization anti-CRH (Guillaume et al. 1992a) and anti-AVP (Guillaume et al. 1992b) led us to conclude that both endogenous CRH and AVP are necessary for a complete ACTH response to stress. Basal and circadian variations of plasma ACTH and cortisol depend upon endogenous CRH. Indeed, immunoneutralization of AVP did not affect these parameters (Guillaume et al. 1993 a,b).

The characterization of neurotansmitters which participate in the control of CRH and AVP neurons has also been extensively studied. The PVN is innervated by noradrenergic and adrenergic fibers. Synaptic contacts between these fibers and CRH and/or AVP neurons have been demonstrated. The stimulating action of norepinephrine and epinephrine has been recently recognized (Plotsky et al.1989). The innervation of CRH^+/AVP^+ and CRH^+/AVP^- neurons has not been studied yet, but recent pharmacological data suggest that α_1-adrenergic stimulation of CRH^+/AVP^+ neurons is a significant component of ACTH response to stress. In addition, the hypothalamic pituitary axis is activated by 5-HT receptors (Van de Kar 1991). ACTH response to stress exposure is lowered after brain serotonin depletion or administration of a 5-HT-antagonist, tianeptine, (Delbende et al. 1991) suggesting that endogenous 5-HT plays a role in hormonal response to stress. Several pharmacological studies indicate that 5-HT stimulation of ACTH release is mediated by 5-HT_{1A}, 5-HT_{1C} and 5-HT_2 receptors (review in Chaouloff, 1993).

Stress and somatotropic function

GH secretion is controlled by two hypothalamic neuropeptides GH-RH which acts as a stimulatory factor and SRIH which is an inhibitory factor. In human as well as in other species including monkeys and sheep, physical and psychological stress conditions stimulate GH secretion. However, the stimulation of GH release is not constant and its amplitude is variable. In the rat, under several stressful conditions (ether stress, insulin-induced hypoglycemia), GH secretion is blunted. Few direct investigations of GH-RH and SRIH secretion during stress are available. In the sheep, an isolation-contention stress stimulates GH secretion which is associated with an increased release of GH-RH and SRIH into HPB (Cataldi et al.1993). In the rat, using a push-pull perfusion of the hypothalamus, Aguila et al.(1991) have also found an augmentation of GH-RH and SRIH release which is associated with a decrease of GH release. Thus, it appears that stress induces in both species an increase in hypothalamic GH-RH and SRIH secretion. In the sheep, the action of GH-RH on the somatotrophs is predominant and plasma GH increases , the opposite being observed in the rat.

Central neurotransmitters participate in the control of GH secretion. α_2-adrenergic and cholinergic stimulatory effects as well as β-adrenergic and serotoninergic inhibiting effects have been documented. However, their role in stress-induced changes in GH secretion is undetermined yet. The role of 5-HT in the regulation of GH secretion is controversial. Several studies indicate that 5-HT agonists increase plasma GH concentration while others found that they are ineffective or even lower it (Van de Kar 1991). For example serotonin has been shown to inhibit hypoglycemia-induced GH release in dog (Muller et al. 1976). Opposite findings have been reported in the rat (Willoughby et al. 1982).

Effect of stress on the activity of the hypothalamic-pituitary-gonadal axis

The ability of stress to interfere with mammalian reproductive functions has long been recognized by investigators. The early observation by Selye (1939) showed that stress is accompanied by both an increase in the activity of the HPA axis and a decrease in the reproductive function. This author attributed this phenomenon to the necessity, in case of emergency, of preserving adrenal cortex function at the expense of gonadal activity. Indeed, CRH, ACTH and corticosterone play a very important role in modulating the effect of stress on reproductive functions (Rivier & Rivest 1991). In counter part, the changes in gonadotropic activity modify the pituitary-adrenal response to stress (Viau & Meaney 1991).

LH response to acute stressors in normal rats is biphasic with an initial increase followed by a decrease. This decrease is only observed if the intensity of the stressor is high enough and the exposure to it lasts for more than 60 min (Mc Grady, 1984). This phenomenon can also be detected in castrated rat that shows high LH levels (Yen, 1986). Thus, chronic restraint stress decreases gonadotropins as well as testosterone secretion. (Lopez-Calderon et al. 1991). In chronically stressed rats there is a decrease in hypothalamic LHRH content and the response of plasma gonadotropins to LHRH administration is enhanced. The inhibitory effect of chronic stress on plasma LH and FSH levels does not seem to be due to a reduction in pituitary responsiveness to LHRH but rather to a decrease of LHRH secretion.

The mechanisms responsible for the stress-induced inhibitory effect on reproductive function could involve peripheral sites (pituitary and/or adrenal) and CNS (CRH, POMC-derived peptides, monoamines). However, it appears that the CNS is probably the most important site that mediates the early response to stress. Indeed, the stress-induced decrease of plasma LH levels is comparable in adrenalectomized rats and in control animals (Rivier and Rivest, 1991).

CRH is one of the main factor known to exert a potent inhibitory control on LHRH secretion. This response could be linked to the close anatomical proximity of CRH and LHRH neurons (McLusky et al. 1988). Direct anatomical connections between CRH axon terminals and dendrites of LHRH neurons have been described. On the other hand, CRH could also act directly on LHRH nerve terminals in the median eminence (Gambacciani et al. 1986). However, complete destruction of the PVN fails to interfer with the inhibitory effect of stress on LH surge in male rat (Rivest & Rivier, 1991). Thus, afferents from other hypothalamic or extrahypothalamic CRH neurons could also be involved in the regulation of LHRH release. CRH neurons located in the medial preoptic area (Sawchenko et al. 1990) or in the central amygdaloid nucleus (Gray, 1990) may act on the stress-induced inhibitory effect.

The inhibitory effect of opiate peptides on LHRH release into HPB is now well accepted (Weiner et al. 1988). Noneless chronic stress does not modify hypothalamic and pituitary β-endorphin content whereas an increase in plasma β-endorphin concentration is observed. However, naltrexone treatment does not modify the decrease in LH or FSH plasma concentrations (Lopez-Calderon et al. 1991). Similar results have been obtained using anti-dynorphin antiserum (Petraglia et al. 1986). This suggests that opioids are not involved in the stress-induced inhibitory effects on levels of gonadotropins. Finally, these results indicate that the effect of CRH on LHRH neurons may be due to a direct action and not to a prior activation of opiate systems.

Stress and thyreotrope axis

The secretion of TSH is stimulated by TRH and inhibited by SRIH (Morley, 1981). The TRH neurons are located in several hypothalamic nuclei, mainly in the peri and paraventricular nuclei (parvocellular part) (Lechan & Jackson 1982). Their axon terminals project onto the median eminence. Exposure to cold environment (1 to 6° C) induces an increase of TSH release. This adaptative response to an increased energetic metabolism induces thermogenesis. This stress-induced effect could be due to an increased TRH release associated with a decreased SRIH secretion (Arancibia et al. 1983, 1987).

Stress and prolactin secretion

A variety of stressors stimulates prolactin release in experimental animals. (see Van de Kar et al. 1991 for review). The responses of prolactin to stress is characterized by a rapid increase reaching a maximum value at 3 min followed by a slow decline, control concentrations being reached after 60 min. The physiological significance of this phenomenon remains unclear. However, plasma prolactin levels are elevated in humans during the peak of panic attack. Interestingly, prolactin enhancement correlates better than plasma cortisol and growth hormone with the degree of panic attack (Cameron et al. 1987).

The pathways involved in the stress-induced prolactin secretion are not known. The question seems to be more complicated than for stress-induced ACTH and corticosterone secretion. Dopaminergic neurons do not represent the primary step for stress-induced prolactin secretion (Negro-Vilar, 1983). Different neuronal pathways could be involved to mediate the effect of distinct stressors on prolactin and corticosterone secretion. During psychological stress, PVN is not involved in stimulating prolactin release (Richardson-Morton et al. 1989) although it plays a role during restraint stress (Minamitani et al. 1987).

SEROTONIN AND NEUROENDOCRINE RESPONSES TO STRESS

Depletion of brain 5-HT induced by electrolytic lesions of dorsal and median raphe nuclei or by 5,7-DHT intraventricular injection or by PCPA treatment inhibited the effect of various stressors-induced increase in ACTH or corticosterone (Ixart et al. 1985) and prolactin (Makara et al. 1986) secretion. Serotoninergic fibers originating from the DRN project mainly in the parvocellular area of the PVN (Liposits et al. 1987). Injection of 5,7-DHT into the PVN inhibits the stress-induced increase of ACTH (Beaulieu et al. 1985), corticosterone and prolactin (Minamitani et al. 1987) release. These findings suggest that 5-HT nerve terminals in the PVN mediate the effect of stress on these hormones.

It is noteworthy that hypothalamic-pituitary-adrenal responses (ACTH and corticosterone) to restraint stress are modified during estrous cycle in the rat, although no differences are found in either basal ACTH and corticosterone levels across the cycle phases (Viau and Meaney 1991). These data may be explained either by intrahypothalamic connections (LHRH/CRH) or by influence of steroids on monoaminergic systems that regulate the threshold of hormone response to stress.

Serotonin released from axons originating from the DRN acts directly on 5-HT receptors located on LHRH neurons (Kiss & Halasz 1985ab). Under basal conditions 5-HT may play either a facilatory or an inhibitory role on LH release, depending on the steroid environment (Weiner et al. 1988). Recently, a blocking effect of PCPA treatment on stress-induced LH release has been reported, suggesting that 5-HT could be necessary to enhance LH secretion during short period of stress (Armario et al. 1993). The 5-HT antagonists mianserin and methiothepin are also able to block the stress-induced LH release. Interestingly, methiothepin has been reported to block the afternoon LH surge observed in castrated female rats primed with estradiol (Héry et al. 1976) as well as LHRH release (Vitale et al. 1986). Although the specific subtype of 5-HT receptor involved is not known, the greater efficacy of methiothepin among the 5-HT antagonists would suggest that $5-HT_1$ rather than $5-HT_2$ receptors could be involved.

Serotonin could also play a role on TSH secretion. Systemic treatments with various serotoninergic agonists reduce the increase of TSH release induced by exposure to cold environment (Toivonen et al. 1990 a). However, the involvement of 5-HT systems in the control of the thyreotrope axis appears to be more complex. Indeed, it is known that 5-HT injection in the anterior part of the 3rd ventricle enhances the release of TSH induced by cold whereas similar injection in the posterior ventricular part inhibits this response. This dual response on TSH secretion can be explained by recent data showing that $5-HT_2$ receptors are involved in the inhibitory effect of 5-HT while $5-HT_1$ receptors are involved in the stimulatory effect of 5-HT (Toivonen et al. 1990 b). Stress-induced changes in thyreotrope axis activity are mediated through an action of 5-HT at the PVN level (Toivonen et al. 1990 c). Administration of the $5-HT_{1A}$ receptor agonist ipsapirone induces a decrease of cold-induced TSH secretion (Broqua et al. 1993). In vitro experiments performed on hypothalamic slices suggest that this effect could be mediated by $5-HT_{1A}$ receptors located on TRH neurons (Chen and Ramirez, 1981).

STRESS, HORMONES AND 5-HT - RELATED ANXIOLYTICS

Several lines of evidence indicate that 5-HT may be involved in generating anxiety. Indeed lesions of 5-HT pathways or inhibition of 5-HT synthesis, causing a disruption of serotoninergic function, increased behavioural responses in conflict procedures. (Iversen 1984 ; Chopin & Briley 1987). The most convincing hypothesis is that increased serotoninergic transmission is associated with increased anxiety and, on the opposite, a decrease in serotoninergic activity leads to a decrease of anxiety. In 1974, Thierry et al. showed that stress (electric footshocks) induced an increase of 5-HT metabolism. Additional evidence is provided by the increased 5-HT release in the hippocampus detected during immobilization stress. There are convincing evidence that anxiolytic drugs of the benzodiazepine class inhibit serotoninergic transmission and that benzodiazepine binding sites within the DRN are implicated in the anxiolytic action of benzodiazepine drugs (Thiebot et al. 1982, Becquet et al. 1990a).

A new class of pyrimidinyl piperazine derivatives such as buspirone, gepirone and ipsapirone appears to be selective $5-HT_{1A}$ agonists and anxiolytic drugs. Moreover, 8-OH-DPAT, the prototype of $5-HT_{1A}$ receptor agonist, has an anxiolytic profile. From several anatomical studies it appears that $5-HT_{1A}$ receptors are always located on somato dendritic neuronal elements in non-serotoninergic neurons (heteroreceptor), for example in hippocampal CA3 area, and on serotoninergic neurons in the DRN (autoreceptor) (Sotelo et al. 1991). Anxiolytic effects induced by $5-HT_{1A}$ agonists are mediated through $5-HT_{1A}$ autoreceptors located within the DRN. Anticonflict effects of buspirone and gepirone are blocked after destruction of brain serotoninergic neurons (Eison et al. 1986). Buspirone (Urban et al. 1986) and ipsapirone (Lorens et al. 1989) inhibit the effect of stress on corticosterone and prolactin secretion.

Serotonin released from nerve endings is dependent on nerve activity (Héry et al. 1979) and local application of 5-HT within the DRN inhibits the firing rate of serotoninergic neurons. However, Descarries et al. (1982) reported that no 5-HT nerve terminals can be detected in the DRN. Thus, what is the origin of the 5-HT released in DRN ? In 1985, we showed, using "in vitro" experiments performed on cat nodose ganglia, that 5-HT was directly released from the serotoninergic cell bodies (Fuéri et al. 1984; Héry et al. 1986). More recently, we demonstrated, by "in vivo" experiments carried out in unanaesthetized cat, that a somatic release of 5-HT within the DRN controls the amine release from nerve endings in the caudate nucleus (Becquet et al. 1990a). The increase of somatic 5-HT release induced by local parachloroamphetamine application within the DRN induced a decrease of 5-HT release in caudate nucleus. This inhibitory effect was blocked by previous local administration of a 5-HT_1 receptor antagonist metitepine in the DRN. Buspirone, gepirone and ipsapirone inhibited the firing rate of dorsal raphe serotoninergic neurons (Schechter et al. 1990) inducing a decrease of 5-HT release from nerve ending. Thus their anxiolytic actions are consecutive to a reduction of 5-HT release detected after acute or chronic treatments (Hamon et al. 1988).

The 5-HT_{1A} receptors may not be the only serotoninergic receptor type involved in anxiety. Intrahippocampal injection of m-CPP, a 5-HT_{1C} receptor agonist, is anxiogenic and on the opposite the 5-HT_{1C}/5-HT_2 antagonists such as LY 53857 and mianserine are anxiolytics. Evidence that 5-HT_3 receptor antagonists have an anxiolytic profile in animal models of anxiety have been reported (Costall & Naylor 1991). It could be suggested that an alteration in 5-HT transmission at different 5-HT receptors could have numerous consequences. Nevertheless, there is no evidence to suggest that such changes act in concert to reduce anxiety.

STRESS, HORMONES, SEROTONIN AND DEVELOPMENT

During the perinatal period in the rat, the pattern of pituitary-adrenal secretion is peculiar. Corticosterone secretion is very high during the late fetal period, and decreases around birth. In the early postnatal period, basal and stress-induced corticosterone release are greatly reduced. From about postnatal day 2 until second week of life rats fail to respond or respond weakly to various stressors that usually induce a large increase in ACTH and corticosterone levels in adult rat. This period has been called "stress hyporesponsive period" (SHRP). The mechanisms responsible for SHRP are still unclear (Grino et al. 1991 for review). Nevertheless, the low circulating glucocorticoid levels during SHRP are believed to be essential for normal brain development and behaviour. Indeed, rats treated with glucocorticoids during the first week of life have permanent reduced brain weights, neuronal, glial and myeline alterations (Sapolski et Meaney 1986 for review).

It is well known that environmental stress during pregnancy in rats interferes with sexual differentiation of the fetal brain and affects the reproductive system of both male and female offspring (Gotz et al. 1989). Prenatal stress can also affect the development of serotoninergic neurons. Peters (1986) reported that various maternal stress enhance the ^{3}H-5-HT and ^{3}H-spiperone binding sites measured in cerebral cortex of 60 day-old male rats.

In rats, an environmental manipulation (handling) during early in life results in changes in the adrenocortical axis for the entire life. Early postnatal handling of rat pups permanently increases hippocampal type II, but not type I, corticosteroid receptor binding sites (Meaney et al. 1989). Handling induces also a transient increase in 5-HT turnover and, the effect of handling on type II corticosteroid receptor binding is blocked by concurrent administration of ketanserine, a 5-HT_2 receptor antagonist (Mitchell et al. 1990 a). Morever, these authors showed, using hippocampal cells in primary cultures, that the effect of 5-HT is exerted directly on hippocampal cells (Mitchell et al. 1990 b). Finally, the higher concentration of type II receptors as compared with type I in the hippocampus leads to an enhanced feedback inhibition of adrenocortical activity. In 24 months-old nonhandled rats basal glucocorticoid levels are higher than in handled ones. Morever, hippocampal cell loss and pronounced spacial memory deficit emerging with age in the nonhandled rats but were almost absent in the handled rats. Glucocorticoid hyper- secretion, hippocampal neuron death and cognitive impairments form a complex degenerative cascade of aging in the rat. Thus the Meaney's data show that subtle manipulation early in life can retard the emergence of this cascade (Meaney et al. 1988).

CONCLUSION

Neuroendocrine reactions in response to stress are part of the biological reaction of the organism that include also behavioural and neurovegetative adaptative changes. There is now increasing evidence for a common involvement of hypothalamic neuropeptides in all three reactions. Endocrine changes during stress can be accurately quantified and therefore may be used to explore neurochemistry of stress and to develop new drugs. These drugs will be helpful for treatment of not only acute biological reactions to stress but also pathological changes induced by chronic stress i.e. anxiety and depression.

REFERENCES.

Aguila, M.C., Pickle, R.L., Yu, W.H., & Mc Cann, S.M. (1991) Roles of somatostatin and growth hormone-releasing factor in ether stress inhibition of growth hormone release. Neuroendocrinology 54, 515-520.

Antoni, F.A. (1986) Hypothalamic control of adrenocotticotropin secretion : advances since the discovery of 41-residue corticotropin-releasing factor. Endocr. Rev. 7, 351-378.

Arancibia, S., Tapia-Arancibia, L., Assenmacher, I. & Astier, H. (1983) Direct evidence of short-term cold-induced TRH release in the median eminence of unanesthetized rats. Neuroendocrinology 37, 225-228.

Arancibia, S., Tapia-Arancibian, L., Astier, H. & Assenmacher, I. (1987) Effect of acute exposure to cold on SRIF release in unanesthetized rats and its temporal correlationship with the cold-induced TRH peak. Exp. Clin. Endocrinol. 6, 265-272.

Armario, A., Marti O., Gavolda, A., & Lopez-Calderon, A. (1993) Evidence for the involvement of serotonin in acute stress-induced release of luteinizing hormone in the male rat. Brain Res. Bull. 31, 29-31.

Beaudet, A. & Descarries, L. (1979) Radioautographic characterization of a serotonin-accumulating nerve cell group in adult rat hypothalamus. Brain Res. 160: 231-241.

Beaulieu, S., Paolo, T., Cote, J., & Barden N. (1985) Implication of the serotonergic system in the decreased ACTH response to stress after lesion of the amygdaloid central nucleus. Prog. Neuro-Psychopharmacol. Biol. Psychopharmacol. biol. Psychiat. 9: 665-669.

Becquet, D., Faudon, M., & Héry, F. (1990a) The role of serotonin release and autoreceptors in the dorsalis raphe nucleus in the control of serotonin release in the cat caudate nucleus. Neuroscience, 39: 639-647.

Becquet, D., François-Bellan, A.M., Boudouresque, F., Faudon, M., Héry, F., Guillaume, V. & Héry, M. (1990b) Serotonin synthesis from tryptophan by hypothalamic cells in serum-free medium culture. Dev. Brain Res., 54: 142-146.

Bosler, O. & Beaudet A. (1985) VIP neurons as a prime synaptic targets for serotonin afferents in rat suprachiasmatic nucleus: a combined radioautographic and immunocytochemical study. J. Neurocytol. 14: 749-763.

Boulenguez, P., Segu, L., Chauveau, J., Morel, A., Lanoir, J. & Delaage, M. (1992) Biochemical and pharmacological characterization of serotonin-o-carboxymethylglycyl. (^{125}I) iodotyrosinamide, a new radioiodinated probe for 5-HT$_{1B}$ and 5-HT$_{1D}$ binding sites. J. Neurochem. 5, 951-959.

Broqua, P., Laude, D., Bluet-Pajot, M.T., Schmidt, B., Baudrie, V. et Chaouloff, F. (1993) Are 5-HT1A autoreceptors involved in the inhibitory effect of ipsapirone on cold-elicited thyrotropin secretion ? Neuroendocrinology, in press.

Cameron, O.G., Lee, M.A., Curtis, G.C. & Mc Dan, D.S. (1987) Endocrine and physiological changes during 'spontaneous' panic attacks. Psychoneuroendocrinology 12: 321-331.

Cannon, W.B. (1914) The emergency function of the adrenal medulla in pain and the major emotions. Am. J. Physiol. 33, 356-372.

Cataldi, M., Magnan, E., Guillaume, V., Dutour, A., Mazzocchi, L., Conte-Devolx, B., & Oliver, C. (1993) Acute stress stimulates secretion of GH-RH and somatostatin into hypophysial portal blood of conscious sheep. Acta Endocrinologica (in press).

Chaouloff, F. (1993) Physiopharmacological interactions between stress hormones and central serotoninergic systems. Brain Res. Rev. 18,1-32.

Chen, Y.F. & Ramirez, V.D. (1981) Serotonin stimulates thyrotropin-releasing hormone release from superfused rat hypothalami. Endocrinology 108: 2359-2366.

Chopin, P., Briley, M. (1987) Animal models of anxiety: The effect of compounds that modify 5-HT neurotransmission. Trends Pharmacol. Sci. 8: 383-388.

Costall, B., & Naylor, R.J. (1991) Anxiolytic effects of 5-HT$_3$ antagonists in animals. In: 5-HT$_{1A}$ agonists, 5-HT$_3$ antagonists and benzodiazepines: Their comparative behavioural pharmacology. Eds. R.J. Rodgers & S.J. Cooper. John Wiley & Sons Ltd. 133-157.

Delbende,C., Contesse, V., Mocaer, E., Kamoun,A. & Vaudry, H. (1991) The novel antidepressant tianeptine reduces stress-evoked stimulation of the hypothalamo-pituitary-adrenal axis. Eur. J. Pharmacol. 202,391-396.

Descarries, L., Watkins, K.C., Garcia, S. & Beaudet, A. (1982) The serotonin neurons in nucleus raphe dorsalis of adult rat : a light and electron microscope autoradiographic study. J. Comp. Neurol. 207, 239-254.

Dunn, A.J., Berridge, D.W. (1990) Physiological and behavioral responses to corticotropin-releasing factor administration : is CRF a mediator of anxiety or stress respopnses ? Brain Res. Reviews 15, 71-100.

Eison, A.S., Eison, M.S., Stanley, M. & Riblet, L.A. (1986) Serotonergic nechanisms in the behavioral effects of buspirone and gepirone. Pharmacol. Biochem. Behav. 24: 701-707.

Fuéri, C., Faudon, M., Héry, M. & Héry, F. (1984) Release of serotonin from perikarya in cat nodose ganglia. Brain Res. 304, 173-177.

Gambacciani, M., Yen, S.S.C. & Rasmussen, D.D. (1986) GnGH release from the mediobasal hypothalamus : *in vitro* inhibition by corticotropin-releasing factor. Neuroendocrinology 43 : 533-536.

Gotz, F., Ohkawa, T., Rohde, W., Stahl, F., Tonjes R., Arai, K. and Dorner G. (1989) Influence of prenatal stress on the fetal neuroendocrine system in rats.In: Stress: Neurochemical and Humoral Mechanisms. Eds. G.R. Van Loon and J. Axelrod. Gordon & Breach Science Publishers, New York., 299-309.

Gray, T.S. (1990) The organization and possible function of amygdaloid corticotropin-releasing factor pathways. In : DeSouza E.B., Nemeroff CB (eds), Corticotropin-releasing Factor : Basic and Clinical of a Neuropeptide. Boca Raton, Florida : CRC Press, Inc : 53-68.

Grino,M., Boudouresque,F., Chautard, T., Becquet, D. Guillaume, V., Strbak V. and Oliver,C. (1991) Developmental aspects of the hypothalamic-pituitary-adrenal-axis in the rat. Endocrine Regul. 25, 36-43.

Guillaume, V., Conte-Devolx, B., Magnan, E., Boudouresque, F., Grino, M., Cataldi, M., Muret, L., Priou, A., Figaroli, J.C., & Oliver, C. (1992b) Effect of chronic active immunization with arginine vasopressin on pituitary-adrenal function in sheep. Endocrinology 130, 3007-3015.

Guillaume, V., Conte-Devolx, B., Magnan, E., Boudouresque, F., Grino, M., Cataldi, M., Muret, L., Priou, Deprez A., Figaroli, J.C., & Oliver, C. (1992a) Effect of chronic active immunization anti-corticotropin-releasing factor on pituitary-adrenal function in sheep. Endocrinology 130, 2291-2298.

Hamon, M., Fattaccini, C.M., Adrien, J., Galissot, M.C., Martin, P. and Gozlan,H. (1988) Alterations of central serotonin and dopamine turnover in rats treated with ipsapirone and other 5-hydroxytryptamine1A agonists with potential anxiolytic properties. J. Pharmacol. Exp. Ther. 246,745-752.

Héry, F., Faudon, M. & Fuéri, C. (1986) Release of serotonin in structures containing serotoninergic nerve cell bodies : dorsalis raphe nucleus and nodose ganglia of the cat. In : Annals New York Academy of Sciences, Vol. 473, 239-255.

Héry, F., Simonnet, G., Bourgoin, S., Soubrié, P., Artaud, F., Hamon, M. & Glowinski, J. (1979) Effect of nerve activity on the in vivo release of 3H-serotonin continuously formed from 3H-tryptophan in the caudate nucleus of the cat. Brain Res. 169, 317-334.

Héry, M.,Laplante, E., Kordon, C., (1976) Participation of serotonin in the phasic release of LH. (I) Evidence from pharmacological experiments. Endocrinology 99, 496-503.

Iversen, S.D.. (1984) 5-HT and anxiety. Neuropharmacol. 23, 1553-1560.

Ixart, G., Szafarczyk, A., Malaval, F., Assenmacher, I. (1985) Impairment of the ether stress-induced ACTH surge in rats by ablation of the suprachiasmatic nuclei or by i.p. injections of p-chlorophenylalanine. Neuroendocrinol. Lett. 7: 171-174.

Kiss, J. & Halasz, B. (1985a) Demonstration of serotoninergic axons terminating on luteinizing hormone-releasing hormone neurons in the preoptic area of the rat using a combination of immunocytochemistry and high resolution autoradiography. Neuroscience 14 : 69-78.

Kiss, J. & Halasz B. (1985b) Synaptic connections between serotoninergic axon terminals and tyrosine hydroxylase-immunoreactive neurons in the arcuate nucleus of the rat hypothalamus. A combination of electron microscopic autoradiography and immunocytochemistry. Brain Res. 364: 284-292.

Lechan, R. & Jackson, I.M.D. (1982) Immunohistochemical localization of thyrotropin-releasing hormone in the rat hypothalamus and pituitary. Endocrinology 111: 55-65.

Liposits, Zs., Phelix, C. & Paull, W.K. (1987) Synaptic interaction of serotonergic axons and corticotropin releasing factor (CRF) synthesizing neurons in the hypothalamic paraventricular nucleus of the rat. A light and electron microscopic immunocytochemical study. Histochemistry 86: 541-549.

Lopez-Calderon, A., Ariznavaretta, C., Gonzalez-Quijana M.J., Tresguerres A.F. & Calderon M.D. (1991) Stress induced changes in testis function. J. Steroid Biochem. Molec. Biol. 40 : 473-479.

Lorens, S.A., Mitsushio H., Van de Kar, L.D. (1989) Effects of the 5-HT$_{1A}$ agonist ipsapirone on the behavioral, endocrine and neurochemical resposes to conditioned fear; in Bevan, cools, Archer, Behavioral pharmacology of 5-HT, pp. 360-370.

Makara, G.B., Kvetnansky, R., Jezova, D., Jindra, A., Kakucska, I., Oprasalova, Z. (1986) Plasma catecholamines do not participate in pituitary adrenal activation by immobilization stress in rats with transection of nerve fibers to the median eminence. Endocrinology 119: 1757-1762.

Manrique, C., Segu, L., Héry, M., Faudon, M. & François-Bellan, A.M. (1993) Increase of central 5-HT1B binding sites following 5,7-dihydroxytryptamine axotomy in the adult rat. Brain Res. (in press).

Mc Grady, A.V. (1984) Effects of physiological stress on male reproduction: a rewiew. Archives of Andrology 13 : 1-7.

McLusky, N.J., Naftolin, F. & Leranch C (1988) Immunocytochemical evidence for direct synaptic connections between corticotropin-releasing factor (CRF) and gonadotropin-releasing hormone (GnRH)-condaining neurons in the preoptic area of the rat. Brain Res 439 : 391-395.

Meaney, M.J., Aitken, D.H., Berkel, C.,Bhatnagar, S. and Sapolsky R.M. (1988) Effect of neonatal handling on age-related impairments with the hippocampus. Science, 239, 766-768.

Meaney, M.J., Aitken, D.H., Viau, V., Sharma, S. and Sarrieau A. (1989) Neonatal handling alters adrenocortical negative feedback sensivity and hippocampal type II glucorticoid receptor binding in the rat. Neuroendocrinology, 50, 597-604.

Minamitani, N., Minamitani, T., Lechan, R.M., Bollinger-Gruber, J. & Reichlin, S. (1987) Paraventricular nucleus mediates prolactin secretory responses to restraint stress, ether stress, and 5-hydroxy-1-tryptophan injection in the rat. Endocrinology 120: 860-867.

Mitchell, J.B., Iny, L.J. and Meaney M.J. (1990a) The role of serotonin in the development and environmental regulation of type II corticosteroid receptor binding in rat. Dev. Brain Res. 55,231-235.

Mitchell, J.B., Rowe, W., Boksa, P. and Meaney M.J. (1990b) Serotonin regulates type II corticosteroid receptor binding in hippocampal cell cultures. J. Neurosc. 10, 1745-1752.

Morley, J.E. (1981) Neuroendocrine control of thyrotropin secretion. Endocrine Rev. 2: 396-403.

Müller, E.E., Udeschini, G., Secchi, C., Zambotti, F., Vicentini, L., Panerai, A.E., Cocola, F., & Mantegazza, P. (1976) Inhibitory role of the serotoninergic system in hypoglycemia-induced growth hormone release in the drog. Acta Endocrinol. 82, 71-91.

Negro-Vilar, A. (1983) Maturation of stress-induced prolactin release in male rats: Involvement of the tuberohypophysial dopaminergic system. neuroendocrinol. Lett. 8: 79-85.

Pazos, A., & Palcios, J.M. (1985) Quantitative autoradiographic mapping of serotonin receptors in the rat brain. I. Serotonin-1 receptors. Brain Res. 346: 205-230.

Pazos, A., Cortes, R. & Palacios, J.M. (1985) Quantitative autoradiographic mapping of serotonin receptors in the rat brain. II. Serotonin-2 receptors. 346: 231-249.

Pertraglia, F., Vale, W. & Rivier C. (1990) Opioids act centrally to modulate stress-induced decrease in luteinizing hormone in the rat. Endocrinology 119 : 2445-2450.

Peters, D.A.V. (1986) Prenatal stress: Effect on development of rat brain serotoninergic neurons. Pharmacol. Biochem. & Behav. 24, 1377-1986.

Plotsky, P.M., Cunningham, Jr.E.T., & Widmaier, E.P. (1989) Catecholaminergic modulation of corticotropin-releasing factor and adrenocorticotropin secretion. Endocrine Reviews 10, 437-458.

Richardson-Morton, K.D., Johnson, M.D., Van de Kar, L.D. Brownfield, M.S., & Bethea, C.L.: (1989) Neuronal cell bodies in the hypothalamic paraventricular nucleus mediate stress-induced renin and corticosterone secretion. Neuroendocrinology 50: 73-80.

Rivier, C. & Rivest S. (1991) Effect of stress on the activity of the hypothalamic-pituitary-gonadal axis : peripheral and central mechanisms. Biology of Reproduction 45 : 523-532.

Sapolsky, R.M. & Meaney, M.J. (1986) Maturation of the adrenocortical stress response: Neuroendocrine control mechanisms and the stress hyporesponsive period. Brain Res. Reviews, 11, 65-76.

Sawchenko, P.E. & Swanson L.W. (1990) Organization of CRF immunoreactive cells and fibres in the rat brain : immunochistochemical studies. In : DeSouza E.B. Nemeroff C.B. (eds), Corticotropin-Releasing Factor : Basic and Clinical Studies of a Neuropeptide Boca Raton. F.L. : CRC Press, Inc : 29-51.

Sawchenko, P.E., Swanson, L.W., Steinbusch, H.W.M. & Verhofstad, A.A.J. (1983) The distribution and cells of origin of serotonergic inputs to the paraventricular and supraoptic nuclei of the rat. Brain Res. 277: 355-360.

Schechter L.E., Bolanos, F.J., Gozlan, H., Lanfumey, L., Haj-Dahmane S., Laporte, A.-M.-, Fattaccini, C.-M. and Hamon, M. (1990) Alterations of central serotoninergic and dopaminergic neurotransmission in rats chronically treated with ipsapirone: Biochemical and electrophysiological studies. J. Pharmacol. Exp. Ther. 255,1335-1347.

Selye, H.A. (1936) A syndrome produced by diverse nocious agents. Nature (London) 138 : 32.

Selye, H. (1939) Effect of adaptation to various damaging agents on the female sex organs in the rat. Endocrinology 25 : 615-624.

Sotelo, C., Cholley, B., El Mestikawy, S., Gozlan, H. & Hamon; M. (1990) Direct immunohistochemical evidence of the existence of $5-HT_{1A}$ autoreceptors on serotonergic neurons in the midbrain raphe nuclei. Eur. J. Neuroscience 2: 1144-1154.

Steinbusch, H.W.M. & Nieuwenhuys, R. (1981) Localization of serotonin-like immunoreactivity in the central nervous system and pituitary of the rat, with special innervation of the hypothalamus. Adv. Med. Biol. Ther. 133, 7-36.

Swanson, L.W. (1987) The hypothalamus. In : Hanbook of Chemical Neuroanatomy, Vol 5 : Integrated systems of the CNS, part I : Hypothalamus, hippocampus, amygdala, retina. Eds. Bjorklund, A., Hökfelt, T. and Swanson, L.W. Elsevier Science Publishers, 1-124.

Thiebot, M.H., Hamon, M., Soubrié, P. (1982) Attenuation of induced-anxiety rats by chlordiazepoxide: Role of raphe dorsalis benzodiazepine binding sties and serotoninergic neurons. Neuroscience 7: 2287-2294.

Thierry, A.M., Fekete, M & Glowinski, J. (1968) Effects of stress on the metabolism of noradrenaline, dopamine and serotonin in the CNS of the rat. (II) Modifications of serotonin metabolism. Eur. J. Pharmacol. 4, 384-389.

Toivonen, M., Rauhala, P. & Männistö, P.T. (1990a) Complex actions of serotonergic agonists on cold-stimulated TSH secretion in male rats. Eur. J. Pharmacol. 180: 91-102.

Toivonen, M., Rauhala, P. & Männistö, P.T. (1990b) Site-dependent action of intracerebroventricular 5-Hydroxytryptamine on the cold-stimulated thyrotropin secretion in male rats. Neuroendocrinolgy 51: 45-50.

Toivonen, M., Tuomainen, P. & Männistö, P.T. (1990c) Effects of hypothalamic paraventricular nucleus lesion on the cold-stimulated TSH response to 5-HT in male rats. Acta Physiol. Scand. 139: 233-239.

Urban, J.H., Van de Kar, L.D., Lorens, S.A. & Bethea, C.L. (1986) Effect of the anxiolytic drug buspirone on prolactin and corticosterone secretion in stresses and unstressed rats. Pharmacol. Biochem. Behav. 25: 457-462.

Van de Kar, L.D. (1991) Neuroendocrine pharmacology of serotoninergic neurons. Ann. Rev. Pharmacol. Toxicol. 31 : 289-320.

Van de Kar, L.D., Richardson-Morton, K.D., and Rittenhouse, P.A. (1991) Stress: Neuroendocrine and Pharmacological Mechanisms. In: Methods and Achievements in Experimental Pathology. Eds. G. Jasmin & M. Cantin. Karger Basel, 14, 133-173.

Viau, V. & Meaney, M.J. (1991) Variations in the hypothalamic-pituitary-adrenal gland response to stress during the estrous cycle in the rat. Endocrinology 129 : 2503-2511.

Vitale, m.L., Parisi, M.N., Chiocchio, S.R. and Tramezzani, J.H.(1986) Serotonin induces gonadotrophin release through stimulation of LHRH release from median eminence. J. Endocrinol. 111, 309-315.

Weiner, R.I., Findell, P.R. & Kordon C. (1988) Role of classic and peptide neuromediators in the neuroendocrine regulation of LH and prolactin. In : Knobil E., Neill J. (eds), The Physiology of Reproduction. New York : Raven Press, 1235-1281.

Whitnall, M.H. (1993) Regulation of the hypothalamic corticotropin-releasing hormone neurosecretory system. Prog. in Neurobiol. 40, 573-629.

Willoughby, J.O., Jervois, P.M., & Menadue, M.F. (1982) Funstion of serotonin in physiologic secretion of growth hormone and prolactin : action of 5,7-dihydroxytryptamine, fenfluramine and p-chlorphenylanine. Brain Research 249, 291-299.

Yen, S.S.C. (1986) Chronic anovulation due to CNS-hypothalamic-pituitary dysfunction In : Yen S.S.C., Jaffe R.B. (Eds), Reproductive Endocrinology : Physiology, Pathophysiology and Clinical Management philadelphia, PA : W.B. Saunders Co : 500-545.

Résumé

L'exposition à une situation de stress conduit l'organisme à la mise en place de réactions adaptatives comportementales, neurovégétatives et neuroendocriniennes. Parmi les réponses hormonales induites par un stress il faut noter la stimulation de l'ACTH et des glucocorticoïdes, ainsi que celle de la prolactine; l'inhibition des hormones gonadotropes et la stimulation et/ou l'inhibition de l'hormone de croissance et de l'hormone thyréotrope suivant la nature du stress et de l'espèce animale étudiée. Les neurotransmetteurs centraux dont la sérotonine sont impliqués dans les réactions adaptatives et particulièrement hormonales déclenchées par un stress. La sérotonine est anxiogène et elle intervient dans le controle de ces mécanismes aussi bien chez le nouveau né que chez l'adulte.

Stress, anxiety and immunity

Robert Dantzer

INRA-INSERM U.176, Laboratoire de Neurobiologie Intégrative, rue Camille Saint-Saëns, 33077 Bordeaux Cedex, France

Summary. Anxiogenic situations are characterized by lack of control and uncertainty. Human and animal studies show that these situations result in changes in many different components of the immune system, in addition to their physiological effects measured by plasma levels of stress hormones or indices of cardiovascular function. Although there has been no systematic studies on the effects of anxiolytics on stress-induced alterations of immunity, benzodiazepine central receptor agonists have been found to affect immune responses in an opposite way to benzodiazepine central receptors antagonists. In addition, benzodiazepine peripheral receptors agonists have profound modulatory effects on immune responses, although their *in vitro* effects do not generalize to *in vivo* conditions. Stress-induced changes in immunity appear to be mediated by a β-adrenergic component, suggesting that under certain conditions, beta blockers can alleviate the effects of stress on imunity. The existence of associations between stress, anxiety and immunity cannot, however, be interpreted as evidence for a causal relationship between stress and disease.

The idea that stress, moods and emotions influence health and disease is not new. It is a recurrent theme in art and literature and it can be found under diverse forms in biology and psychology. Selye's stress theory, with its emphasis on the non specific general adaptation syndrome was one of the first attempts to formulate this hypothesis in scientific terms (Selye, 1956). The development of the field of health psychology is the modern version of the credo in the existence of relationships between psychosocial factors and disease (Rodin and Salovey, 1989).

The understanding of the relationship between stressful experience and health cannot proceed without a full consideration of the different terms of the chain of events, from the perception and representation of psychosocial factors to the pathophysiological mechanisms responsible for functional and structural alterations at the level of the target organ. Concerning this last aspect, a significant step forward has been achieved with the possibility of investigating the effects of stress on immune responses since they represent an important component of the host sensitivity to infection and tumor proliferation. This field of investigation, known as psychoneuroimmunology (Ader, 1981), has been the object of a flurry of research during the last decade, thanks to the availability of quantitative *in vitro* methods for assessing immune responses in humans and animals. The objective of the present chapter is to critically review the progress made in this field and the way it relates to anxiety disorders.

I. Relationship between stress and anxiety

Stress is usually defined as the non specific response to any demand which exceeds the organism's ability to adapt. Anxiety belongs to a different domain since it is used to refer to the negative feelings and physical symptoms which are experienced by someone confronted with unpredictable and uncontrolable events. However, the distinction between these two concepts is not as marked as it appears *a priori*. Ample evidence indicates that the increased reactivity of the sympathetic-adrenal medullary system and the pituitary-adrenal axis, which characterizes the stress response, is not an ineluctable and invariable outcome of the physical properties of the stressor but a function of the ability of the subject to predict and control the situation (Dantzer, 1989). From a cognitive-behavioural perspective, the stress response is modulated by the coping strategies the subject interposes between the stressor and himself. The affective components of these coping strategies are diverse. Anxiety shoud be predominent in situations which are perceived as difficult to control and of which the evolution appears to be uncertain. In terms of hormonal concomitants, such situations are likely to be characterized by high levels of pituitary-adrenal hormones and sympathetic and adrenal medullary hormones corresponding respectively to lack of control and enhanced arousal with readiness for action (Henry, 1986).

II. Effects of stress on immunity

A wide variety of stressors have been found to influence immune responses in animals and humans (Dantzer and Kelley, 1989; Dantzer, 1994). In animals they include painful electric shock, restraint, forced exercise, exposure to cold, change in housing conditions (crowding or social isolation) and social stress. In humans, the effects of stress on immunity has been assessed in experimental settings and in clinically oriented studies. In the first case, volunteers are submitted to well controlled stressful procedures (e.g., mental arithmetic task) or to techniques for inducing specific emotions. In the case of clinically oriented studies, the emphasis has been mainly on negative life events (e.g., death of a spouse, difficulties in marital life, problems with a sick parent) and negative affective states (mainly depression).

The immune variables which are usually considered in the studies of the influence of stress on immunity include proliferative responses of blood lymphocytes or splenocytes to mitogens, cytotoxic activity of natural killer cells, antibody titers to T cell-dependent or independent antigen. *In vivo* measures of immunity (e.g., contact sensitivity, delayed-type hypersensitivity) which were used in the early days of these studies tend to be replaced by *in vitro* assays.

In acordance with what is known concerning the importance of predictability and controllability on the neurochemical and hormonal consequences of stressors (Dantzer, 1989), these two factors have been found to be determinant for the influence of stress on immunity. The rate of tumour growth was found to be accelerated in mice exposed to a single session of inescapable shock 24 hours following tumour cell transplantation, whereas mice exposed to escapable shock did not differ from non-shocked mice in tumour size and time of tumour appearance (Sklar and Anisman, 1979). This detrimental effect of uncontrollability on tumour development was no longer apparent, however, in animals exposed chronically to the stressor (Sklar et al, 1981). In rats, a single session of inescapable but not of escapable shock significantly reduced the incidence of rejection of transplanted non-syngeneic tumour cells (Visintainer et al, 1982). The possibility that such changes are mediated by suppression of the immune system was suggested by studies showing that inescapable shock delivered in an intermittent manner decreased NK cell activity (Shavit et al, 1984). In addition, inescapable but not escapable shock has been found to decrease cellular immune responses. Rats submitted to inescapable electric shocks on the first day and re-exposed to a few 'reminder' shocks on the second day displayed a lower proliferative response of blood lymphocytes to T-cell mitogens than rats submitted to escapable electric shocks or apparatus-control animals (Laudenslager et al, 1983). This impairment of lymphoproliferative response due to inescapable electric shock appears to carry over to chronic conditions, since it was also observed in yoked rats paired with rats exposed to ten sessions of free-operant avoidance learning in a shuttle box (Mormède et al, 1988). In the same manner, rats exposed to unsignalled electric shocks displayed decreased lymphoproliferative responses whereas rats exposed to signalled electric shocks did not differ from non-shocked animals (Mormède et al, 1988).

It would be wrong to conclude from the previous findings that uncontrollability and unpredictability always result in immunosuppressive effects. The primary antibody response against sheep red blood cells was depressed in rats exposed to free-operant avoidance in a shuttle-box but not in yoked rats and apparatus-control animals (Mormède et al, 1988). In human beings exposed to mild electric shock and loud white noise administered over a 30-min period in an unpredictable intermittent manner, subjects with control displayed a lowered lymphoproliferation to mitogens whereas subjects who could not control the stressor were not affected, despite increased anger and frustration (Weisse et al, 1990).

Besides uncontrollability and uncertainty, situations that can be considered as anxiogenic are those in which individuals are presented with cues previously associated with aversive stimuli. In animal studies, cues that had been explicitely paired with electric shock were found to depress lymphoproliferative responses to a mitogen much like that provoked by the stressor itself (Lysle et al, 1988). In the same manner, exposure to apparatus cues that had been associated with a stressor influenced the humoral immune response in mice inoculated with sheep red blood cells, the nature of the effect (immunosuppression or immunoenhancement) depending on time at which the initial stressor treatment was applied relative to antigenic inoculation (Zalcman et al, 1988). Mice exposed for 24 h to odors from shocked donors displayed a decrease in interleukin-2 production by splenocytes stimulated with a T cell mitogen, a reduction in NK cell activity and an increase in IgM and IgG antibody titers against the keyhole limpet hemocyanin antigen, in comparison to the response of home cage or apparatus control animals (Cocke et al, 1993). In humans, the immune concomitants of experimentally induced anxiety or anxiety disorders have not been studied in a systematic way.

III. Immune effects of drugs acting on benzodiazepine receptors

Based on the previous findings and assuming that anxiolytic drugs are able to reduce the somatic concomitants of stress and anxiety, it can be anticipated that anxiolytics should block the effects of stress on immune responses. In contrast, anxiogenic drugs should mimic the effects of stress on immunity. The few studies which have been carried out suggest that this might be so, but it is difficult to generalize, due to an insufficient database. Most of the work in this area has focused on the effects of compounds acting on peripheral benzodiazepine receptors which have been found to be present on accessory immune cells.

III.1. Central benzodiazepine receptors

There are relatively few studies on the effects of benzodiazepine receptor agonists or inverse agonists on immune responses in normal individuals and in anxious or stressed subjects.

Injections of alprazolam, a benzodiazepine agonist mainly used for its efficacy in patients with panic attack, enhanced lymphoproliferative responses to mitogens and the mixed lymphocyte reaction in mice (Fride et al, 1990). However, the same compound had immunosuppressive effects when tested *in vitro* on both lymphoproliferative responses to mitogens and production of proinflammatory cytokines by activated peritoneal macrophages (Chang et al, 1991).

Benzodiazepine receptor inverse agonists of the β-carboline family which induce anxiety-like symptoms have been found to depress lymphoproliferative responses to mitogens and allogeneic cytotoxic T lymphocyte activity. Central injections of these molecules into the locus coeruleus and the hippocampus reduced NK cell activity and production of IL-2 by splenocytes (Libri et al, 1991).

III.2. Peripheral benzodiazepine receptors

In accordance with the high density of peripheral benzodiazepine receptors found on blood mononuclear cells, ligands with high affinity for these receptors have a number of effects on immune responses ranging from stimulation of monocyte chemotaxis (Ruff et al, 1985) to enhanced production of proinflammatory cytokines by activated monocytes (Taupin et al, 1991). It is interesting to note that the *in vivo* effects of these compounds are opposed to those observed *in vitro*. Peritoneal and spleen cells collected from mice treated with various peripheral benzodiazepine receptor agonists produced less reactive oxygen species than cells collected from placebo treated mice. The same treatment had an inhibitory effect on the production of proinflammatory cytokines by activated accessory immune cells (Zavala et al, 1990).Such effects are specific to compounds acting at the level of peripheral benzodiazepine receptors since centrally acting benzodiazepines had no effect. The possibility that the *in vivo* immune effects of peripheral benzodiazepine receptor antagonists are mediated by the modulatory effect of these compounds on mitochondrial regulation of neurosteroid and adrenal steroid synthesis (Ferrarese et al, 1993) remains to be tested.

IV. Beta-adrenergic modulation of the immune response

Primary and secondary lymphoid organs have been demonstrated to be innervated by fibers of the sympathetic nervous system (Felten et al, 1987). Since the noradrenaline containing terminals are located in the splenic periarteriolar lymphatic sheath, lymphocytes are likely to be exposed to high local levels of catecholamines. In addition, sympathetic fibers are found in areas containing macrophages and other accessory immune cells. Lymphocytes and macrophages have membrane receptors of the β-adrenergic type (Madden and Livnat, 1991; Roszman and Carlson, 1991). Like in other cell types, these receptors are coupled to an adenylate-cyclase system. In addition to the large body of evidence in favor of a modulatory role of catecholamines on immune functions, recent studies have addressed the possibility of a role for β-adrenergic receptors in the effects of stress on immunity.

In an extensive series of studies, Lysle and colleagues (1993) have shown that the depressed mitogenic responsiveness of splenocytes to mitogens displayed by rats reexposed to the cage in which they had previously been shocked but without shock, was attenuated by administering propranolol, a nonselective β-adrenergic receptor antagonist, atenolol, a β1 selective antagonist and ICI-118,551, a β2 selective antagonist prior to reexposure to the cage conditioned cues. These treatments had no effect on the depression of NK cell activity and reduction of IL-2 production observed in the situation. Since similar effects were observed after administration of the opiate receptor antagonist naltrexone but not its quaternary derivative which does not cross the blood-brain barrier, they interpreted these findings to suggest that exposure to conditioned fear cues activate central opioid mechanims resulting in activation of the peripheral β-adrenergic system. It is interesting to note that a similar relationship between central opioid systems and β-adrenergic activity has been noted by Ben-Eliyahu et al (1993) in their studies on the effects of stress on tumor metastasis on rats.

V. Immunologic effects on behaviour and mood

The interactions between the nervous and immune systems are not unidirectional but fully bidirectional (Dantzer and Kelley, 1989). There is growing evidence that nervous influences on immunity correspond to the efferent arm of a regulatory pathway. The afferent pathway is represented by communication signals from the immune system to the brain. These signals are represented by the same cytokines which already serve to regulate the proliferation and differentiation of immunocytes. The attention has mainly focused on interleukin-1 (IL-1) and tumor necrosis factor (TNF) which are released by activated accessory immune cells and have potent neurotropic effects, in the form of fever, increased slow-wave sleep, depressed behavioural activities and increased activity of the pituitary-adrenal axis (Rothwell, 1991; Kent et al, 1992). These molecules play a key role in the coordination of the host response to infection and inflammation. In particular, cytokines are responsible for the profound behavioural and psychic changes which take place in sick individuals (Dantzer et al, 1992). However, in terms of mood changes, the observed effects are closer to depressed mood than to anxiety. Terminally ill cancer patients have been reported to respond to infusion of IL-1 with symptoms of fear and anxiety (Dinarello, personal communication) but their pathological condition is certainly more important in these effects than the cytokine itself.

VI. Conclusions

We all hold the belief of a strong association between anxiety and depression on one hand and illness on the other hand. However, whether the relationship is at the level of objective or subjective symptomatology can be debated (Dantzer, 1993). This issue tends to be overlooked by those who, by emphasizing the biological aspects of anxiety, would like to find in this new discipline called psychoneuroimmunology the ultimate mechanistic evidence for a relationship between stress and disease. However, as outlined by health psychologists, the existence of such a relationship can be questioned since it is known to be strongly distorted by the high prevalence of neuroticism in the population displaying somatic complaints (Costa and McCrae, 1987; Watson and Pennebaker, 1989). Neuroticism refers to a broad dimension of individual differences in the tendency to express negative, distressing emotions, and to possess associated behavioural and cognitive traits. These traits include fearfulness, irritability, low self-esteem, social anxiety, poor inhibition of impulses and helplessness. Neurotic subjects differ from normal subjects in their perception and attentiveness to symptoms and their likelihood of using health care resources, but not in their objective symptomatology (Krantz and Hedges, 1987).

This does not mean that it is useless to consider possible associations between stress and immunity. It just warrants caution in the elaboration of attractive theories on the causal role of these associations.

REFERENCES

Ader, R. ed. (1981) : Psychoneuroimmunology. New York: Academic Press.

Arora, P.K., Hanna, E.E., Paul, S.M. & Skolnick, P. (1987) : Suppression of the immune response by benzodiazepine receptor inverse agonists. J. Neuroimmunol. 15: 1-9.

Ben-Eliyahu, S., Page, G.G., Yirmiya, R., Taylor, A.N. & Liebeskind, J.C. (1993) : Sympathetic modulation of natural killer cell activity and metastatic growth: a role for adrenal epinephrine. In Proc. 4th Research Perspectives in Psychoneuroimmunology, Abstract # 23, Boulder.

Chang, M.P., Castle, S.C. & Norman, D.C. (1991) : Suppressive effects of alprazolam on the immune response of mice. Int. J. Immunopharmacol. 13: 259-266.

Cocke, R., Moynihan, J.A., Cohen, N., Grota, L.J. & Ader, R. (1993) : Exposure to conspecific alarm chemosignals alters immune responses in BALB/c mice. Brain Behav. Immun. 7: 36-46.

Costa, P.T., McCrae, R.R. (1987) : Neuroticism, somatic complaints, and disease: is the bark worse than the bite? J. Personality 55: 299-316.

Dantzer, R. (1989) : Neuroendocrine correlates of control and coping. In Stress, Personal Control and Health, eds A. Steptoe & A. Appels, pp. 277-294. Chichester: Wiley.

Dantzer, R. (1993) : The Psychosomatic Delusion. New York: The Free Press.

Dantzer, R. (1994) : Psychoneuroimmunology of stress. In Stress, The Immune System and Psychiatry, eds B.E. Leonard & K. Miller. Chichester: Wiley. (In press).

Dantzer, R. & Kelley, K.W. (1989) : Stress and immunity: an integrated view of relationships between the brain and immune system. Life Sci. 44: 1995-2008.

Felten, D.L., Felten, S.Y., Bellinger, D.L., Carlson, S.L., Ackerman, K.D., Madden, K.S., Olschowka, J.A. & Livnat, S. (1987) : Noradrenergic sympathetic neural interactions with the immune system: structure and function. Immunol. Rev. 100: 225-260.

Ferrarese, C., Appolinio, I., Bianchi, G., Frigo, M., Marzorati, C., Pecora, N., Perego, M., Pierpaoli, C. & Frattola, L. (1993) : Benzodiazepine receptors and diazepam binding inhibitor: a possible link between stress, anxiety and the immune system. Psychoneuroendocrinology 18: 3-22.

Fride, E., Skolnick, P. & Arora, P.K. (1990) : Immunoenhancing effects of alprazolam in mice. Life Sci., 47: 2409-2420.

Henry, J.P. (1986) : Neuroendocrine patterns of emotional response. In Emotion: Theory, Research and Experience, Vol. 3: Biological Foundations, eds R. Plutchik & H. Kellerman, pp. 37-60. Orlando: Academic Press.

Kent, S., Bluthé, R.M., Kelley, K.W. & Dantzer, R. (1992) : Sickness behaviour: a new target for drug development. Trends Pharmacol. Sci. 13: 24-28.

Krantz, D.S. & Hedges, S.M. (1987) : Some cautions for research on personality and health. J. Personality 55: 351-357.

Laudenslager, M.L., Ryan, S.M., Drugan, R.C., Hyson, R.L. & Maier, S.F. (1983) : Coping and immunosuppression: inescapable but not escapable shock suppresses lymphocyte proliferation. Science 221: 568-570.

Libri, V., Del Gobbo, V., Villani, N., Agosto, R., Calio, R. & Nistico, G. (1991) : Microinfusion of ethyl-β-carboline-3-carboxylate into the locus coeruleus reduces both interleukin-2 production and natural killer cell activity. Progr. NeuroendocrinImmunol. 4: 79-85.

Lysle, D.T., Cunnick, J.E., Fowler, H. & Rabin, B.S. (1988) : Pavlovian conditioning of shock-induced suppression of lymphocyte reactivity. Acquisition, extinction and preexposure effects. Life Sci. 42: 2185-2194.

Lysle, D.T., Coussons, M.E., Fecho, K., Perez, L., Maslonek, K.A. & Dykstra, L.A. (1993) : Conditioned alterations of immune status: evidence for the involvement of endogenous opioid activity and the β-adrenergic system. In Proc. 4th Research Perspectives in Psychoneuroimmunology, Abstract # 31, Boulder.

Madden, K.S. & Livnat, S. (1991) : Catecholamine action and immunologic reactivity. In Psychoneuroimmunology, eds R. Ader, D.L. Felten. & N. Cohen, pp. 283-310. San Diego: Academic Press.

Mormède, P., Dantzer, R., Michaud, B., Kelley, K.W. & Le Moal, M. (1988) : Influence of stressor predictability and behavioral control on lymphocyte reactivity, antibody response and neuroendocrine activation in rats. Physiol. Behav. 43: 577-583.

Rodin, J. & Salovey, P. (1989) : Health psychology. Ann. Rev. Psychol. 40: 533-579.

Roszman, T.L. & Carlson, S.L. (1991) : Neurotransmitters and molecular signaling in the immune response. In Psychoneuroimmunology, eds R. Ader, D.L. Felten. & N. Cohen, pp. 311-335. San Diego: Academic Press.

Ruff, M.R., Pert, C.B., Weber, R.J., Wahl, L.M., Wahl, S.M. & Paul, S.M. (1985) : Benzodiazepine receptor mediated chemotaxis of human monocytes. Science 229: 1281-1283.

Selye, H. (1956) The Stress of Life. New York: McGraw Hill

Shavit, Y., Lewis, J.M., Terman, G.W., Gale, R.P. & Liebeskind, J.C. (1984) : Opioid peptides mediate the suppressive effects of stress on natural killer cell cytotoxicity. Science 223: 188-190.

Sklar, L.S. & Anisman, H. (1979) : Stress and coping factors influence tumor growth. Science 205: 513-515.

Sklar, L.S., Bruto, V. & Anisman, H. (1981) : Adaptation to the tumor-enhancing effects of stress. Psychosom. Med. 43: 331-342.

Taupin, V., Herbelin, A., Descamps-Latscha, B. & Zavala, F. (1991) : Endogenous anxiogenic peptide, ODN-diazepam binding inhibitor and benzodiazepines enhance the production of interleukin-1 and tumor necrosis factor by human monocytes. Lympokine Cytokine Res. 10: 7-13.

Visintainer, M.A., Volpicelli, J.R. & Seligman, M.E.P. (1982) : Tumor rejection after inescapable or escapable shock. Science 216: 1185-1192.

Watson, D. & Pennebaker, J.W. (1989) : Health complaints, stress and distress: exploring the central role of negative affectivity. Psychol. Rev. 96: 234-254.

Weisse, C.S., Pato, C.N., McAllister, C.G., Littman, R., Breier, A., Paul, S.M. & Baum, A. (1990) : Differential effects of controllable and uncontrollable acute stress on immune function in humans. Brain Behav. Immun. 4: 339-351.

Zalcman, S., Minkiewiccz-Janda, A., Richter, M. & Anisman, H. (1988) : Critical periods associated with stressor effects on antibody titers and on the plaque-forming-cell repsonse to sheep red blood cells. Brain Behav. Immun. 2: 254-256.

Zavala, F., Taupin, V. & Descamps-Latscha, B. (1990) : In vivo treatment with benzodiazepines inhibits murine phagocyte oxidative metabolism and production of interleukin 1, tumor necrosis factor and interleukin 6. J. Pharmacol. Exp. Therap. 255: 442-450.

Résumé De nombreuses données indiquent que des situations anxiogènes caractérisées entre autres par l'absence de contrôle et l'incertitude ont, en plus de leurs effets sur les concentrations circulantes des hormones du stress et divers indicateurs des fonctions cardio-vasculaires, de profondes conséquences sur les réponses immunes, aussi bien chez l'homme que chez l'animal. Pour autant, ces effets n'ont pas encore servi de base à l'appréciation du pouvoir anxiolytique de médicaments. Les antagonistes des récepteurs centraux des benzodiazépines ont, en règle générale, des effets propres sur les réponses immunes et ces effets sont à l'opposé de ceux des agonistes de ces récepteurs. Les agonistes des récepteurs périphériques des benzodiazépines ont également d'importants effets modulateurs sur diverses fonctions immunes, mais leur activité n'est pas la même *in vitro* et *in vivo*. Dans un certain nombre de cas, les effets du stress sur l'immunité comportent une composante β-adrénergique, si bien que l'administration de bêta-bloquants peut s'avérer efficace dans ces conditions. Ces relations entre stress, anxiété et immunité ne peuvent toutefois être utilisées comme un argument en faveur de l'existence d'une relation causale entre stress et maladie.

III. Neuropharmacological aspects - molecular targets of anxiolytic drugs

III. Aspects neuropharmacologiques - les cibles moléculaires des anxiolytiques

Anxiety: Neurobiology, Clinic and Therapeutic Perspectives. Eds M. Hamon, H. Ollat, M.-H. Thiébot. Colloque INSERM/ John Libbey Eurotext Ltd. © 1993, Vol. 232, pp. 107-118.

GABA$_A$/BZ receptors: recent advances in molecular biology

Hartmut Lüddens

Laboratory for Molecular Neuroendocrinology, Center for Molecular Biology, Im Neuenheimer Feld 282, D-69120 Heidelberg, Germany

1 SUMMARY AND CONCLUSION

Multiple GABA$_A$ receptors exist in the brain that show differential distribution and developmental pattern. Their regulation by BZ receptor ligands, neurosteroids, GABA and its analogs differs dramatically with the α variant present in the complex, whereas the EC$_{50}$ and K$_i$ for the GABA analog [^{3}H]muscimol do not seem to be affected accordingly. Additional variation of the GABA$_A$Rs comes with the exchange of the γ subunits, though the actual bearing on the *in vivo* system has still to be resolved. No clear picture exists for the role of the β subunits, though they may play an important part at least during development.

Parts of the putative binding site for BZ ligands have been identified, but it will take considerable effort before the BZ binding pocket has been analyzed in full. Only first steps have been taken towards the identification of the domains involved in the binding of the neurotransmitter itself.

Large progress has been made in the characterization of the GABA$_A$ neurotransmitter receptor systems, but here as elsewhere it seems that more questions arise the more have been resolved.

2 ARCHITECTURE OF LIGAND-GATED ION CHANNELS

Ligand-gated ion channels mediate excitatory and inhibitory fast synaptic neurotransmission in the central nervous system (Dingledine, et al., 1988). The family of ligand gated ion channels now comprises nicotinic acetylcholine receptors (AChR), γ-aminobutyric acid type A receptors (GABA$_A$R), glycine receptors (GlyR), the serotonin receptor 5-HT$_3$ and possibly some members of the glutamate receptor family (GluR) (Betz, 1990; Maricq, et al., 1991; Monyer, et al., 1992; Moriyoshi, et al., 1991; Schofield, et al., 1987).

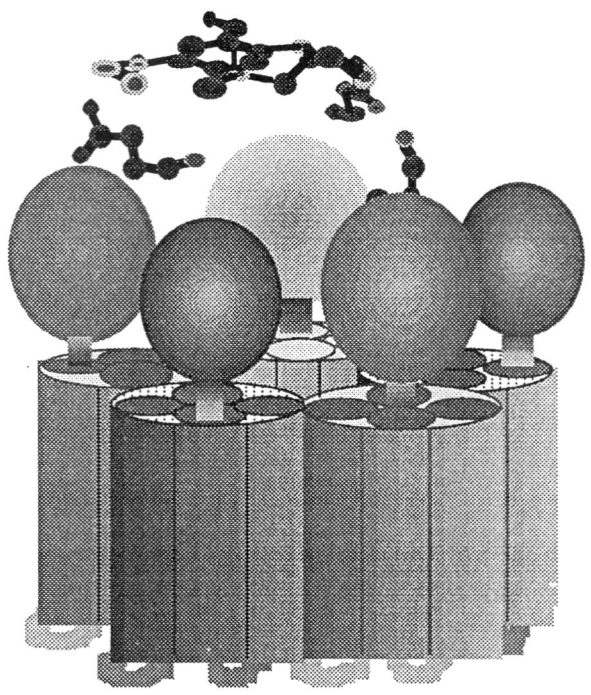

Figure 1: Model of a GABA$_A$ receptor with five subunits surrounding the integral channel pore. GABA and Ro 15-453 molecules are shown on at the extracellular domains of the receptor

The ligand-gated ion channels form by the assembly of presumably five subunits (figure 1). The channels are either homo-oligomers (5-HT$_3$) or hetero-oligomers of up to four different subunits (peripheral nAChR). Each of the five peptides in a ligand-gated ion channel/receptor spans the plasma membrane four times (Unwin, 1989). The second transmembrane regions (TM 2) of the five subunits arrange around a central channel pore, thus providing the hydrophilic environment essential for the selectivity and passage of ions (Unwin, 1989). It was common knowledge that the TM regions exist in an α-helical form (Unwin, 1989), but some recent findings support the idea that they transverse the plasma membrane as β-sheets (Akabas, et al., 1992).

GABA transmits the majority of the inhibiting signals in the mammalian brain. An obvious question is how a single receptor type can specifically regulate brain functions, given the diverse circuitry's in the various brain areas.

3 SUBUNIT HETEROGENEITY OF GABA$_A$ RECEPTORS

All families in the group of the ligand gated ion channels besides the 5-HT$_3$ receptor are multimembered. As the functional complex assembles from five subunits this provides a means to build an array of different receptors from a limited number of proteins. The GABA$_A$R is a prime example of this feature.

Early pharmacological and biochemical data provided clues to the existence of receptor subtypes, but the diversity of GABA$_A$R subunits was not anticipated until the cloning of now 15 different proteins detected in the mammalian CNS and the retina (Cutting, et al., 1991; Lüddens and Wisden, 1991; Seeburg, et al., 1990). The subunits were grouped into five classes with one to six variants (α1–6, β1–3, γ1–3, δ and ρ1,2) according to the degree of AA identity. One further β subunit was identified in chick brain (β4) (Bateson, et al., 1991). Whereas the classes α to δ constitute classical GABA$_A$Rs, a functional proof for the membership is missing for the ρ variants (Shimada, et al., 1992). Though originally an arbitrary classification, the AA identity measure turned out to reflect functional similarities as well.

Two of the subunits exist in splice variants (Bateson, et al., 1991; Kofuji, et al., 1991; Sikela, et al., 1991; Whiting, et al., 1990). The best studied example is the γ2' form that contains an eight AA long insert between TM3 and TM4 as compared to the γ2 variant. It adds a potential phosphorylation site to the γ2 subunit that may be involved in the ethanol sensitivity of GABA$_A$ receptors expressed in *Xenopus* oocytes (Wafford, et al., 1991). The chicken β4 subunit isoforms β4 and β4' differ by a 12 base pair long insert, again into the intracellular loop between TM3 and TM4 (Bateson, et al., 1991).

Without the diversity added by the splice variants and the ρ subunits, 72 GABA$_A$R combinations of the form $\alpha x_2 \beta x_2 \gamma x$ or $\alpha x_2 \beta x_2 \delta$ may exist in the mammalian brain. The possibility of different variants of one class in a single receptor, e.g., $\alpha x \alpha y \beta x \beta y \gamma x$ or other subunit stoichiometries, e.g., $\alpha x_3 \beta x_2$, increases the theoretically possible number of different receptors manifold. However, this number is restricted by the subunit co-distribution in the brain.

The mRNAs coding for α1-6, β1-3, γ1-3 and δ all display unique distribution in the mammalian CNS. Some neuronal cell populations, as the dentate granule cells, contain all mRNA species besides the α6 mRNA (Laurie, et al., 1992; Wisden, et al., 1992). Other areas, as the Purkinje cells of the cerebellum, express a limited number of $GABA_AR$ mRNAs (Laurie, et al., 1992; Shivers, et al., 1989). The α1 mRNA is the most prominent $GABA_AR$ subunit in the rodent brain and is widely codistributed with the β2 mRNA (Khrestchatisky, et al., 1989; Laurie, et al., 1992; Malherbe, et al., 1990b; Sequier, et al., 1988; Wisden, et al., 1992). The γ2 variant mRNA often colocalizes with these two mRNA species (Laurie, et al., 1992; Malherbe, et al., 1990b; Shivers, et al., 1989; Wisden, et al., 1992). This triple combination constitutes the vast majority of $GABA_AR$ mRNA in a number of cell populations. α2β1(β3) and α5β1(β3) combinations are the most abundant $GABA_AR$ mRNA species in the hippocampus (Laurie, et al., 1992; Wisden, et al., 1992) and could form constituents of the majority of the $GABA_ARs$ in this brain area.

The intracellular location of a mRNA in a neuron may drastically differ from the area where the protein inserts into the plasma membrane. For a number of $GABA_A$ R subunits and in most parts of the brain the protein and mRNA distribution pattern overlap (Benke, et al., 1991; Laurie, et al., 1992; Shivers, et al., 1989; Wisden, et al., 1992; Zimprich, et al., 1991), leaving a few exemptions like the intensities of the γ2 signals in the hippocampus, which is high for the mRNA signal but low for the immunoreactivity (Malherbe, et al., 1990b; Shivers, et al., 1989; Wisden, et al., 1992).

4 ROLE OF SUBUNITS

Coexpression of the α1 and β1 subunits in *Xenopus laevis* oocytes resulted in Cl⁻ channels opened by GABA (Schofield, et al., 1987). Furthermore, the α2, α3 and α5 variants coexpressed in *Xenopus laevis* oocytes with β1, and α1 together with β1, β2 or β3 all assemble to GABA gated ion channels (Levitan, et al., 1988; Ymer, et al., 1989; Ymer, et al., 1989). The exchange of one α variant for another in an αxβ1 combination shifted the dose-response curve for GABA, but it did not affect the overall pharmacological properties of the resulting channels (Levitan, et al., 1988). These heteromeric recombinant GABA channels were positively modulated by pentobarbital and blocked by picrotoxinin and bicuculline, classifying them as $GABA_ARs$. However, the GABA response of *Xenopus laevis* oocytes expressing $α_1β_1$ subunits was only inconsistently modified by benzodiazepines (Malherbe, et al., 1990a; Schofield, et al., 1987).

5 BENZODIAZEPINE RECEPTORS

Only when the $\gamma2$ subunit was coexpressed in the human embryonic kidney cell line 293 with an α and a β variant, GABA$_A$ channels were formed, which consistently responded to BZ ligands, i.e., the receptors resembled the GABA$_A$/BZ receptors described for the mammalian brain (Pritchett, et al., 1989). The coexpression of the $\alpha1$, $\beta2$ and $\gamma3$ in 293 cells leads to GABA$_A$ receptors recognizing BZ ligands with reduced affinities for agonistic acting BZ ligands as compared to antagonists or inverse agonists (Herb, et al., 1992; Knoflach, et al., 1991). Replacement of the $\gamma2$ by the $\gamma1$ subunit in an $\alpha x\beta x\gamma x$ combination (Ymer, et al., 1990) leaves BZ receptors with a pharmacology reminiscent of the peripheral type BZ acceptor site (Lueddens and Skolnick, 1987).

Autoradiographic studies on rat brain sections indicate mismatches between the binding of GABA$_A$ receptor ligands and different BZ ligands (Olsen and Tobin, 1990). Most benzodiazepines bind to the GABA$_A$/BZ receptors with similar affinities throughout the brain, but the binding properties of several compounds, most notably Cl 218 872 (Nielsen and Braestrup, 1980; Sieghart, 1983; Squires, et al., 1979) and 2-oxoquazepam (Corda, et al., 1988), demonstrated the heterogeneity of GABA$_A$/BZ receptors. Type I receptors have greater affinity to the triazolopyridine Cl 218 872 than type II receptors and constitute the predominant GABA$_A$ receptor class in the CNS. The lower affinity type II receptors are enriched in hippocampus, striatum, and spinal cord (Lo, et al., 1983; Sieghart, et al., 1985).

Coexpression of the $\alpha1$, $\beta1$, and $\gamma2$ subunits in 293 cells leads to the assembly of functional GABA$_A$ receptors that display the characteristics of BZ type I receptors (Pritchett, et al., 1989). Exchange of the $\beta1$ by any other β variant does not alter the affinity of any BZ ligand to the receptor complex (Pritchett, et al., 1989). On the other hand, replacing the $\alpha1$ subunit by any other α variant dramatically effects the affinity of the formed GABA$_A$/BZ receptor complex to selected BZ ligands (Pritchett, et al., 1989).

The pharmacological and electrophysiological properties of the GABA$_A$/BZ I receptors can only be mimicked by recombinant receptors of the $\alpha1\beta x\gamma2$ type. BZ II receptors assemble in 293 cells from the $\alpha 2$, $\alpha 3$ or $\alpha 5$ variants together with the $\beta x \gamma 2$ combination (Pritchett, et al., 1989; Pritchett and Seeburg, 1990). The $\alpha 2 \beta x \gamma 2$ and $\alpha 3 \beta x \gamma 2$ receptors display both the characteristics of the "classical" BZ type II receptors. Transiently expressed $\alpha 5 \beta 2 \gamma 2$ receptors have affinities for CL 218,872 and 2-oxoquazepam similar to $\alpha 2$ or $\alpha 3$ containing $\alpha x \beta x \gamma 2$ receptors. However, the binding properties for imidazopyridines like zolpidem and alpidem differ from conventional $GABA_A$/BZ II receptors (Pritchett & Seeburg, 1990), so that they constitute a subtype of the BZ II receptors.

BZ I and BZ II receptors distribute unevenly over the rat brain. BZ I receptors predominate in the cerebellum, but are rare in the hippocampus (Faull and Villiger, 1988; Faull, et al., 1987; Olsen, et al., 1990). On the other hand, BZ II receptors are strongly expressed in the hippocampus and nearly absent from the cerebellum, whereas both receptor subtypes are similarly expressed in the cortical layers (Faull & Villiger, 1988; Faull, et al., 1987; Olsen, et al., 1990). Data derived from ligand binding to brain membranes or brain slices are in good agreement with the mRNA distribution of the α subunits (see above). These data strongly indicate that transiently expressed $\alpha 1 \beta x \gamma 2$, $\alpha 2 \beta x \gamma 2$, $\alpha 3 \beta x \gamma 2$ or $\alpha 5 \beta 2 \gamma 2$ BZ receptors reflect properties of their counterparts in the brain. This view is supported by immunopurification of $GABA_A$ receptor subtypes solubilized from rat brain that display affinities comparable to those measured in transiently transfected cells (McKernan, et al., 1991). Already previously it had been shown by sequential immunoprecipitation using antibodies specific for the $\alpha 1$, $\alpha 2$ and $\alpha 3$ variants that iso-oligomers of the $GABA_A$ receptor exist in bovine brain (Duggan and Stephenson, 1990).

The $\alpha 6$ variant confers several striking features. It is the subunit with the most restricted distribution as it is limited to the cerebellar granule cells (Lüddens, et al., 1990). Recombinant receptors expressing $\alpha 6$ in 293 cells together with $\beta 2$ and $\gamma 2$ bind with high affinity the GABA agonist [^{3}H]muscimol and the imidazo-1,4-benzodiazepine [^{3}H]Ro 15-4513. Other benzodiazepines and two β-carbolines are either not recognized by this receptor or at an affinity two to three orders of magnitude lower than that of $\alpha 1$, $\alpha 2$, $\alpha 3$ or $\alpha 5$ containing receptors (Lüddens, et al., 1990; Pritchett, et al., 1989; Pritchett & Seeburg, 1990). Several but not all BZ receptor ligands displace all [^{3}H]Ro 15-4513 binding from cerebellar membranes in a two-step manner. The affinities of these ligands correspond well with the data obtained from recombinant receptors: In two alcohol tolerant and non-tolerant rat lines (Uusi-Oukari and Korpi, 1990) as well as in membranes derived from Sprague-Dawley rat, bovine or human cerebellum (Lüddens, et al., 1990; Turner, et al., 1991; Wong and Skolnick, 1992) inhibition of [^{3}H]Ro 15-4513 binding was best fitted to two-site curves in which the low affinity site was present in a relative abundance of 20-30% and most likely α6 containing receptors.

After construction of N-terminal chimeras between the α1 and α6 variants a single arginine^{100} to histidine^{100} substitution in α6 was shown to be responsible for the insensitivity of α6β2γ2 receptors to diazepam (Wieland, et al., 1992). Furthermore, diazepam insensitivity could be transferred to α1 receptors by replacing the corresponding his^{101} with an arginine (Wieland, et al., 1992). The importance of this amino acid residue for BZ agonist binding is underlined by the fact that all diazepam sensitive receptors, i.e., α1(α2, α3, α5)β2γ2, contain a histidine at the corresponding

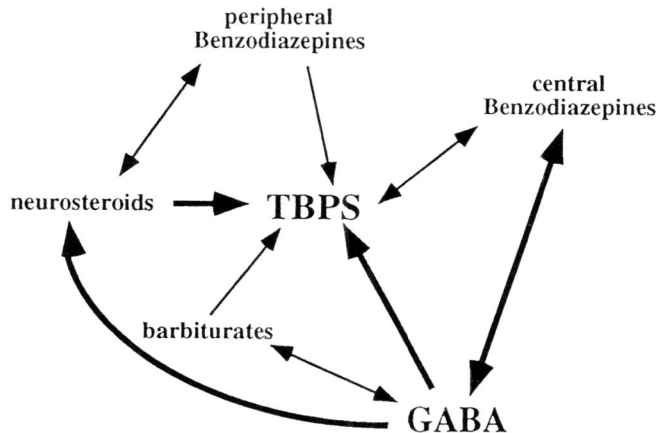

Figure 2: Interactions of ligands at the GABA$_A$ receptor.
Multiple regulatory sites on GABA$_A$ receptors are shown with the ways the act on each other. The graph does not necessarily claim to be complete. The interactions indicated by bold arrows are discussed in the text.

position whereas it is replaced by an arginine in the diazepam insensitive receptor types α4(α6)β2γ2. Recently, a natural point mutation in α6 (arg^{101} to gln^{101}) was shown to occur in the alcohol non-tolerant ANT rat strain (Korpi, et al., 1993). The gln^{101} induces an increase of affinity for diazepam as compared to the wild type α6 without reaching the high affinity of α1, α3 or the mutant α6his[101] BZ receptors. As it was the case for the glycine/glutamate exchange involved in BZ I/ BZ II selectivity the diazepam insensitivity may reflect selective steric hindrance of agonist binding.

6 [^{35}S]TBPS RECEPTORS

GABA modulates the convulsant binding site on GABA$_A$ receptors labeled by [^{35}S]t-butylbicyclophophorothionate ([^{35}S]TBPS). The modulation varies between different brain regions, reflecting the molecular heterogeneity of the GABA$_A$ receptors. In rat brain cryostat sections, the main sensitivity difference to GABA between brain regions was observed within the cerebellum (Korpi, et al., 1992). [^{35}S]TBPS binding in the granule cell layer was more sensitive to GABA than that in the molecular layer, and was detected only after blockade of the GABA agonist sites by the specific GABA$_A$ antagonists 95531, RU 5135 or bicuculline (Korpi and Lüddens, 1993). This indicates that the [^{35}S]TBPS binding sites in cerebellar granule cells were blocked by endogenous GABA. Expression in human embryonic kidney cells of α6β2γ2 produced [^{35}S]TBPS binding sites that were 10-fold more sensitive to inhibition by GABA than those inherent to α1β2γ2 receptors, tracing the sensitivity difference to the α subunits of the GABA$_A$ receptor (Korpi & Lüddens, 1993). Similar results were obtained for the regulation of [^{35}S]TBPS binding of α1β2γ2 and α6β2γ2 receptors by the neurosteroid 5α-pregnan-3α-ol-20-one (Korpi & Lüddens, 1993). These data indicate that the α variants do not only provide differential sensitivity to BZ ligands but to the neurotransmitter itself and to neurosteroids.

7 REFERENCES

Akabas, M. H., Stauffer, D. A., Xu, M., and Karlin, A. (1992): Acetylcholine receptor channel structure probed in cysteine-substitution mutants. *Science* 258, 307-10.

Bateson, A. N., Lasham, A., and Darlison, M. G. (1991): γ-Aminobutyric acid$_A$ receptor heterogeneity is increased by alternative splicing of a novel β-subunit gene transcript. *J. Neurochem.* 56, 1437-40.

Benke, D., Mertens, S., Trzeciak, A., Gillessen, D., and Mohler, H. (1991): Identification and Immunohistochemical Mapping of GABA$_A$ Receptor Subtypes Containing the δ-Subunit in Rat Brain. *FEBS Lett.* 283, 145-149.

Betz, H. (1990): Ligand-gated ion channels in the brain: the amino acid receptor superfamily. *Neuron* 5, 383-92.

Corda, M. G., Giorgi, O., Longoni, B., Ongini, E., Montaldo, S., and Biggio, G. (1988): Preferential affinity of ^{3}H-2-oxo-quazepam for type I benzodiazepine recognition sites in the human brain. *Life Sci* 42, 189-97.

Cutting, G. R., Lu, L., Ohara, B. F., Kasch, L. M., Montroserafizadeh, C., Donovan, D. M., Shimada, S., Antonarakis, S. E., Guggino, W. B., Uhl, G. R., and Kazazian, H. H. (1991): Cloning of the γ-Aminobutyric Acid (GABA) ρ1 cDNA - A GABA Receptor Subunit Highly Expressed in the Retina. *Proc. Natl. Acad. Sci. USA* 88, 2673-2677.

Dingledine, R., Boland, L. M., Chamberlin, N. L., Kawasaki, K., Kleckner, N. W., Traynelis, S. F., and Verdoorn, T. A. (1988): Amino acid receptors and uptake systems in the mammalian central nervous system. *Crit Rev Neurobiol* 4, 1-96.

Duggan, M. J., and Stephenson, F. A. (1990): Biochemical evidence for the existence of γ-aminobutyrate$_A$ receptor iso-oligomers. *J. Biol. Chem.* 265, 3831-5.

Faull, R. L., and Villiger, J. W. (1988): Benzodiazepine receptors in the human hippocampal formation: a pharmacological and quantitative autoradiographic study. *Neuroscience* 26, 783-90.

Faull, R. L., Villiger, J. W., and Holford, N. H. (1987): Benzodiazepine receptors in the human cerebellar cortex: a quantitative autoradiographic and pharmacological study demonstrating the predominance of type I receptors. *Brain Res.* 411, 379-85.

Herb, A., Wisden, W., Lüddens, H., Puia, G., Vicini, S., and Seeburg, P. H. (1992): The third γ subunit of the γ-aminobutyric acid type A receptor family. *Proc. Natl. Acad. Sci. USA*, 1433-37.

Khrestchatisky, M., MacLennan, A. J., Chiang, M. Y., Xu, W. T., Jackson, M. B., Brecha, N., Sternini, C., Olsen, R. W., and Tobin, A. J. (1989): A novel α subunit in rat brain GABA$_A$ receptors. *Neuron* 3, 745-53.

Knoflach, F., Rhyner, T., Villa, M., Kellenberger, S., Drescher, U., Malherbe, P., Sigel, E., and Mohler, H. (1991): The γ3-subunit of the GABA$_A$-receptor confers sensitivity to benzodiazepine receptor ligands. *FEBS Lett.* 293, 191-4.

Kofuji, P., Wang, J. B., Moss, S. J., Huganir, R. L., and Burt, D. R. (1991): Generation of two forms of the γ-aminobutyric acid$_A$ receptor γ2-subunit in mice by alternative splicing. *J. Neurochem.* 56, 713-5.

Korpi, E. R., Kleingoor, C., Kettenmann, H., and Seeburg, P. H. (1993): Benzodiazepine-induced motor impairment linked to point mutation in cerebellar GABA$_A$ receptor. *Nature* 361, 356-359.

Korpi, E. R., and Lüddens, H. (1993): Regional GABA Sensitivity of [^{35}S]TBPS Binding Depends on GABA$_A$ Receptor α subunit. *Mol. Pharmacol.* in press.

Korpi, E. R., Lüddens, H., and Seeburg, P. H. (1992): GABA$_A$ antagonists reveal binding sites for [^{35}S]TBPS in cerebellar granular cell layer. *Eur. J. Pharmacol.* 211, 427-428.

Laurie, D. J., Seeburg, P. H., and Wisden, W. (1992): The distribution of 13 GABA$_A$ receptor subunit mRNAs in the rat brain. II. Olfactory Bulb and Cerebellum. *J. Neurosci.* 12, 1063-76.

Levitan, E. S., Schofield, P. R., Burt, D. R., Rhee, L. M., Wisden, W., Köhler, M., Fujita, N., Rodriguez, H. F., Stephenson, F. A., Darlison, M. G., Barnard, E., and Seeburg, P. H. (1988): Structural and functional basis for GABA$_A$ receptor heterogeneity. *Nature* 335, 76-79.

Lo, M. M., Niehoff, D. L., Kuhar, M. J., and Snyder, S. H. (1983): Differential localization of type I and type II benzodiazepine binding sites in substantia nigra. *Nature* 306, 57-60.

Lüddens, H., Pritchett, D. B., Köhler, M., Killisch, I., Keinänen, K., Monyer, H., Sprengel, R., and Seeburg, P. H. (1990): Cerebellar GABA$_A$ receptor selective for a behavioural alcohol antagonist. *Nature* 346, 648-51.

Lüddens, H., and Wisden, W. (1991): Function and Pharmacology of Multiple GABA$_A$ Receptor Subunits. *Trends Pharmacol. Sci.* 12, 49-51.

Lueddens, H. W., and Skolnick, P. (1987): 'Peripheral-type' benzodiazepine receptors in the kidney: regulation of radioligand binding by anions and DIDS. *Eur J Pharmacol* 133, 205-14.

Malherbe, P., Draguhn, A., Multhaup, G., Beyreuther, K., and Möhler, H. (1990a): GABA$_A$-receptor expressed from rat brain α- and β-subunit cDNAs displays potentiation by benzodiazepine receptor ligands. *Brain Res. Mol. Brain Res.* 8, 199-208.

Malherbe, P., Sigel, E., Baur, R., Persohn, E., Richards, J. G., and Möhler, H. (1990b): Functional characteristics and sites of gene expression of the α1, β1, γ2-isoform of the rat GABA$_A$ receptor. *J. Neurosci.* 10, 2330-7.

Maricq, A. V., Peterson, A. S., Brake, A. J., Myers, R. M., and Julius, D. (1991): Primary structure and functional expression of the 5HT3 receptor, a serotonin-gated ion channel. *Science* 254, 432-7.

McKernan, R. M., Quirk, K., Prince, R., Cox, P. A., Gillard, N. P., Ragan, C. I., and Whiting, P. (1991): GABA$_A$ Receptor Subtypes Immunopurified from Rat Brain with a Subunit-Specific Antibodies Have Unique Pharmacological Properties. *Neuron* 7, 667-676.

Monyer, H., Sprengel, R., Schoepfer, R., Herb, A., Higuchi, M., Lomeli, H., Burnashev, N., Sakmann, B., and Seeburg, P. H. (1992): Heteromeric NMDA Receptors: Molecular and Functional Distinction of Subtypes. *Science* 256, 1217-21.

Moriyoshi, K., Masu, M., Ishii, T., Shigemoto, R., Mizuno, N., and Nakanishi, S. (1991): Molecular cloning and characterization of the rat NMDA receptor [see comments]. *Nature* 354, 31-7.

Nielsen, M., and Braestrup, C. (1980): Ethyl ß-carboline-3-carboxylate shows differential benzodiazepine receptor interaction. *Nature* 286, 606-607.

Olsen, R. W., McCabe, R. T., and Wamsley, J. K. (1990): GABA$_A$ receptor subtypes: autoradiographic comparison of GABA, benzodiazepine, and convulsant binding sites in the rat central nervous system. *J. Chem. Neuroanat.* 3, 59-76.

Olsen, R. W., and Tobin, A. J. (1990): Molecular biology of GABA$_A$ receptors. *FASEB J.* 4, 1469-80.

Pritchett, D. B., Lüddens, H., and Seeburg, P. H. (1989): Type I and type II GABA$_A$-benzodiazepine receptors produced in transfected cells. *Science* 245, 1389-92.

Pritchett, D. B., and Seeburg, P. H. (1990): γ-aminobutyric acid$_A$ receptor α5-subunit creates novel type II benzodiazepine receptor pharmacology. *J. Neurochem.* 54, 1802-4.

Pritchett, D. B., and Seeburg, P. H. (1991): γ-Aminobutyric acid type A receptor point mutation increases the affinity of compounds for the benzodiazepine site. *Proc. Natl. Acad. Sci. U S A* 88, 1421-5.

Pritchett, D. B., Sontheimer, H., Shivers, B. D., Ymer, S., Kettenmann, H., Schofield, P. R., and Seeburg, P. H. (1989): Importance of a novel GABA$_A$ receptor subunit for benzodiazepine pharmacology. *Nature* 338, 582-5.

Saitoh, S., Kubota, T., Ohta, T., Jinno, Y., Niikawa, N., Sugimoto, T., Wagstaff, J., and Lalande, M. (1992): Familial Angelman syndrome caused by imprinted submicroscopic deletion encompassing GABA$_A$ receptor β3-subunit gene [letter]. *Lancet* 339, 366-7.

Schofield, P. R., Darlison, M. G., Fujita, N., Burt, D. R., Stephenson, F. A., Rodriguez, H., Rhee, L. M., Ramachandran, J., Reale, V., Glencorse, T. A., Reale, V., Seeburg, P. H., and Barnard, E. A. (1987): Sequence and functional expression of the GABA$_A$ receptor shows a ligand-gated receptor superfamily. *Nature* 328, 221-7.

Seeburg, P. H., Wisden, W., Verdoorn, T. A., Pritchett, D. B., Werner, P., Herb, A., Lüddens, H., Sprengel, R., and Sakmann, B. (1990): The GABA$_A$ receptor family: Molecular and functional diversity. *CSH Symp. Quant. Biol.* 55, 29-44.

Sequier, J. M., Richards, J. G., Malherbe, P., Price, G. W., Mathews, S., and Möhler, H. (1988): Mapping of brain areas containing RNA homologous to cDNAs encoding the α and β subunits of the rat GABA$_A$ γ-aminobutyrate receptor. *Proc. Natl. Acad. Sci. U S A* 85, 7815-9.

Shimada, S., Cutting, G. R., and Uhl, G. R. (1992): γ-Aminobutyric Acid A or C Receptor? γ-Aminobutyric Acid ρ1 Receptor RNA Induces Bicuculline-, Barbiturate-, and Benzodiazepine-Insensitive γ-Aminobutyric Acid Responses in *Xenopus* oocytes. *Mol. Pharmacol.* 41, 683-7.

Shivers, B. D., Killisch, I., Sprengel, R., Sontheimer, H., Köhler, M., Schofield, P. R., and Seeburg, P. H. (1989): Two novel $GABA_A$ receptor subunits exist in distinct neuronal subpopulations. *Neuron* 3, 327-37.

Sieghart, W. (1983): Several new benzodiazepines selectively interact with a benzodiazepine receptor subtype. *Neurosci Lett* 38, 73-8.

Sieghart, W., Eichinger, A., Riederer, P., and Jellinger, K. (1985): Comparison of benzodiazepine receptor binding in membranes from human or rat brain. *Neuropharmacology* 24, 751-9.

Sigel, E., Baur, R., Kellenberger, S., and Malherbe, P. (1992): Point mutations affecting antagonist affinity and agonist dependent gating of $GABA_A$ receptor channels. *EMBO J.* 11, 2017-23.

Sikela, J. M., Wilson-Shaw, D., Khan, A. S., Lin, L.-H., Leidenheimer, N., Gambarana, C., and Siegel, R. (1991): A Novel Form of the γ2 Subunit of the $GABA_A$ Receptor: Functional Expression and Localization. *Neuron* 7.

Squires, R. F., Benson, D. I., Braestrup, C., Coupet, J., Klepner, C. A., Myers, V., and Beer, B. (1979): Some properties of brain specific benzodiazepine receptors: new evidence for multiple receptors. *Pharmacol. Biochem. Behav.* 10, 825-830.

Turner, D. M., Sapp, D. W., and Olsen, R. W. (1991): The Benzodiazepine/Alcohol Antagonist Ro-15-4513 - Binding to a GABA Receptor Subtype That Is Insensitive to Diazepam. *J. Pharmacol. Exp. Ther.* 257, 1236-1242.

Unwin, N. (1989): The structure of ion channels in membranes of excitable cells. *Neuron* 3, 665-76.

Uusi-Oukari, M., and Korpi, E. R. (1990): Diazepam sensitivity of an Imidazobenzodiazepine, [^{3}H]Ro 15-4513, in Cerebellar Membranes from Two Rat Lines Developed for High and Low Alcohol Sensitivity. *J. Neurochem.* 54, 1980-7.

Wafford, K. A., Burnett, D. M., Leidenheimer, N. J., Burt, D. R., Wang, J. B., Kofuji, P., Dunwiddie, T. V., Harris, R. A., and Sikela, J. M. (1991): Ethanol sensitivity of the $GABA_A$ receptor expressed in Xenopus oocytes requires 8 amino acids contained in the gamma 2L subunit. *Neuron* 7, 27-33.

Whiting, P., McKernan, R. M., and Iversen, L. L. (1990): Another mechanism for creating diversity in gamma-aminobutyrate type A receptors: RNA splicing directs expression of two forms of gamma 2 phosphorylation site. *Proc Natl Acad Sci U S A* 87, 9966-70.

Wieland, H., Lüddens, H., and Seeburg, P. H. (1992): A Single Histidine in $GABA_A$ Receptors Is Essential for Benzodiazepine Agonist Binding. *J. Biol. Chem.* 257, 1426-9.

Wisden, W., Laurie, D. J., Monyer, H., and Seeburg, P. H. (1992): The distribution of 13 $GABA_A$ receptor subunit mRNAs in the rat brain. I. Telencephalon, Diencephalon, Mesencephalon. *J. Neurosci.* 12, 1040-62.

Wong, G., and Skolnick, P. (1992): High affinity ligands for 'diazepam-insensitive' benzodiazepine receptors. *Eur J Pharmacol* 225, 63-8.

Ymer, S., Draguhn, A., Köhler, M., and Seeburg, P. H. (1989): Sequence and expression of a novel $GABA_A$ receptor α subunit. *FEBS Lett.* 258, 119-122.

Ymer, S., Draguhn, A., Wisden, W., Werner, P., Keinänen, K., Schofield, P. R., Sprengel, R., Pritchett, D. B., and Seeburg, P. H. (1990): Structural and functional characterization of the $γ_1$ subunit of $GABA_A$/benzodiazepine receptors. *EMBO J.* 9, 3261-7.

Ymer, S., Schofield, P. R., Draguhn, A., Werner, P., Köhler, M., and Seeburg, P. H. (1989): $GABA_A$ receptor β subunit heterogeneity: functional expression of cloned cDNAs. *EMBO J.* 8, 1665-1670.

Zimprich, F., Zezula, J., Sieghart, W., and Lassmann, H. (1991): Immunohistochemical Localization of the α1, α2 and α3 Subunit of the $GABA_A$ Receptor in the Rat Brain. *Neurosci Lett.* 127, 125-128.

Résumé

De nombreux récepteurs de type GABA$_A$ existent dans le cerveau. Ils se caractérisent par des distributions régionales distinctes, et leur mise en place au cours du développement est également très variable. La modulation des récepteurs GABA$_A$ par les ligands des sites de liaison des benzodiazépines (BZ), les neurostéroïdes, le GABA et ses analogues dépend étroitement de la nature de la sous unité α au sein du complexe-récepteur. En revanche, les caractéristiques de la liaison du [^{3}H]muscimol sur ce complexe restent sensiblement les mêmes quelle que soit cette sous unité. Des variations dans les propriétés des récepteurs GABA$_A$ sont également observées à la suite de l'échange de la sous unité γ. Le rôle de la sous unité β n'est pas encore clairement défini, mais il pourrait surtout être important au cours du développement.

Certaines zones du site de reconnaissance des benzodiazépines au sein du complexe-recepteur ont été identifiées. Les domaines impliqués dans la liaison du GABA sont moins bien connus. En dépit des données accumulées au cours des dernières années, beaucoup de questions clés concernant la structure et le fonctionnement des récepteurs GABA$_A$ restent sans réponse.

Anxiolytic drugs and cognitive function

David J. Sanger, Danielle Joly and Branimir Zivkovic

Département de Biologie, Synthélabo Recherche (L.E.R.S.), 31, avenue Paul Vaillant-Couturier, B.P. 110, 92225 Bagneux Cedex, France

SUMMARY

It is well known that benzodiazepines can produce anterograde amnesia although the extent to which this creates a significant problem for the clinical use of these drugs as anxiolytics is unclear. It also remains to be established whether memory problems are invariably associated with these drugs' sedative effects. In the animal laboratory benzodiazepines disrupt the acquisition of passive avoidance responding and interfere with place learning. Recent studies of BZ receptor partial agonists suggest that, whereas some of these agents produce similar disruptions of learning, others do not. The BZ_1 (ω_1) selective drugs zolpidem and alpidem also affect learning but only at sedative doses. Further research may be able to provide a clearer definition of the specific role of BZ (ω) receptor subtypes in cognition.

INTRODUCTION

Benzodiazepines have been known to produce amnesia since shortly after their introduction into clinical medicine. Most early studies of the effects of these drugs on learning and memory in human subjects were carried out in the context of their use in surgical premedication. Two of the most important attributes of drugs used for this indication are that they reduce anxiety and interfere with memory; the latter being considered desirable so that patients do not retain vivid memories of pain and other unpleasant aspects of surgical procedures. But, the most widespread use of benzodiazepines is in the treatment of generalised anxiety in general practice and here significant effects on cognitive function would be undesirable. In addition to the literature of experimental research which clearly establishes that benzodiazepine anxiolytics affect memory, there are indications in the clinical literature that such actions may be important side effects of anxiolytic therapy. Thus, in a recent report (Task Force, 1992) it was stated that: "The well-documented side effects of the anxiolytic and hypnotic benzodiazepines are believed to be mainly associated with sedation ... include anterograde amnesia, cognitive dysfunction ...". It is striking, however, that detailed descriptions of side effects associated with benzodiazepines often do not even refer to memory (Edwards, 1981; Ricci et al., 1987). Relatively few studies have attempted the difficult task of objectively evaluating the effects of anxiolytic drugs on cognition in patients during long-term therapy but, in one report it was concluded that: "Since the memory-impairing effects of BZs would be limited only to new information presented during a short critical period of time, one may question whether patients taking BZ medications chronically would suffer from or be aware of any effects on their memory." (Lucki et al., 1986). These same authors also noted, however, that under certain conditions and with certain types of patients, perhaps including the elderly, memory problems could be potentially serious.

EFFECTS OF BENZODIAZEPINES ON HUMAN MEMORY

The storage of information has usually been conceptualised as consisting of three basic processes: an immediate store which serves to maintain perceptual information for very brief periods, a limited capacity short-term memory store which holds information for a few seconds, and a long-term memory store in which information may be permanently held and whose capacity is unlimited. The distinction between short-term and long-term memory is also frequently discussed as involving, on the one hand, a form of working memory which allows the efficient performance of cognitive and psychomotor tasks through a continuous updating of the store, and on the other hand, reference memory which is information stored in a more fixed form. Information may be held in reference memory in various forms and distinctions between semantic and episodic memory and between declarative and procedural memory have been of importance in recent research in cognitive psychology.

In principle, drugs can interfere with learning and memory in a number of different ways. Administration of a drug could affect the acquisition of information, its consolidation in a memory store or its retrieval from the store. Drug effects may also be highly specific, i.e. acting only on the neural mechanisms underlying memory formation, or may affect memory indirectly by interfering with the perceptual or motor processes necessary for the efficient acquisition or retrieval of information.

Many studies involving human subjects have shown that benzodiazepines can produce anterograde amnesia. Thus, information learned in the drugged state is not retrieved during subsequent tests. In general, these drugs do not interfere with the consolidation of memory for information presented before drug administration, i.e. they do not produce retrograde amnesia, and may even facilitate such storage, possibly by producing amnesia for subsequently presented information and thus reducing interference (Lister, 1985). Benzodiazepines generally do not interfere with short-term memory and do not disrupt the retrieval of previously acquired information. Furthermore, there is evidence that the storage of only certain types of information is affected. The acquisition of forms of memory which can be accessed without conscious awareness appears not to be disrupted by benzodiazepines (e.g. Weingartner et al., 1992).

Curran (1986) has pointed out that three major explanations can be proposed for the observed effects of benzodiazepines on memory:
1)   That these drugs selectively impair the consolidation of memory traces, acting on the coding mechanisms involved in the transfer of information from a short-term to a long-term store.
2)   Benzodiazepines produce state-dependent learning. Information is acquired during the drugged state but cannot be retrieved in the non-drug condition.
3)   The effects of benzodiazepines on learning are a "by product" of their sedative actions. Thus, these drugs do not produce selective effects on cognition but rather interfere with the acquisition of information through actions on perception, vigilance or motor performance.

Although Curran (1986) concludes that there is evidence that benzodiazepines can have specific effects on memory consolidation, she also notes that many studies have shown that, in conditions where benzodiazepines affect memory, they also frequently disrupt psychomotor performance and produce other subjective and objective signs of sedation. King (1992) has recently reviewed the literature dealing with the association between amnesia and sedation produced by benzodiazepines and concludes that there is frequently a close relationship which was not taken into account in many early studies. Nevertheless, research exists indicating that certain doses of some benzodiazepines may affect learning without producing sedation (e.g. 0.2 mg/kg diazepam - Ghoneim et al., 1981). However, the extent to which such results can be interpreted as showing specific interference with memory mechanisms rather than differential sensitivity of different test measures remains controversial (King, 1992).

LEARNING AND MEMORY IN THE ANIMAL LABORATORY

Passive avoidance learning

The procedures most frequently used for assessing the effects of benzodiazepines on learning in rats and mice are simple passive avoidance tasks. An animal is allowed to make a simple motor response such as stepping off a raised platform or moving from a brightly lit into a dark box and is given a mild electric shock or other type of aversive stimulus. When the animal is put back into the apparatus one or more days later it will show a relatively long latency before making the same motor response demonstrating that it has learned to fear the aversive situation. Several classes of psychoactive drugs, including anticholinergic agents and benzodiazepines, when administered before the learning trial, interfere with this fear learning. Table 1 illustrates such effects obtained with the benzodiazepine anxiolytics, chlordiazepoxide and clorazepate, and the anticholinergic scopolamine. All three drugs produce dose-related decreases in response latencies on trial 2 indicating that they had interfered with the fear learning during the first, drugged trial.

Table 1. Effects of chlordiazepoxide, clorazepate and scopolamine on passive avoidance learning in rats and mice. Drugs were administered before trial 1 during which animals received electric footshock after making a step-down (rats) or step-through (mice) response. The figures show the mean (±S.E.M.) response latencies during trial 2 which was 24 hrs after trial 1. No drugs were administered before trial 2. * $p<0.05$, ** $p<0.01$ difference from controls.

	Rats		Mice	
	Dose mg/kg	Latency sec	Dose mg/kg	Latency sec
Chlordiazepoxide	0	131 ± 28	0	167 ± 80
	1	105 ± 29	2.5	131 ± 35
	3	106 ± 36	5.0	96 ± 32
	10	45 ± 12 *	10	62 ± 23 *
			20	14 ± 2 **
Clorazepate	0	162 ± 29	0	194 ± 24
	1	161 ± 40	2.5	137 ± 27
	3	121 ± 39	5	98 ± 32 *
	10	54 ± 23 *	10	35 ± 15 **
			20	54 ± 31 **
Scopolamine	0	122 ± 36	0	168 ± 30
	0.3	50 ± 12	0.1	149 ± 32
	1	33 ± 21 **	0.3	111 ± 25
	3	19 ± 11 **	1	48 ± 12 **
			3	35 ± 8 **

A number of studies have reported such effects in rodents and it seems that all benzodiazepines tested produce similar disruptions of passive avoidance learning (Broekkamp et al., 1984; Oishi et al., 1972; Gamzu, 1988; Sanger & Joly, 1985). Most research is consistent in showing that benzodiazepines are active only if administered before the first trial and that the disruption of passive avoidance learning does not represent a form of state-dependent learning. Thus, the results of these animal studies seem to parallel those found in human research. However, there are several reports that benzodiazepines can produce state-dependent learning in passive avoidance (Patel et al., 1979) and appetitively reinforced (Colpaert, 1986) tasks.

Spatial learning

In recent years the role of different pharmacological and physiological mechanisms in spatial learning in rats has been extensively investigated (Barnes, 1988). Two novel and ingenious learning procedures, the Morris water maze (Morris, 1981) and the radial maze (Olton, 1987), have been used in many of these studies. The Morris water maze consists of a large tank of opaque water through which a rat is obliged to swim to find a submerged escape platform. The platform is always in the same place but, as the animal is started from different points on the circumference of the tank on different trials, it is necessary to make use of spatial information concerning the position of the platform in relation to visual landmarks in the laboratory. Other forms of learning can also be studied using this apparatus such as the ability to discriminate between a safe (fixed) and unsafe (floating) platform marked with different visual cues (cue learning).

Several studies have reported that chlordiazepoxide and diazepam interfere with spatial learning in the water maze (McNaughton & Morris, 1987; Brioni & Arolfo, 1992; McNamara & Skelton, 1991, 1992a). Although drug-treated rats may acquire the escape response at a rate similar to controls (e.g. McNamara & Skelton, 1991) their escape latencies are longer than those of controls throughout training and a specific deficit of spatial learning appears to be present. Thus, Brioni & Arolfo (1992) reported that rats trained to escape to a hidden platform while treated with diazepam showed no preference for the target quadrant of the pool when the platform was removed. This indicated that the animals had not acquired spatial information about the position of the platform. Furthermore, diazepam did not interfere with the abilities of rats to learn the escape task when the platform was visible or when they were required to discriminate between a safe and a floating platform. These results, therefore, provide strong evidence that diazepam specifically disrupted the acquisition of spatial learning which may parallel the long-term memory impairments observed in humans.

The radial maze is also a spatial learning apparatus which can be used in a number of ways to evaluate different aspects of learning and memory. In one version of the test food pellets are placed at the ends of all the maze arms (usually eight). Food-deprived rats are allowed to explore the maze until they obtain all the pellets and this they learn to do without re-entering any of the arms they have already visited. To effectively perform this task rats must make use of short-term, working memory (i.e. remember which of the maze arms have already been visited) concerning spatial information about the position of the maze arms in relation to visual landmarks.

As benzodiazepines appear not to produce marked effects on short-term memory performance in humans, except at grossly sedative doses, they would not be expected to affect this form of working memory in rats. Table 2 shows results obtained in rats trained to obtain all eight food rewards in the radial maze. Chlordiazepoxide produced no effect, at the doses tested, on the efficiency of performance even though the time taken to find the food was greatly increased. This later effect probably reflects mild sedation or ataxia produced by the benzodiazepines. In contrast to the results seen with chlordiazepoxide, scopolamine both increased the session time and decreased the efficiency of performance by increasing the number of arm re-entries. These results indicate that whereas scopolamine produced a deficit in working memory, chlordiazepoxide did not.

Table 2. Effects of chlordiazepoxide and scopolamine on working memory performance of rats in an eight-arm radial maze. Rats were placed in the maze and allowed to explore until all 8 pellets had been found and consumed. Measures were taken of the efficiency of performance (N° of arms entered ÷ 8 x 100) and the time required to obtain all the food. * p<0.05, ** p<0.01 difference from control.

Drug	Dose mg/kg	Percent Efficiency	Session Time sec
Chlordiazepoxide	0	95 ± 1	132 ± 10
	2.5	93 ± 3	130 ± 13
	5	84 ± 5	228 ± 38 **
	10	88 ± 5	265 ± 47 **
Scopolamine	0	91 ± 1	95 ± 7
	0.1	79 ± 7	167 ± 35
	0.3	58 ± 7 *	252 ± 55 **
	1.0	55 ± 9 **	345 ± 66 **

In apparent contradiction to these results, Willner & Birbeck (1986) reported that two doses of chlordiazepoxide (2.5 and 7.5 mg/kg) increased the time to complete a working memory, radial maze task and also increased errors. However, in another spatial learning procedure involving the position of a single water bottle in a large arena, a dose of chlordiazepoxide (5 mg/kg) disrupted the performance of both a spatial learning and a cue learning task. Willner & Birbeck therefore concluded that chlordiazepoxide disrupted the performance of the animals in all procedures but probably did not give rise to a specific working memory deficit.

Also using an eight-arm radial maze, Stackman & Walsh (1992) removed rats from the maze after they had obtained four of the eight food pellets and replaced them 1-hour later. In order to find the four remaining pellets efficiently, i.e. without more than a minimum of entries into the no-longer baited arms, the rats clearly needed to remember the arms which they had visited 1-hour before. The authors referred to this as delayed working memory. When chlordiazepoxide was injected systemically or into the medial septum, but not into the amygdala, immediately after the pre-delay trial there was an increase in errors during the post-delay trial 1-hour later. As the errors consisted of entries into the arms already visited during the pre-delay session rather than perseverative errors, Stackman & Walsh concluded that chlordiazepoxide had produced a disruption of the consolidation of delayed working memory. These results therefore seem inconsistent with findings from other animal and human studies demonstrating that benzodiazepines do not produce retrograde amnesia in other long-term memory tasks.

NON-BENZODIAZEPINE ANXIOLYTICS

With increasing concern about potential hazards associated with the treatment of anxiety with benzodiazepines and particularly the possibility that long-term use may lead to physical dependence

(Woods et al., 1992), there has been a resurgence of interest in the development of non-benzodiazepine anxiolytics. Much research has been directed at the anxiolytic-like actions of compounds acting at different subtypes of serotonin receptors following the finding that the anxiolytic agent, buspirone, had affinity for $5HT_{1A}$ receptors (Barrett & Gleeson, 1991; Sanger et al., 1991). However, another successful approach has involved agents which, while distinct from benzodiazepines in chemical structure, act through the BZ (ω) binding sites associated with $GABA_A$ receptors. The imidazopyridine derivative, alpidem, is the first such drug to have entered into clinical use as an anxiolytic (Morselli, 1990; Zivkovic et al., 1990).

Benzodiazepines produce their characteristic pharmacological actions by potentiating the effects of the inhibitory neurotransmitter GABA. They do this by binding to sites called BZ (ω) receptors which are associated with the α subunits of the $GABA_A$ receptors. Benzodiazepines generally exert full agonist activity at BZ (ω) receptors and do not distinguish between subtypes of these receptors. It has been proposed, however, that either BZ (ω) site partial agonists (Haefely et al., 1990) or compounds selective for BZ (ω) receptor subtypes (Langer et al., 1990) would exert anxiolytic effects with fewer side effects than are associated with benzodiazepines. Several partial agonists, including the imidazo-benzodiazepine, bretazenil, have been reported to produce anxiolytic activity and, as noted above, alpidem which has selectivity for BZ_1 (ω_1) sites, is marketed for this indication.

Partial agonists

The different pharmacological effects associated with benzodiazepines (anxiety reduction, sedation, muscle relaxation, etc.) occur at different doses and therefore at different levels of receptor occupation. Partial agonists with relatively low intrinsic activity would produce pharmacological effects normally associated with low doses of full agonists (e.g. anxiety reduction) without giving rise to effects associated with high doses (e.g. sedation). The question of what effects partial agonists would exert on cognitive function is an important one, therefore, as it is possible that such drugs could reduce anxiety without producing memory disturbance.

Several partial agonists have been investigated in tests of passive avoidance learning in rodents. Tang et al. (1991) found that U-78875 had no effect on the acquisition of a step-through response in mice and Wada & Fukuda (1992) reported a similar lack of activity of DN-2327 in rats. However, two other research groups reported that CGS 9896 and ZK 91296 did interfere with passive avoidance learning in mice despite having no sedative activity (Petersen et al., 1984; Sanger & Joly, 1985). Clinical studies with bretazenil and related compounds have also reported some cognitive effects, including disruption of short-term memory, although mild sedation also occurred (Saletu et al., 1989).

Selective agonists

A number of compounds including CL 218,872, alpidem, zolpidem and abecarnil, have been reported to have selective affinity for the BZ_1 (ω_1) subtype of BZ (ω) receptors (Langer et al., 1990; Stephens et al., 1992). It was originally suggested that CL 218,872 was a non-sedative anxiolytic and that BZ_1 (ω_1) receptors were therefore particularly important for mediating anxiolytic activity and BZ_2 (ω_2) sites important for sedation (Lippa et al., 1979). This was subsequently shown not to be the case as zolpidem has hypnotic activity which predominates over other aspects of its pharmacological profile (Depoortere et al., 1986). In relation to cognitive processes, Morselli (1990) proposed that BZ_1 (ω_1) selective drugs might be expected to have relatively little effect on learning and memory because the population of this receptor subtype found in the hippocampus, a brain area with an important role in memory, is relatively small.

The BZ_1 (ω_1) selective compounds zolpidem, alpidem and CL 218,872 have been studied in animal learning tests and the effects of alpidem and zolpidem have also been investigated on human memory. All three drugs disrupted the acquisition of learned fear in mice in a step-through passive avoidance procedure but, with alpidem and zolpidem this effect occurred only at doses which greatly decreased locomotion during the learning trial (Sanger et al., 1986; Zivkovic et al., 1990). These results are presented in Table 3 which shows that ratios between the doses affecting fear learning and those decreasing locomotion were considerably greater for alpidem and zolpidem than for the benzodiazepines diazepam and triazolam. It has also been reported that CL 218,872 interfered with spatial learning in the Morris water maze but similar doses of the drug produced a deficit in rotarod performance (McNamara & Skelton, 1992b).

Table 3. Comparison of the activities of BZ_1 (ω_1)-selective and nonselective drugs on the acquisition of conditioned fear in mice. MEDs are the smallest doses which produced a statistically significant decrease in the number of crossings between the black and white compartments of the two-compartment box on the first day or gave rise to statistically significant increases in time spent in the black compartment on the second day. Alpidem was administered orally and the other drugs by i.p. injection. For experimental details, see Sanger et al. (1986).

Drug	Minimal effective dose (MED) mg/kg		
	Fear learning	Exploration	Ratio
Alpidem	40	10	4
Zolpidem	2	0.5	4
Diazepam	0.5	0.5	1
Triazolam	0.025	0.05	0.5

Zolpidem has also been found to have effects on delayed recall in humans in doses between 10 and 45 mg (Cashman et al., 1987; Evans et al., 1990; Berlin et al., 1993) although this drug does not always produce effects on memory in conditions where benzodiazepines are active (Balkin et al., 1992). As the clinically recommended dose of this drug for sleep-induction is 10 mg, it seems likely that cognitive effects, when they occur, are secondary to sedation. Alpidem can similarly produce disruption in tests of recall and recognition but at doses higher than those recommended for the treatment of anxiety. Curran et al. (1987) found that 100 mg of alpidem produced some amnesia but also affected psychomotor skills indicating some sedation. Lower doses had little effect. In one study involving anxious patients under treatment with either alpidem or the benzodiazepine, lorazepam, it was found that while lorazepam produced a recall deficit, alpidem did not (Morton & Lader, 1992).

Both animal and human data therefore show that while the BZ_1 (ω_1) selective drugs alpidem and zolpidem do interfere with learning they do so only at sedative doses. It is thus difficult to draw conclusions about the role of BZ (ω) receptor subtypes in cognition. In order to investigate the hypothesis outlined earlier, that benzodiazepine-induced amnesia is related to activity at BZ_2 (ω_2) sites in the hippocampus, more selective compounds may be necessary together with research involving intracerebral injection of currently available drugs.

REFERENCES

Balkin, T.J., O'Donnell, V.M., Wesensten, McCann & Belenky, G. (1992): Comparison of the daytime sleep and performance effects of zolpidem versus triazolam. *Psychopharmacology* 107, 83-88.

Barnes, C.A. (1988): Spatial learning and memory processes: the search for their neurobiological mechanisms in the rat. *Trends Neurosci.* 11, 163-169.

Barrett, J.E. & Gleeson, S. (1991): Anxiolytic effects of $5HT_{1A}$ agonists, $5HT_3$ antagonists and benzodiazepines: conflict and drug discrimination studies. In *$5HT_{1A}$ agonists, $5HT_3$ antagonists and benzodiazepines. Their comparative behavioural pharmacology*, eds R.J. Rodgers & S.J. Cooper, pp. 59-105. Chichester: Wiley.

Berlin, I., Warot, D., Hergueta, T., Moliner, P., Bagot, C. & Puech, A.J. (1993): Comparison of the effects of zolpidem and triazolam on memory functions, psychomotor performances, and postural sway in healthy subjects. *J. Clin. Psychopharmacol.* 13, 100-106.

Brioni, J.D. & Arolfo, M.P. (1992): Diazepam impairs retention of spatial information without affecting retrieval or cue learning. *Pharmacol. Biochem. Behav.* 41, 1-5.

Broekkamp, C.L., LePichon, M. & Lloyd, K.G. (1984): The comparative effects of benzodiazepines, progabide and PK 9084 on acquisition of passive avoidance in mice. *Psychopharmacology* 83, 122-125.

Cashman, J.N., Power, S.J. & Jones, R.M. (1987): Assessment of a new hypnotic imidazo-pyridine (zolpidem) as oral premedication. *Brit. J. Clin. Pharmacol.* 24, 85-92.

Colpaert, F.C. (1986): A method for quantifying state-dependency with chlordiazepoxide in rats. *Psychopharmacology* 99, 144-146.

Curran, H.V. (1986): Tranquillising memories: a review of the effects of benzodiazepines on human memory. *Biol. Psychol.* 23, 179-213.

Curran, V., Allen, D. & Lader, M. (1987): The effects of single doses of alpidem (SL 80.0342-00), lorazepam and placebo on memory and psychomotor performance in healthy human volunteers. *J. Psychopharmacol.* 1, 81-89.

Depoortere, H., Zivkovic, B., Lloyd, K.G., Sanger, D.J., Perrault, G., Langer, S.Z. & Bartholini, G. (1986): Zolpidem, a novel non-benzodiazepine hypnotic. I. Neuropharmacological and behavioral effects. *J. Pharmacol. Exp. Ther.* 237, 649-658.

Edwards, J.G. (1981): Adverse effects of antianxiety drugs. *Drugs* 22, 495-514.

Evans, S.M., Funderburk, F.R. & Griffiths, R.R. (1990): Zolpidem and triazolam in humans: behavioral and subjective effects and abuse liability. *J. Pharmacol. Exp. Ther.* 255, 1246-1255.

Gamzu, E.R. (1988): Animal model studies of benzodiazepine-induced amnesia. In *Benzodiazepine receptor ligands, memory and information processing*, eds I. Hindmarch & H. Ott, pp. 218-229. Berlin: Springer-Verlag.

Ghoneim, M.M., Mewaldt, S.P., Berie, J.L. & Hinrichs, J.V. (1981): Memory and performance effects of single and 3-week administration of diazepam. *Psychopharmacology* 73, 147-151.

Haefely, W., Martin, J.R. & Schoch, P. (1990): Novel anxiolytics that act as partial agonists at benzodiazepine receptors. *Trends Pharmacol. Sci.* 11, 452-456.

King, D.J. (1992): Benzodiazepines, amnesia and sedation: theoretical and clinical issues and controversies. *Human Psychopharmacol.* 7, 79-87.

Langer, S.Z., Arbilla, S., Tan, S., Lloyd, K.G., George, P., Allen, J. & Wick, A.E. (1990): Selectivity for omega-receptor subtypes as a strategy for the development of anxiolytic drugs. *Pharmacopsychiatry* 23 (Suppl.), 103-107.

Lippa, A.S., Coupet, J., Greenblatt, E.N., Klepner, C.A. & Beer, B. (1979): A synthetic non-benzodiazepine ligand for benzodiazepine receptors: a probe for investigating neuronal substrates of anxiety. *Pharmacol. Biochem. Behav.* 11, 99-106.

Lister, R.G. (1985): The amnesic action of benzodiazepines in man. *Neurosci. Biobehav. Rev.* 9, 87-94.

Lucki, I., Rickels, K. & Geller, A.M. (1986): Chronic use of benzodiazepines and psychomotor and cognitive test performance. *Psychopharmacology* 88, 426-433.

McNamara, R.K. & Skelton, R.W. (1991): Diazepam impairs acquisition but not performance in the Morris water maze. *Pharmacol. Biochem. Behav.* 38, 651-658.

McNamara, R.K. & Skelton, R.W. (1992a): Assessment of a cholinergic contribution to chlordiazepoxide deficits of place learning in the Morris water maze. *Pharmacol. Biochem. Behav.* 41, 529-538.

McNamara, R.K. & Skelton, R.W. (1992b): Like diazepam, CL 218,872, a selective ligand for the benzodiazepine ω_1 receptor subtype, impairs place learning in the Morris water maze. *Psychopharmacology* 107, 347-351.

McNaughton, N. & Morris, R.G.M. (1987): Chlordiazepoxide, an anxiolytic benzodiazepine, impairs place navigation in rats. *Behav. Brain Res.* 24, 39-46.

Morris, R.G.M. (1981): Spatial localization does not require the presence of local cues. *Learn Motiv.* 12, 239-260.

Morselli, P.L. (1990): On the therapeutic action of alpidem in anxiety disorders: an overview of european data. *Pharmacopsychiatry* 23, 129-134.

Morton, S. & Lader, M. (1992): Alpidem and lorazepam in the treatment of patients with anxiety disorders: comparison of physiological and psychological effects. *Pharmacopsychiatry* 25, 177-181.

Oishi, H., Iwahara, S., Yang, K.M. & Yogi, A. (1972): Effects of chlordiazepoxide on passive avoidance responses in rats. *Psychopharmacologia* 23, 373-385.

Olton, D.S. (1987): The radial arm maze as a tool in behavioral pharmacology. *Physiol. Behav.* 40, 793-797.

Patel, J.B., Ciofalo, V.B. & Iorio, L.C. (1979): Benzodiazepine blockade of passive-avoidance task in mice: a state-dependent phenomenon. *Psychopharmacology* 61, 25-28.

Petersen, E.N., Jensen, L.H., Honore, T., Braestrup, C., Kehr, W., Stephens, D.W., Wachtel, H., Seidelman, D. & Schmiechen R. (1984): ZK 91296, a partial agonist at benzodiazepine receptors. *Psychopharmacology* 83, 240-248.

Ricci, S., Elisei, S. & Quartesan, R. (1987): Side effects of benzodiazepines: a review. *Drugs of Today* 23, 525-537.

Saletu, B., Grunberger, J. & Linzmayer, L. (1989): On the central effects of a new partial benzodiazepine agonist RO 16-6028 in man: pharmaco-EEG and psychometric studies. *Int. J. Clin. Pharmacol. Ther. Tox.* 27, 51-65.

Sanger, D.J. & Joly, D. (1985): Anxiolytic drugs and the acquisition of conditioned fear in mice. *Psychopharmacology* 85, 284-288.

Sanger, D.J., Joly, D. & Zivkovic, B. (1986): Effects of zolpidem, a new imidazopyridine hypnotic, on the acquisition of conditioned fear in mice. Comparison with triazolam and CL 218,872. *Psychopharmacology* 90, 207-210.

Sanger, D.J., Perrault, G., Morel, E., Joly, D. & Zivkovic, B. (1991): Animal models of anxiety and the development of novel anxiolytic drugs. *Prog. Neuro-Psychopharmacol. Biol. Psychiat.* 15, 205-212.

Stackman, R.W. & Walsh, T.J. (1992): Chlordiazepoxide-induced working memory impairments: site specificity and reversal by flumazenil (RO 15-1788). *Behav. Neural Biol.* 57, 233-243.

Stephens, D.N., Turski, L., Hillman, M., Turner, J.D., Schneider, H.H. & Yamaguchi, M. (1992): What are the differences between abecarnil and conventional anxiolytics? In *GABAergic synaptic transmission*, eds G. Biggio, A. Concas & E. Costa, pp. 395-405. New York: Raven Press.

Tang, A.H., Franklin, S.R., Himes, C.S. & Ho, P.M. (1991): Behavioral effects of U-78875, a quinoxalinone anxiolytic with potent benzodiazepine antagonist activity. *J. Pharmacol. Exp. Ther.* 259, 248-254.

Task Force of the Collegium Internationale Neuro-Psychopharmacologicum (CINP) (1992): Impact of neuropharmacology in the 1990s - treatment strategies for anxiety disorders and insomnia. *Eur. Neuropsychopharmacol.* 2, 167-169.

Wada, T. & Fukuda, N. (1992): Effect of a new anxiolytic, DN-2327, on learning and memory in rats. *Pharmacol. Biochem. Behav.* 41, 573-579.

Weingartner, H.J., Hommer, D., Lister, R.G., Thompson, K. & Wolkowitz, O. (1992): Selective effects of triazolam on memory. *Psychopharmacology* 106, 341-345.

Willner, P. & Birbeck, K.A. (1986): Effects of chlordiazepoxide and sodium valproate in two tests of spatial behaviour. *Pharmacol. Biochem. Behav.* 25, 747-751.

Woods, J.H., Katz, J.L. & Winger, G. (1992): Benzodiazepines: use, abuse, and consequences. *Pharmacol. Rev.* 44, 151-347.

Zivkovic, B., Morel, E., Joly, D., Perrault, G., Sanger, D.J. & Lloyd, K.G. (1990): Pharmacological and behavioral profile of alpidem as an anxiolytic. *Pharmacopsychiatry* 23 (Suppl.), 108-113.

Résumé

Il est bien connu que les benzodiazépines produisent une amnésie antérograde, bien que l'on ne sache pas dans quelle mesure cela pose un problème significatif dans l'utilisation clinique de ces composés. Il reste aussi à établir si les problèmes de mémoire sont invariablement associés aux effets sédatifs de ces médicaments. Chez l'animal de laboratoire, les benzodiazépines bloquent l'acquisition d'une réponse d'évitement passif et interfèrent avec la mémoire spatiale. L'étude récente des agonistes partiels des benzodiazépines suggère que certains de ces agents stoppent l'apprentissage tandis que d'autres non. Le zolpidem et l'alpidem, sélectifs pour les récepteurs BZ_1 (ω_1) affectent aussi l'apprentissage mais seulement à des doses très sédatives. La poursuite des recherches devrait permettre de mieux définir le rôle spécifique des sous-types des récepteurs des benzodiazépines (ω) dans les fonctions cognitives.

Anxiety: Neurobiology, Clinic and Therapeutic Perspectives. Eds M. Hamon, H. Ollat, M.-H. Thiébot. Colloque INSERM/ John Libbey Eurotext Ltd. © 1993, Vol. 232, pp. 129-139.

In vivo study of central-type benzodiazepine receptors in humans by means of positron emission tomography

J.-C. Baron* and P. Abadie

* INSERM U.320, Centre Cycéron, Université de Caen, boulevard Henri Becquerel, B.P. 5027, 14021 Caen, France

SUMMARY

In vivo study of the central benzodiazepine receptor (cBZR) - GABA- A complex in the human brain may be of potential interest to assess the pathophysiology and pharmacology of anxiety. Such an investigation is now possible with the use of Positron Emission Tomography (PET) and the labeled specific cBZR antagonist, 11C-Flumazenil (11C-FLU). After its intravenous administration, 11C-FLU is heterogeneously distributed in brain structures ; displacement and inhibition studies documented a large specific, and a negligible non-specific binding, of 11C-FLU, characteristics which have allowed the development of quantitative methods. Both "Pseudoequilibrium" and "Dynamic" approaches have been described. Pseudoequilibrium methods are based on i) the assumption of a pharmacological quasi-equilibrium between free (F) and specifically bound (B) radioligand; and ii) the determination of F to estimate B, and, in turn, Bmax and Kd values. A pseudo-equilibrium approach is presented, comparing, to establish F in healthy unmedicated volunteers, three "reference" brain structures, devoid of cBZR (pons, hemispheric white matter, corpus callosum). This work shows that pons is a structure of choice, and documents the feasibility of estimating Bmax and Kd values in different brain regions in a clinical paradigm.

Dynamic quantification methods, which entail a complex mathematical analysis of 11C-FLU blood and brain kinetics, have not been implemented for clinical research as yet.

INTRODUCTION

Since its discovery in 1977 by Squires and Braestrup, and by Möhler and Okada, the central-type benzodiazepine receptor (cBZR) has attracted considerable interest because of its implication in the mediation of the sedative, anticonvulsant and anxiolytic properties of benzodiazepines (BDZ). It is now well established that the cBZR is functionally and structurally linked to the GABAergic system (GABA A receptor associated with the chloride channel), the main inhibitory system in the central nervous system, as part of a postsynaptic supramolecular complex.

Alterations in the density (B_{max}), affinity (K_d) and/or regional brain distribution of the cBZR may be associated with anxiety disorders. This hypothesis would be supported by

a - the efficacy of BDZ in the treatment of such disorders;

b - acute and chronic stress studies in animals where modifications have been found in the cBZR itself or in related parts of the GABA A receptor complex (Braestrup et al., 1979; Medina et al., 1983; Inoue et al., 1985; Havoudjian et al., 1986, Miller et al., 1987). However, no cBZR study in post-mortem brains of anxious patients have been reported to date. First, this presumably reflects the problems with obtaining this material from subjects naive from BZD treatment. Second, agonal conditions may in itself after brain tissue environment, and in turn, cBZR.

In vivo investigations of the cBZR associated with a detailed assessment of the clinical characteristics pertaining to anxiety disorders, by means of quantitative scales, would be ideal to assign changes in cBZR, if any, to clinical dimensions (e.g. "State" or "Trait" dimensions, Spielberger et al, 1983). Furthermore, with a 3 - dimensional method to assess the cBZR, the opportunity arises to simultaneously probe brain regions which may be especially implicated in behavioral experiences related to anxiety (e.g. fear, stress, anticipation, poor inhibitory capacity), such as the amygdala, the hippocampus, the prefrontal cortex or the nucleus accumbens.

Positron Emission Tomography (PET) with the cBZR antagonist 11C-Flumazenil now allows both imaging and quantification of the cBZR in the living human brain. This would represent the method of choice to non-invasively investigate the relationships between anxiety disorders and the cBZR (for review : Abadie and Baron, 1990).

Flumazenil (RO-15-1788) is an imidazo-benzodiazepine which lacks the aromatic cycle in position 5 of the C cycle that is typical of the benzodiazepines. It is a highly specific, selective cBZR antagonist which has been clinically used for several years in toxicology and anesthesia. It can be labeled with ^{11}C at high specific radioactivity (SRA) (0.5 to 1.8 Ci/μmol) by methylation of its nor-precursor using ^{11}C-methyl iodide derived from ^{11}C-CO$_2$ (Mazière et al, 1983; Halldin et al, 1988).

A number of investigations have shown Flumazenil to be a better radioligand than agonists (e.g., flunitrazepam) for the *in vivo* study of cBZR (Mazière et al, 1983 ; Hantraye et al, 1984 ; Samson et al, 1985). First, its *in vitro* dissociation from the receptor is much slower, and its binding to the cBZR is not GABA-dependent (Möhler and Richards, 1981; Brown and Martin, 1984). Second, it has no pharmacological effect and displacing doses can be used without risk of inconvenience. Third, *in vivo* studies in rodents with ^{3}H-flumazenil have shown i) a highly detectable specific binding, ii) a regional tracer distribution similar to that obtained in *in vitro* binding studies, iii) no binding to the peripheral BZR, and iiii) negligible non-specific binding (in contrast, ³H-flunitrazepam showed a very low specific *in vivo* binding) (Goeders and Kuhar, 1985), while brain radioactivity represented, almost exclusively, unchanged Flumazenil (Inoue et al, 1985). Finally, plasma protein binding of ³H-flumazenil in mice was favorably low (around 45% of total).

11C-FLUMAZENIL PET STUDIES IN HUMANS

Following extensive validation in baboons (Hantraye et al, 1984), initial PET studies in humans, which employed intravenous bolus injections, were published in 1985 (Samson et al, 1985).

a - *Tracer-dose experiments*

Since brain penetration of 11C-Ro-15-3890, the almost exclusive labeled metabolite of 11C-Flumazenil, is negligible (Halldin et al, 1988; Persson et al, 1989a; Barré et al, 1990) the cerebral 11C kinetics after 11C-Flumazenil injection represent unchanged ligand. In all brain regions a rapid uptake of ¹¹C-FLU is observed, which reflects an easy transfer across the blood-brain-barrier. A slower rise is seen in gray matter regions until about 10 min after the tracer injection, followed by a quasi-plateau of about 5 min and then a slow decline. In white matter, the maximum uptake, lower than in gray matter regions, occurs earlier (2 to 7 min). While the initial uptake is grossly proportional to perfusion, with all gray matter structures having a somewhat identical uptake, there is a rapid redistribution in favor of the cerebral cortex, followed in order by the cerebellar cortex and the basal ganglia-thalamus (Persson et al, 1989; Samson et al, 1985) in agreement with known differences in cBZR densities as determined for the human brain *in vitro*. (Figure)

b - *Displacement and inhibition studies*

Intravenous administration of cold loads of Flumazenil 10 to 20 min following trace amounts of 11C-Flumazenil, induced an immediate, abrupt, dose-dependent displacement of radioligand from gray matter structures (around 90% for a dose of 20mg). Inhibition of specific binding of 11C-Flumazenil was achieved either by pretreatment with or by coinjection of cold Flumazenil with the radioligand (Shinotoh et al, 1986; Pappata et al, 1988). These studies demonstrated a dose-dependent inhibition of 11C-Flumazenil uptake in gray matter structures, the maximum of which being close to 90% of control for doses of 10mg or 0.1mg/Kg, documenting a very large specific binding (B) of 11C-Flumazenil in the human brain *in vivo*, and a negligible non-specific (NS) binding.

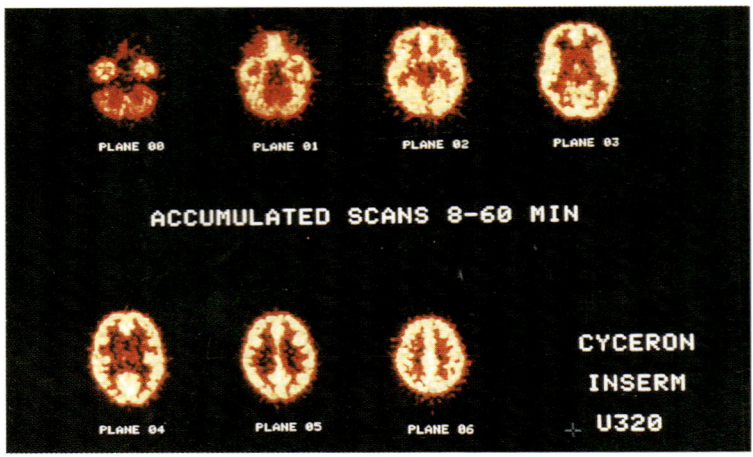

Figure : ^{11}C-Flumazenil high-resolution PET brain images from a healthy subject, obtained according to seven axial planes parallel to the Glabella-Inion (GI) line, and -4, +8, +20, +32, +44, +56 and +68 mm relative to this line, respectively. The data were acquired on a TTV Ø 3 device (LETI, Grenoble), with lateral and axial resolutions of 5.5 mm and 9 mm, respectively. The images shown are oriented so that anterior is up and left side is on the right. They represent accumulated counts from T_0 to T_{+60min} following the intravenous injection of tracer amounts of ^{11}C-labeled Flumazenil. Areas with high count rates (shown in yellow) indicate brain regions with highest ^{11}C-Flumazenil binding, while orange or red-colored areas have low binding. Binding is highest in all neocortical areas, intermediate in cerebellar cortex (plane ØØ), low in basal ganglia and thalamus (plane Ø 3), and lowest in pons (plane ØØ), where specific binding in assumed negligible. This regional distribution of ^{11}C-Flumazenil binding *in vivo* reflects the distribution of central-type benzodiazepine receptors in the adult human brain known from previous *in vitro* studies.

c - *quantification of regional brain cBZR in vivo*

Up until recently, determination of Bmax and Kd of the cBZR in human brain regions with 11C-Flumazenil and PET has almost exclusively relied upon "pseudo-equilibrium" approaches.

"Pseudo-equilibrium" quantitative methods have been developed to measure the density (B_{max}) and affinity (K_d) of cBZR in the human brain with 11C-Flumazenil (Pappata et al, 1988; Persson et al, 1989b; Iyo et al, 1991; Abadie et al, 1992). All these methods require the estimation of free radioligand concentration (F) in brain tissue, thereby allowing the measurement of specifically bound ligand (B) in gray matter structures of interest by subtraction of free radioligand concentration from total radioligand concentration (T).

With PET determinations of in vivo specific binding, however, true pharmacological equilibrium is unlikely to be reached because of the elimination and disposition of the externally administered radioligand. True equilibrium would exist only if the concentration of specifically bound radioligand was stable, indicating no net flux in the association/ dissociation reaction. In human PET studies with 11C-Flumazenil, Pappata et al (1988) showed that the B/F ratio progressively increased for about 15-20 min and was essentially stable until 60 min; in most regions, however, this ratio slightly declined after 40 min. Persson et al (1989b), using pons or corona radiata to determine F, found that the B/F ratio for the neocortex rose until about 25 min and was essentially stable thereafter, but with a larger variability after 40 min. Savic et al (1988, 1990) documented the stability of the B/F ratio for the parietal cortex between 18 and 54 min. Thus, a "pseudo-equilibrium" interval between 15 and 40 min has been assumed to be an acceptable time period for determination of F and B (Savic et al, 1988).

Using this paradigm and Scatchard transformation, Pappata et al. (1988) and Persson et al. (1989) were able to calculate regional B_{max} and K_d values. In the former study, these variables were obtained in 4 different regions from 13 healthy volunteers, each subject contributing to one value. In the latter, they were obtained in a single large area of neocortex, but measured in five healthy volunteers, each of them subjected to four or five PET 11C-Flumazenil studied at different SRAs. Pappata et al. (1988) have estimated the free radioligand (F) in each anatomical region, as the non-displaceable radioactivity in coinjections studies; Persson et al. (1989b) estimated F from the radioactivity measured in a "reference" brain structure, theoretically devoid of cBZR (e.g. pons, hemispheric white matter).

In both studies, linearity of the Scatchard plots was demonstrated, with Hill coefficients >0.98, indicating that Flumazenil apparently binds to a single class of receptors in vivo, as it also does in vitro. Both studies reported Bmax and Kd values in the neocortex that were comparable to earlier in vitro studies performed at physiological temperature (Bmax = 40-90nM; Kd = 7-9nM) (Kopp et al, 1990).

However, application of such methods to clinical investigations is logistically cumbersome because several PET sessions, for the repeated administration of 11C-Flumazenil at different specific radioactivities, are required for each subject . To investigate epileptic patients, Savic et al (1988, 1990) used a simplified approach that required only two injections of the radioligand (and the "reference structure paradigm" to estimate the parameter F). This method is based on the 2-point Scatchard procedure pioneered by Farde et al (1986) for striatal D_2 receptors, and relies on the use of well-defined, extreme SRA values such that the two data pairs in the Scatchard plot are widely apart and in a sense "anchor" the plot.

Although Savic's results were encouraging, this approach lacked a systematic investigation of its limitations when measuring Bmax and Kd in multiple brain regions. To this end, we have evaluated, in seven unmedicated healthy volunteers, the relative merits of three "reference" structures (pons, hemispheric white matter and corpus callosum) in which the free radioligand concentration in brain tissue was estimated 15-40 min after i.v. injection of the radioligand (Abadie et al, 1992) by means of high-resolution PET. Bmax and Kd were calculated for each subject in 18 gray matter structures, based on a two-point Scatchard plot. We showed that the use of the corpus callosum as reference often resulted in spurious Bmax and Kd values. The pons, the easiest region to sample on PET images, was the best reference structure because it provided satisfactory Bmax values (closest to in vitro data) and most consistent Kd values. The pattern of regional Bmax was consistent with that expected from *in vitro* studies, with highest values in the cerebral cortex, intermediate in the cerebellum, and lowest in striatum and thalamus. The Kd values were uniform among regions and consistent with earlier *in vitro* and *in vivo* data. Furthermore, coefficients of variation (COVs) of such measurements were acceptable (around 15% for Bmax and 20% for Kd), except in areas with low density of cBZR such as the striatum and thalamus, where larger COVs were obtained (Table 1). This work documented the feasibility of estimating Bmax and Kd of cBZR in multiple brain regions for clinical research.

Table 1 : Quantitative positron emission tomography in healthy volunteers Bmax and Kd determination using pons as "reference structure"

	B_{max} (nM) *	K_d (nM) *
Medial frontal cortex	78 ± 13	12 ± 2
Cingulate Gyrus	92 ± 18	16 ± 4
Medial occipital cortex	103 ± 15	14 ± 2
Lateral frontal cortex (left)	72 ± 9	13 ± 2
Lateral temporal cortex (left)	76 ± 11	13 ± 3
Mesial temporal cortex (left)	49 ± 14	10 ± 2
Occipital cortex (left)	83 ± 13	14 ± 3
Parietal cortex (left)	75 ± 4	14 ± 3
Cerebellum	55 ± 11	14 ± 2
Striatum (left)	44 ± 8	12 ± 4
Thalamus (left)	25 ± 15	9 ± 5

* mean ± SD, N = 7

DYNAMIC APPROACHES

Because PET allows images to be obtained dynamically, it is possible to subject the radioactivity time-activity data from a brain region of interest to a multi-compartmental model in order to express receptor binding in terms of Bmax and Kd. However, this requires both a minimum of two injections of the radioligand at different SRAs to solve for the two unknowns, and an accurate determination (i.e., uncontaminated by labeled metabolites) of the arterial plasma input function (Delforge et al, 1993). Major issues in these "dynamic" studies are their complexity in terms of computer science, difficulties in validating the models used, the statistical assessment of the obtained parameters, and the limited regional capability of the measurement due to inadequate count rate. Therefore, these methods are not well suited for clinical research.

More simple paradigms using a single-injection approach allow to determine a cBZR binding index which should be related to Bmax if one assumes Kd is constant across regions and across subjects (Koeppe et al, 1991). But the need to obtain arterial blood, and the added complexity of determining unmetabolized 11C-Flumazenil in plasma (Barré et al, 1991; Debruyne et al, 1992) reduce the applicability of this method in clinical research.

Although a two-injection method with pixel-by-pixel estimation of Bmax and Kd of the cBZR and without requirement for arterial input function has been proposed (Blomqvist et al, 1990), it has so far not received adequate validation and therefore must remain of uncertain applicability.

IN VIVO STUDIES OF cBZR OCCUPANCY BY AGONISTS

In addition to regional studies of the cBZR density and affinity, PET with 11C-Flumazenil allows the *in vivo* assessment of receptor occupancy by agonist drugs in humans.

In this respect, Shinotoh et al (1989) studied cBZR occupancy by orally given clonazepam (30 µg/kg in six subjects and 50 µg/kg in one); 11C-Flumazenil-PET was performed before clonazepam and 1.5h after the drug administration. Receptor occupancy was estimated by simply calculating the percentage reduction of the 11C-Flumazenil normalized uptake measured in the cerebral cortex 30 min after tracer injection, assuming negligible NS binding and equilibrium conditions. In the treated conditions, tracer uptake was reduced 15.3 - 23.5% (depending on the cortical region studied) in the low dose study (N=6) and around 30% in the high-dosage study (N=1). Clinically, this level of receptor occupancy was accompanied by drowsiness, ataxia, and significant delay of the P 300 (late auditory evoked potential). These results clearly demonstrated that clinical effects of benzodiazepines do not require a large occupancy of the cBZR. Similar results have been recently obtained by Pauli et al (1991) using diazepam. This paradigm has been also applied to study the acute effects of alcohol (Pauli et al, 1992).

REFERENCES

Abadie, P. & Baron, J.C. (1990) : In vivo studies of the central benzodiazepine receptors in the human brain with positron emission tomography. in : *Radiopharmaceuticals and Brain Pathology Studied with PET and SPECT*, eds M. Diksic and R.C. Reba, pp 357-379. CRC Press.Boca Raton.

Abadie, P., Baron, J.C., Bisserbe, J.C., Boulenger, J.P., Rioux, P., Travère, J.M., Barré, L., Petit-Taboue, M.C. & Zarifian, E. (1992) : Central benzodiazepine receptors in human brain : estimation of regional Bmax and Kd values with positron emission tomography. *Eur.J. Pharmacol.* 213,107-115.

Barré, L., Debruyne, D., Abadie, P., Moulin, M. & Baron, J.C. (1990) : Methods for 11C Ro 15-1788 radioactive metabolite assay in rabbit, baboon and human blood. *Appl. Rad. Isot.* 42, 435-439.

Blomqvist, G., Pauli, S., Farde, L.E., Persson, A., & Halldin, C. (1990) : Maps of receptor binding parameters in the human brain : a kinetic analysis of PET measurements. *Euro. J. Nucl. Med.*, 16, 257-265.

Braestrup, C., Nielsen, M., Nielsen, E.B., & Lyon, M. (1979) : Benzodiazepine receptors in the brain as affected by different experimental stress : the changes are small and not unidirectional. *Psychopharmacology.* 65, 273-277.

Brown, C.L. & Martin, I.L. (1984) : Kinetics of 3H RO15-1788 binding to membrane bound rat brain benzodiazepine receptors. *J. Neurochem.* 42, 918-923.

Delforge, J., Syrota, A., Bottlaender, M., Varastet, M., Loc'h, C., Bendriem, B., Crouzel, C. Brouillet, E. & Maziere, M. (1993) : Modeling analysis of 11C-Flumazenil kinetics studied by PET : application to a critical study of the equilibrium approaches. *J.Cereb.Blood Flow Metab.* 3, 454-468.

Debruyne, D., Abadie P,., Barré, L., Albessard, F., Moulin, M., Zarifian, E., & Baron J.C. (1993) : Plasma pharmacokinetics and metabolism of the benzodiazepine antagonist 11C Ro 15-1788 (Flumazenil) in baboon and human during positron emission tomography studies. *Eur.J. Drug Metabol. Pharmacol.*16,141-152.

Farde, L., Hall, H., Ehrin, E., & Sedvall, G. (1986) : Quantitative analysis of D2 dopamine receptor binding in the living brain by PET. *Science.* 231, 258-261.

Goeders, N.E. & Kuhar, M.J. (1985) : Benzodiazepine receptor in vivo with 3H RO 15-1788. *Life Sci.* 37, 345-355.

Halldin, C., Stone-Elander, S., Thorell, J.O., Persson, A., Sedvall G. (1988) : ^{11}C-labelling of Ro 15 1788 in two different positions, and also ^{11}C-labelling of its main metabolite Ro15-3890 for PET studies of benzodiazepine receptors. *Int. J. Radiat. Appl. Instrum.* 39,933-997.

Hantraye, P., Brouillet, E., Fukuda, H., Chavoix, C., Guibert, B., Dodd, R.H., Prenant, C., Crouzel, M., Naquet, R., & Mazière, M. (1984) : Central type benzodiazepine binding sites : a positron emission tomography study in the baboon's brain. *Neurosci. Lett.* 48, 115-120.

Havoudijan, H., Paul, S.M. & Skolnick, P. (1986) : Acute stress induced changes in the benzodiazepine-Aminobutyric acid receptor complex are confined to the chloride ionophore. *J. Pharmacol. Exp. Ther.* 237, 787-793.

Inoue, O., Akimoto, Y., Mashimoto, K. & Yamasaki, T. (1985) : alterations in biodistribution of 3H RO 15 1788 in mice by acute stress : possibly changes in *in vivo* binding availability to brain benzodiazepine receptor. *Int. J. Nucl. Med. Biol.* 12, 369-374.

Iyo, M., Itoh, T., Yamasaki, T., Fukuda, H., Inoue, O., Shinotoh, H., Suzuki, K., Fukui, S., & Tateno, Y. (1991) : Quantitative in vivo analysis of benzodiazepine binding sites in the human brain using positron emission tomography. *Neuropharmacology.* 30, 207-215.

Koeppe, R.A., Holthoff, V.A., Frey, K.A., Kilbourn, M.R., Kuhl, D.E. (1991) : Compartmental analysis of ^{11}C-Flumazenil kinetics for the activation of ligand transport rate and receptor distribution using positron emission tomography. *J. Cereb. Blood Flow Metab.* 11, 735-744.

Kopp, J., Hall, H. Persson, A. & Sedvall, G. (1990) : Temperature dependence of 3H-Ro 15-1788 bindings to benzodiazepine receptors in human postmortem brain homogenates. *J. Neurochem.* 55, 1310-1315.

Mazière, M., Prenant, C., Sastre, J., Crouzel, M., Comar, D., Hantraye, P., Kaijima, M., Guibert, B., & Naquet, R. (1983) : C11-Ro 15-1788 et C11-flunitrazepam, deux coordinats pour l'étude par tomographie par émission de positons des sites de liaison des benzodiazépines. *C.R. Acad. Sci. Paris.* 293, 871-876.

Medina, J.H., Novas, M.L. & De Robertis, E. (1983) : Change in benzodiazepine receptors by acute stress : different effect of diazepam or RO 15 1788 treatment. *Eur. J. Pharmacol.* 96, 181-185.

Miller, L.G., Thompson, M.L., Greenblatt, D.J., Deutsch, S.I., Shader, R.I. & Paul, S.M. (1987) : Rapid increase in brain benzodiazepine receptor binding following defeat stress in mice. *Brain Res.* 414, 395-400.

Möhler, H. & Okada, T. (1977) : Benzodiazepine receptor : demonstration in the central nervous system. *Science.* 198, 849-851.

Möhler, H., & Richards, J.G. (1981) : Agonist and antagonist receptor interaction in vitro. *Nature.* 294, 763-765.

Pappata, S., Samson, Y., Chavoix, C., Prenant, C., Mazière, M. & Baron, J.C. (1988) : Regional specific binding of 11C RO 15-1788 to central type benzodiazepine receptors in human brain : quantitative evaluation by PET. *J. Cereb. Blood Flow Metab.* 8, 304-313.

Pauli, S., Farde, L., Halldin, C. & Sedvall, G. (1991) : Occupancy of the central benzodiazepine receptors during benzodiazepine treatment determined by PET. *Eur. Neuropsychopharmacol.* 1, S-3-4, 229-232.

Pauli, S., Liljequist, S., Farde, L., Swahn, C.G., Halldin, C., LItton, J.E. & Sedvall, G. (1992) : PET analysis of alcohol interaction with the brain disposition of 11C flumazenil. *Psychopharmacology.* 107, 180-185.

Persson, A., Pauli, S., Halldin, C., Stone-Ellander, S., Farde, L., Sjögren, I., & Sedvall, G. (1989b) : Saturation analysis of specific 11C RO 15-1788 binding to the human neocortex using positron emission tomography. *Human Psychopharmacol.* 4, 21-31.

Persson, A., Pauli, S., Swahn, C.G., Halldin, C., & Sedvall, G. (1989a) : Cerebral uptake of 11C RO 15-3890 : a PET study in healthy volunteers. *J. Cereb. Blood Flow Metab.* 9, S122.

Samson, Y., Hantraye, P., Baron, J.C., Soussaline, F., Comar, D., & Mazière, M. (1985) : Kinetics and displacement of 11C RO 15-1788, a benzodiazepine antagonist studied in human brain in vivo by positron emission tomography. *Eur. J. Pharmacol.* 110, 247-251.

Savic, I., Lennart, J.O., Thorell, G., Blomqvist, G., Ericson, K., & Roland P. (1990) : Cortical benzodiazepine receptor binding in patients with generalized and partial epilepsy. *Epilepsia,* 31, 724-730.

Savic, I., Roland, P., Sedvall, G., Persson, A., Pauli, S. & Widen, L. (1988) : In vivo demonstration of reduced benzodiazepine receptor binding in human epileptic foci. *Lancet.* II, 863-866.

Shinotoh, H., Yamasaki, T., Inoue, O., Itoh, T., Suzuki, K., Tatano, Y. & Ikehira, H. (1986) : Visualisation of specific binding sites of benzodiazepine in human brain. *J. Nucl.Med.* 27, 1593-1599.

Shinotoh, H., Iyo, M., Yamada, T., Inoue, O., Suzuk,i K., Fukuda, H., Yamasaki, T., Tateno, Y. & Hirayama, K. (1989) : Detection of benzodiazepine receptor occupancy in the human brain by positron emission tomography. *Psychopharmacology.* 99, 202-207.

Spielberger, C.D., Gorsuch, R.L., Lushene, R., Vagg, P.R., & Jacobs, G.A. (1983) : Inventaire d'anxiété Etat-Trait, Manuel. Ed : Consulting Psychologist Press Inc, Adaptation franc. : Bruchon-Schweitzer M., Laboratoire de psychologie génétique et différentielle de l'Université de Bordeaux II (1988-89).

Squire, R.F. & Braestrup, C. (1977) : Benzodiazepine receptors in rat brain. *Nature.* 266, 732-734.

Résumé

L'étude *in vivo*, chez l'homme, du complexe : récepteur aux benzodiazépines de type central (cBZR)-récepteur GABA-A est d'un intérêt certain pour la physiopathologie et la pharmacologie de l'anxiété. Ceci est possible en Tomographie par Emission de Positons (TEP), et grâce à l'utilisation d'un antagoniste spécifique, radioactif, des cBZR, le C11-Flumazenil (C11-FLU). Après injection intraveineuse, le C11-FLU se fixe au niveau des structures cérébrales de façon hétérogène. Les études de déplacement et d'inhibition ont montré une liaison spécifique importante avec une liaison non-spécifique négligeable. Ces caractéristiques du C11-FLU permettent le développement de méthodes de quantification. Des approches "à l'équilibre" et "dynamiques" sont décrites.

Les méthodes "à l'équilibre" s'appuient sur les hypothèses : i) de l'établissement dans le cerveau d'un quasi-équilibre pharmacologique entre radioligand libre (F) et radioligand spécifiquement lié (B) ii) de la possibilité de déterminer F, et ainsi d'estimer B, puis Bmax et Kd. Une méthode de quantification "à l'équilibre" est présentée ici et consiste à comparer chez sept volontaires sains, trois régions cérébrales "de référence" dépourvues de cBZR, définies afin de déterminer F (pont, substance blanche hémisphérique, corps calleux). Ce travail montre que le pont est la région de choix et souligne la faisabilité de cette méthode en recherche clinique pour l'estimation des valeurs de densité et d'affinité des cBZR au niveau de multiples structures cérébrales. Les méthodes dynamiques de quantification de Bmax et Kd, nécéssitant une analyse mathématique complexe des pharmacocinétiques sanguines et cérébrales du C11-FLU, sont actuellement inapplicables en recherche clinique.

Pharmacology and molecular biology of central 5-HT receptors

Henri Gozlan and Michel Hamon

INSERM U.288, Faculté de Médecine Pitié-Salpêtrière, 91, boulevard de l'Hôpital, 75634 Paris Cedex 13, France

SUMMARY

Recent progress in molecular neurobiology has confirmed the concept of the heterogeneity of neurotransmitter receptors, especially in the case of serotonin (5-HT) receptors. To date, four main classes of pharmacologically defined serotonin receptors, named $5\text{-}HT_1$, $5\text{-}HT_2$, $5\text{-}HT_3$ and $5\text{-}HT_4$, have been identified, and at least the first two classes contain several receptor subtypes. Except the $5\text{-}HT_3$ receptor which corresponds to a ligand-gated cation channel, the other 5-HT receptors belong to the G protein-coupled receptor superfamily and are linked to different transduction systems: positive ($5\text{-}HT_4$) and negative ($5\text{-}HT_{1A}$, $5\text{-}HT_{1B}$, $5\text{-}HT_{1D}$, $5\text{-}HT_{1E}$) coupling to adenylate cyclase; positive coupling to phospholipase C ($5\text{-}HT_{1C}$ and $5\text{-}HT_2$), positive ($5\text{-}HT_{1A}$) and negative ($5\text{-}HT_{1C}$, $5\text{-}HT_2$) coupling to K^+ channels. All the pharmacologically defined 5-HT receptors, except the $5\text{-}HT_4$, have been cloned, confirming that they correspond to distinct proteins. Evidence for a further heterogeneity of 5-HT receptors has recently been provided by both pharmacological experiments with newly developed ligands and the cloning of additional 5-HT receptors unrelated to those already described. With the use of the powerful PCR technique, the number of 5-HT receptors will undoubtedly continue to grow and the development of new pharmacological tools is an urgent need for a better understanding of their functional properties.

The main contribution of molecular neurobiology over the past 5 years has been the classification of neurotransmitter receptors into two distinct superfamilies, the G protein-coupled receptors (GPCR) and the ligand-gated ion channel receptors (LGICR). Receptors in the first superfamily are made of a single protein whereas those in the second one are complexes composed of several protein subunits. Interestingly, most of the 5-HT receptors belong to the GPCR superfamily and only the $5\text{-}HT_3$ receptor is a LGICR.

1. G-PROTEIN COUPLED RECEPTORS

With the introduction of the binding techniques, two types of 5-HT binding sites have been distinguished on the basis of their respective affinity for serotonin itself. Thus, $5\text{-}HT_1$ sites were characterized by a high affinity (Kd nanomolar), and $5\text{-}HT_2$ sites by a low affinity (Kd micromolar) for the indoleamine. The subsequent discovery of central 5-HT$_3$ and 5-HT$_4$ receptors with micromolar affinity for 5-HT further contributed to caracterize 5-HT$_1$ sites as the only ones with a high affinity for the endogenous ligand. However, 5-HT$_1$ sites are now recognized as a heterogeneous family with 5 different subtypes called 5-HT$_{1A}$, 5-HT$_{1B}$, 5-HT$_{1C}$, 5-HT$_{1D}$ and 5-HT$_{1E}$ (Fig.1). Except the 5-HT$_{1E}$ site, all the others also exhibit a high affinity (nanomolar) for 5-carboxamidotryptamine (5-CT).

1.1. 5-HT$_{1A}$ receptors

The 5-HT$_{1A}$ subtype is characterized by its unique high (nanomolar) affinity for the non-indolic agonist 8-hydroxy-2-(di-n-propylamino)tetralin (8-OH-DPAT, Gozlan et al., 1983). Autoradiographic studies with radioactive ([^{3}H], [^{125}I]) derivatives of this molecule allowed the visualization of 5-HT$_{1A}$ receptor binding sites, especially in the limbic system (hippocampus, septum, entorhinal cortex, amygdala) and the anterior raphe nuclei. Further investigations in 5,7-dihydroxytryptamine (5,7-DHT)-treated rats (Vergé et al., 1986) and with specific anti-5-HT$_{1A}$ receptor antibodies (Sotelo et al., 1990) indicated that 5-HT$_{1A}$ receptors within the dorsal and median raphe nuclei are in fact autoreceptors located on the somas and dendrites of serotoninergic neurons. In other structures, these receptors are located postsynaptically with respect to afferent serotoninergic projections. The stimulation of 5-HT$_{1A}$ autoreceptors by specific agonists induces a dramatic reduction in the firing rate of 5-HT neurons (Sprouse and Aghajanian, 1987) and the release of 5-HT from their terminals. Thus, agonists acting at these autoreceptors exert an inhibitory influence on central serotoninergic neurotransmission. This action is very probably responsible for the anxiolytic-like effects of the azapirones (buspirone, gepirone, ipsapirone) and other more recently developed 5-HT$_{1A}$ receptor agonists (Griebel et al., 1992).

On the postsynaptic neuronal targets of serotoninergic projections, 5-HT$_{1A}$ receptors are negatively coupled to adenylate cyclase (Fig.1) via a pertussis toxin (PTX)-sensitive Gi protein. Expression of the cloned gene confirmed the negative coupling to adenylate cyclase but when the expression was performed in various cells types, a coupling to phospholipase C could also occur, probably due to the unusual interaction of the 5-HT$_{1A}$ receptor protein with Gq proteins in some of these cells (Raymond et al., 1992).

In line with the aminoacid sequence homology between the 5-HT$_{1A}$ receptor and the ß$_2$-adrenergic receptor, some ß-antagonists bind the 5-HT$_{1A}$ receptor with a relatively high affinity. Interestingly, a single aminoacid residue (Asn^{385}) in the 7th transmembrane domain (TM7) of the 5-HT$_{1A}$ receptor seems to be responsible for this property (Guan et al., 1992).

Extensive studies on the respective biochemical and pharmacological properties of pre- (i.e. on the somas and dendrites of 5-HT neurons) and postsynaptic 5-HT$_{1A}$ receptors have shown that they are nearly identical. However, differences in their functional expression and regulation have been reported. Thus, some compounds (buspirone...) are full agonists at somatodentritic 5-HT$_{1A}$ autoreceptors but act as partial agonists at postsynaptic 5-HT$_{1A}$ receptors. In addition, some antagonists (NAN-190, BMY 7378) are able to completely inhibit postsynaptic responses but stimulate -partially- somatodentritic 5-HT$_{1A}$ autoreceptors. Among the hypotheses which have been put forward to explain these differences, the existence of a 5-HT$_{1A}$ receptor reserve on the somas and dendrites of 5-HT neurons but not on their postsynaptic targets (Meller et al., 1990) is probably one of the more plausible possibilities. In addition, Boddeke et al. (1992) have shown that the intrinsic activity of a ligand not only depends on its chemical structure but also on the number of receptors expressed at the cell surface. Potent and selective 5-HT$_{1A}$ receptor ligands (notably antagonists such as WAY-100135 and WAY-100635) have recently been developed. They

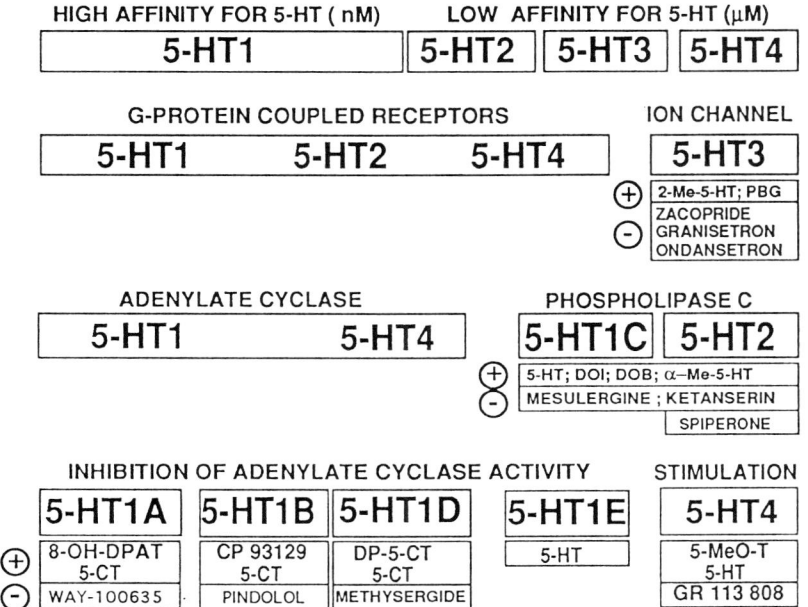

Fig. 1: Main properties of pharmacologically identified 5-HT receptors in the central nervous system. (+) : agonists ; (-) : antagonists.

Table 1: Characteristics of the cloned 5-HT receptors

Receptor	Species	aa	introns	Chromosomic localization	mRNA (kb)
$5\text{-}HT_{1A}$	man	421	no	5q11.2-2-q13	6.0
	rat	422	no		3.3-3.9
$5\text{-}HT_{1B\alpha}$	rat	374-377	no		
$5\text{-}HT_{1B\beta}$	rat	386	no		6.0-6.8
	mouse	386	no		6.0
$5\text{-}HT_{1D\alpha}$	man	377	no	1p34.3-36.3	
$5\text{-}HT_{1D\beta}$	man	390	no	6q12-q13	5.5-5.6
$5\text{-}HT_{1EA}$	man	365	no		5.3
$5\text{-}HT_{1EB}$	man	366	no		
$5\text{-}HT_{1C}$	man	458	yes	X	5.2
	rat	460	yes		
	mouse	459	yes	X	
$5\text{-}HT_2$	man	471	yes	13q14-q21	5.0-6.0
	rat	471	yes		
$5\text{-}HT_3$	mouse	487	yes		2.2
$5\text{-}HT_{5A}$	mouse	357	yes	7q36	
$5\text{-}HT_{5B}$	mouse	370	yes	2q11-13	
$5\text{-}HT_6$	rat	437	yes ?		4.2

aa: number of aminoacid residues in the coded protein; introns: "yes" for the presence and "no" for the absence of introns in the gene; chromosomic localization of the encoding gene.

should help to understand the actual reasons for the differences between the actions of ligands at somatodendritic and postsynaptic 5-HT$_{1A}$ receptors.

1.2. 5-HT$_{1B}$ and 5-HT$_{1D}$ receptors

The 5-HT$_{1B}$ subtype was originally described in the rat brain as a 5-HT$_1$ site having a low affinity for spiperone and 8-OH-DPAT. This site is also characterized by a high affinity (nM) for some β-adrenergic antagonists. The density of 5-HT$_{1B}$ sites is high in extrapyramidal areas (substantia nigra, globus pallidus), the superior colliculus and the dorsal subiculum. In addition, these sites also exist in the hippocampus, cerebral cortex and cerebellum. A 5-HT$_1$ site with the same regional distribution but different pharmacological properties (i.e. low affinity for β-adrenergic antagonists) was subsequently found in the brain of other species. This site was called 5-HT$_{1D}$ and was initially thought to be the species homologue of the 5-HT$_{1B}$ receptor (Hoyer and Middlemiss, 1989).

However, 5-HT$_{1D}$ sites were also found in the rat brain (Herrick-Davis and Titeler, 1988) and further binding studies clearly indicated that they correspond to a heterogeneous class (Mahle et al., 1991). Evidence for heterogeneity also derived from biochemical investigations aimed at identifying the transduction mechanisms of 5-HT$_{1B}$ and 5-HT$_{1D}$ receptors. Thus, both receptor types are negatively coupled to adenylate cyclase (Fig.1) in the substantia nigra of the rat (Bouhelal et al., 1988) and the calf (Hoyer and Schoeffter, 1988). However, this coupling was not found in the calf striatum (Waeber et Palacios, 1990) and one report indicated that 5-HT$_{1B}$ receptors in the rat hippocampus were affected neither by PTX nor by cholera toxin (Blier, 1991), in contrast to that expected for receptors coupled to adenylate cyclase.

Therefore, both 5-HT$_{1B}$ and 5-HT$_{1D}$ receptors, and even subtypes of each, probably exist in the brain of all mammalian species, where they may interact with different transduction mechanisms.

The recent cloning of two genes encoding distinct 5-HT$_{1D}$ receptors in the human brain and of two other genes coding for 5-HT receptors with some 5-HT$_{1D}$-like properties (Matthes et al., 1993), in addition to the cloning of two distinct 5-HT$_{1B}$ receptor genes in rodents (Bach et al., 1993), provided an elegant and clearcut demonstration of the 5-HT$_{1B}$/5-HT$_{1D}$ receptor heterogeneity (Table 1).

Thus, a human, intronless, 5-HT$_{1D\beta}$ gene has been cloned and claimed to correspond to the rat 5-HT$_{1B\beta}$, with which it shares 93% identity (Adham et al., 1992). However, some pharmacological differences exist and especially, the affinity of the 5-HT$_{1D\beta}$ receptor for ß-adrenergic antagonists is markedly less than that of the 5-HT$_{1B\beta}$ receptor. Apparently, a single amino acid residue is responsible for this difference as the replacement of Thr^{355} by an asparagine renders the pharmacological properties of the 5-HT$_{1D\beta}$ receptors identical to those of the 5-HT$_{1B\beta}$ receptor (Oksenberg et al., 1992). Interestingly, this asparagine naturally exists in the 5-HT$_{1A}$ and 5-HT$_{1B\beta}$ receptors, where this residue plays a key role in their affinity for some ß-adrenergic antagonists.

In addition to the 5-HT$_{1D\beta}$ receptor gene, a second gene encoding another 5-HT$_{1D}$ receptor called 5-HT$_{1D\alpha}$, has also been cloned in the human brain (Hartig et al., 1992). Despite a relatively low degree of homology between their amino sequences, the 5-HT$_{1D\alpha}$ and 5-HT$_{1D\beta}$ receptors exhibit nearly identical pharmacological properties. Very recently, Bach et al. (1993) described the successful cloning of a new gene encoding another 5-HT$_{1B}$ receptor in the rat, i.e. the 5-HT$_{1B\alpha}$. So far, very little is known about this second 5-HT$_{1B}$ receptor, but preliminary data indicated that its pharmacological properties are markedly different from those of the 5-HT$_{1B\beta}$ receptor. The latter receptor seems to be the most abundant within the 5-HT$_{1B}$ family (Voigt et al., 1991). As expected from previous studies on brain tissues, the cloned 5-HT$_{1D\alpha}$, 5-HT$_{1D\beta}$ and 5-HT$_{1B\beta}$ receptors were found to be negatively coupled to adenylate cyclase in competent cells transfected with their genes (Hartig et al., 1992).

In vitro as well as in vivo studies have shown that the 5-HT autoreceptor which is responsible for the negative control that 5-HT exerts on its own release from nerve endings has pharmacological properties typical of 5-HT$_{1B}$ receptors in the rat and of 5-HT$_{1D}$ receptors in non-rodent species (Hoyer and Middlemiss, 1989). Therefore, 5-HT$_{1B}$/5-HT$_{1D}$ autoreceptors probably exist on 5-HT terminals, although binding studies with appropriate radioligands failed to provide a direct demonstration of this location. Recently, Doucet et al. (1993) found that the in situ hybridization signal corresponding to 5-HT$_{1B\beta}$ mRNA within the dorsal raphe nucleus disappeared after the selective lesion of 5-HT neurons by 5,7-DHT in the rat. Accordingly, the 5-HT$_{1B\beta}$ receptor is very probably synthesized by these neurons, as expected from their autoreceptor function at the level of 5-HT terminals.

To date, selective ligands for each 5-HT$_{1B}$/5-HT$_{1D}$ receptor subtype are not available. However, the high affinity of the 5-HT$_{1B\beta}$ receptor for some ß-adrenergic antagonists ((-)pindolol, (-)penbutolol, (-)propranolol) is especially helpful in distinguishing this receptor from 5-HT$_{1D}$ receptors. Recently, a more selective compound, CP 93129, was found to have a much higher affinity for 5-HT$_{1B}$ binding sites (Ki = 8.1 nM) than for 5-HT$_{1D}$ sites (Ki = 1100 nM) in brain tissues (Koe et al., 1992). Conversely, dipropylamino-5-CT (DP-5-CT), methysergide and some α_2 adrenergic receptor antagonists (idazoxan, rauwolscine) have a better affinity for 5-HT$_{1D}$ than for 5-HT$_{1B}$ sites. The development of specific ligands for each class of 5-HT$_{1B}$/5-HT$_{1D}$ receptors will undoubtedly be of great interest for identifying their functional implications. In addition, much can be expected from such drugs as potential therapeutic agents if one considers, for instance, the marked improvement in the acute treatment of migraine which has been achieved with the introduction of sumatriptan. This drug is a rather selective 5-HT$_{1D}$ receptor agonist, but the receptor subtype at which it acts to stop migraine has not yet been identified.

1.3. 5-HT$_{1E}$ receptors:

Leonhardt et al. (1989) were the first to report that the occupancy of 5-HT$_{1A}$, 5-HT$_{1B}$/5-HT$_{1D}$ and 5-HT$_{1C}$ sites by selective unlabeled ligands in membranes from the human brain still allows [^{3}H]5-HT to recognize an additional high affinity binding site, that they named 5-HT$_{1E}$. Subsequently, additional studies demonstrated that these sites also exist in the brain of various animal species, especially in the caudate nucleus and putamen. The 5-HT$_{1E}$ binding sites are clearly distinct from other 5-HT$_1$ receptors, as they are the only ones within this family to display a low (Ki in the micromolar range) affinity for 5-CT. No selective radioligand is presently available for the specific labeling of 5-HT$_{1E}$ sites, and 5-HT itself is the only high affinity ligand (Fig.1). Studies with brain membranes indicated that the specific binding of [^{3}H]5-HT to 5-HT$_{1E}$ sites can be inhibited by GppNHp and GTP-γ-S, as expected of receptors from the GPCR superfamily (Leonhardt et al., 1989). However, only studies with cells transfected with the 5-HT$_{1E}$ receptor gene allowed the demonstration of its negative coupling to adenylate cyclase (Mc Allister et al., 1992; Adham et al., 1993).

In fact, two genes apparently code for receptors with 5-HT$_{1E}$-like pharmacological properties in the mouse brain, which led to the distinction of 5-HT$_{1E\alpha}$ and 5-HT$_{1E\beta}$ receptors (Table 1). Sumatriptan, yohimbine and 5-MeO-DMT are better recognized by 5-HT$_{1E\beta}$ than 5-HT$_{1E\alpha}$ receptors, whereas the reverse is true for 5-HT and methiothepin (Adham et al., 1993). In situ hybridization studies revealed that large pyramidal cells in the frontal and piriform cortices contain the 5-HT$_{1E\beta}$ receptor mRNA. In addition, this mRNA is also found in large neurons of the dorsal raphe nucleus, and, to a lesser extent, in pyramidal cells of the CA1-CA3 fields of the Ammon horn and the dentate gyrus of the hippocampus (Adham et al., 1993). The brain distribution of 5-HT$_{1E}$ binding sites and 5-HT$_{1E\beta}$ receptor mRNA suggests that these receptors may participate in the control of various functions and behaviors, but only pharmacological studies with selective 5-HT$_{1E\alpha/1E\beta}$ ligands would provide clearcut data in this respect. Unfortunately, no such ligands have yet been developed.

1.4. 5-HT$_{1C}$ and 5-HT$_2$ receptors

5-HT$_{1C}$ receptors were first identified as [^{3}H]5-HT high affinity binding sites with a unique pharmacological profile in the rat choroid plexus (Palacios et al., 1990). Although the affinity of 5-HT$_{1C}$ receptors for 5-HT is about two orders of magnitude higher than that of 5-HT$_2$ receptors (identified with a selective antagonist radioligand), extensive studies with numerous agonists and antagonists have shown that both receptor types have very similar pharmacological properties. Nevertheless, some drugs allow their distinction as, for instance, spiperone has a 1000-fold higher affinity for 5-HT$_2$ than for 5-HT$_{1C}$ sites. Conversely, mianserin is a more potent antagonist at 5-HT$_{1C}$ than 5-HT$_2$ receptors. 5-HT$_{1C}$ sites are particularly abundant in the choroid plexus of all mammalian species, and they can also be detected in limbic and extrapyramidal areas (Palacios et al., 1990). Epithelial cells are the only cell type expressing 5-HT$_{1C}$ receptors within the choroid plexus. At this level, the stimulation of 5-HT$_{1C}$ receptors by endogenous 5-HT (that is naturally present in the cerebral ventricles) might influence the secretion of specific proteins into the cerebrospinal fluid.

The 5-HT$_2$ receptor in fact corresponds to the D receptor which was initially identified by Gaddum and Picarelli (1957) in the guinea pig ileum. High densities of 5-HT$_2$ receptor binding sites, usually labeled with [^{3}H]ketanserin, exist in the cerebral cortex, especially its frontal zone where they are probably located (in part) on GABAergic interneurons. The claustrum, hippocampus (subiculum), basal ganglia (caudate putamen) and nucleus accumbens also contain 5-HT$_2$ receptors, but at a generally lower density (Palacios et al., 1990).

Cloning of the 5-HT$_{1C}$ and 5-HT$_2$ receptor genes confirmed that these receptors are closely related. Thus, a 78% homology exists between their aminoacid sequences within the transmembrane domains. Both genes contain introns, in contrast to those encoding 5-HT$_{1A}$, 5-HT$_{1B}$ and 5-HT$_{1D}$ receptors (Table 1). Because of these similarities regarding their molecular features and pharmacological properties, 5-HT$_{1C}$ and 5-HT$_2$ receptors are currently considered as two members of the same subfamily of 5-HT receptors. A further confirmation of their close relationships derives from the functional properties of 5-HT$_{1C}$ and 5-HT$_2$ receptors as both are positively coupled to phospholipase C (Fig.1) and negatively coupled to K$^+$ channels in the brain as well as in cells transfected with the corresponding genes.

5-HT$_2$ receptors seem to be involved in several behavioral processes, but, as suggested by Leysen (1990), their stimulation by endogenous 5-HT might occur solely under pathological conditions. 5-HT$_2$ antagonists exhibit potential therapeutic interest in the treatment of sleep disorders, schizophrenia, depression and anxiety, possibly through functional interactions between 5-HT$_2$ receptors and 5-HT$_{1A}$ receptors in the CNS.

1.5. 5-HT$_4$ and related receptors

These receptors were first characterized by their positive coupling to adenylate cyclase in brain neurons (Bockaert et al., 1992; Fig.1). In all cells where they have been found, the stimulation of 5-HT$_4$ receptors produces an increased accumulation of intracellular cyclic AMP which ends with the closure of specific K$^+$ channels due to phosphorylation by protein kinase A. Among drugs that recognize (with a moderate affinity) 5-HT$_4$ receptors are some 5-HT$_3$ antagonists which can act either as agonists (zacopride) or antagonists (tropisetron) at 5-HT$_4$ receptors. The recent availability of selective ligands will probably contribute to a better knowledge of these receptors. In particular, an indolic compound, GR 113808, has recently been shown to be a competitive antagonist with a high affinity and selectivity for 5-HT$_4$ receptors (Fig.1). Autoradiographic studies with its tritiated derivative revealed that these receptors are present mainly in extrapyramidal areas (substantia nigra, caudate-putamen, globus pallidus, olfactory tubercles) and hippocampus in the rat, guinea pig and man (Dumuis, personal communication).

The structure of the 5-HT$_4$ receptor is not yet known. However, Monsma et al. (1993) recently cloned another receptor, called 5-HT$_6$ (Table 1), which might be related to the 5-HT$_4$ type as it is also positively coupled to adenylate cyclase. Nevertheless, marked differences exist between the respective pharmacological properties of these two receptor types. Interestingly, the 5-HT$_6$ receptor has a rather high affinity for tricyclic antidepressant and antipsychotic drugs (Monsma et al., 1993).

1.6. 5-HT$_5$ Receptors

The discovery of the 5-HT$_5$ receptors only derives from the application of molecular biology techniques to the mouse brain (Matthes et al., 1993). Indeed, two genes, with one intron each, have been cloned (Table 1). Their expression in transfected Cos-7 cells results in the GPCR-like receptor binding sites called 5-HT$_{5A}$ and 5-HT$_{5B}$ with high affinity for 5-HT and 5-CT, and low affinity for sumatriptan, indicating pharmacological profiles different from those of 5-HT$_{1E}$ and 5-HT$_{1D}$ receptors, respectively. To date, the coupling mechanisms of the 5-HT$_5$ receptors is not known, as neither adenylate cyclase nor phospholipase C could be modulated by 5-HT in Cos-7 cells transfected with the corresponding genes. The distinction between 5-HT$_{5A}$ and 5-HT$_{5B}$ receptors is based on differences not only in their aminoacid sequences but also in their pharmacological properties and regional distributions of encoding mRNAs. Thus, the 5-HT$_{5A}$ receptor has a low (micromolar) affinity for 8-OH-DPAT, whereas the 5-HT$_{5B}$ receptor binds this ligand with a high (nanomolar) affinity. In situ hybridization histochemistry showed that 5-HT$_{5A}$ mRNA exists in the cerebral cortex, hippocampus, olfactory bulb and the granular layer of the cerebellum, but not in the basal ganglia. 5-HT$_{5B}$ mRNA is located in the habenula, CA1 area of the hippocampus, dorsal raphe nucleus and cerebellum (Matthes et al., 1993).

The functional roles of these receptors are completely unknown. Selective agonists and antagonists are urgently needed to provide some keys to this pending problem.

2. LIGAND-GATED ION CHANNEL: 5-HT$_3$ RECEPTORS

5-HT$_3$ receptors were initially discovered at the periphery, where they correspond to the M receptor described 36 years ago by Gaddum and Picarelli (1957). As soon as selective 5-HT$_3$ receptor antagonists were available, studies in rats and mice revealed their potential anxiolytic, promnesic and antipsychotic properties, as expected of drugs acting in the CNS.

The direct proof of the existence of 5-HT$_3$ receptors in brain was provided by Kilpatrick et al. (1987) who used the selective radioligand [^{3}H]GR 65630 for their specific labeling in rat brain membranes. At present, numerous selective and potent 5-HT$_3$ antagonists such as ondansetron, tropisetron, granisetron and zacopride are available (Fig.1). In contrast, only few agonists have been developed so far (2-methyl-5-HT, phenylbiguanide, 3-chlorophenyl-biguanide).

5-HT$_3$ receptors are located in limbic areas (entorhinal cortex, hippocampus, amygdala), but they are especially abundant in the nucleus of the solitary tract (NTS) within the dorso-vagal complex. At this level, 5-HT$_3$ receptors are almost exclusively located on the terminals of vagal afferent fibres. Indirect evidence of the preferential location of these receptors on axon terminals has also been reported for other brain areas, therefore suggesting that 5-HT$_3$ receptors may be involved in the presynaptic modulation of the release of various neurotransmitters in brain (Hamon, 1992).

The functional responses triggered by the stimulation of 5-HT$_3$ receptors have been investigated mainly using electrophysiological techniques. The activation of 5-HT$_3$ receptors induces a rapid depolarization due to cation influx through the receptor-channel (Fig.1). The ionic selectivity of this channel is limited, since in addition to Na$^+$ and K$^+$, organic cations such as Tris are able to pass through the opened channel. Continuous exposure to agonists leads to rapid desensitization of 5-HT$_3$ receptors.

Heterogeneity of 5-HT$_3$ receptors has frequently been evoked, but it is usually proposed that species differences in the same receptor type rather than distinct receptors account for the variations noted in their pharmacological properties from one tissue to another (Kilpatrick and Tyers, 1992). However, this explanation seems incompatible with the fact that an antisense probe which binds the mRNA encoding a 5-HT$_3$ receptor subunit in brain (Table 1) does not allow its detection in the intestine, where, however, 5-HT$_3$ receptors are especially abundant (Maricq et al., 1991).

To date, only the antiemetic properties of 5-HT$_3$ receptor antagonists are firmly established, and these drugs are regularly used for preventing nausea and emesis in patients subjected to anti-cancer therapy. In contrast, the anxiolytic-like effects of 5-HT$_3$ antagonists, as well as their antipsychotic-like properties that have been reported in relevant animal models, are still the matter of debate because no such effects have been observed in man. Nevertheless, some promnesic effects have been reported for 5-HT$_3$ antagonists in rats, monkeys and also in man (Preston et al., 1992), suggesting that these drugs may still have potential therapeutic application(s) in addition to the prevention of nausea associated with anti-cancer therapy.

REFERENCES

Adham, N., Kao, H.-T., Schechter, L.E., Bard, J., Olsen, M., Urquhart, D., Durkin, M., Hartig, P.R., Weinshank, R.L. & Branchek, T.A. (1993): Cloning of another human serotonin receptor (5-HT$_{1F}$): A fifth 5-HT$_1$ receptor subtype coupled to the inhibition of adenylate cyclase. *Proc. Natl. Acad. Sci. USA* 90, 408-412.

Adham, N., Romanienko, P., Hartig, P., Weinshank, R.L. & Branchek, T. (1992): The rat 5-hydroxytryptamine$_{1B}$ receptor is the species homologue of the human 5-hydroxytryptamine$_{1D\beta}$ receptor. *Mol. Pharmacol.* 41, 1-7.

Bach, A.W.J., Unger, L., Sprengel, R., Mengod, G., Palacios, J., Seeburg, P.H. & Voigt, M.M. (1993): Structure, functional expression and spatial distribution of a cloned cDNA encoding a rat 5-HT$_{1D}$-like receptor. *J. Recept. Res.* 13, 479-502.

Blier, P. (1991): Terminal serotonin autoreceptor function in the rat hippocampus is not modified by pertussis and cholera toxins. *Naunyn-Schmiedeberg's Arch. Pharmacol.* 344, 160-166.

Bockaert, J., Fozard, J.R., Dumuis, A. & Clarke, D.E. (1992): The 5-HT$_4$ receptor: A place in the sun. *Trends Pharmacol. Sci.* 13, 141-145.

Boddeke, H.W.G.M., Fargin, A., Raymond, J.R., Schoeffter, P. & Hoyer, D. (1992): Agonist/antagonist interactions with cloned human 5-HT$_{1A}$ receptors: Variations in intrinsic activity studied in transfected HeLa cells. *Naunyn-Schmiedeberg's Arch. Pharmacol.* 345, 257-263.

Bouhelal, R., Smounya, L. & Bockaert, J. (1988): 5-HT$_{1B}$ receptors are negatively coupled with adenylate cyclase in rat substantia nigra. *Eur. J. Pharmacol.* 151, 189-196.

Doucet, E., Emerit, M.B., Pohl, M., El Mestikawy, S., Adrien, J., Berger, B. & Hamon, M. (1993): In situ hybridization evidence of the synthesis of 5-HT$_{1B}$ receptors in central serotoninergic neurons. *Soc. Neurosci.* (in press).

Gaddum, J.H. & Picarelli, Z.P. (1957): Two kinds of tryptamine receptors. *Br. J. Pharmacol.* 12, 323-328.

Gozlan, H., El Mestikawy, S., Pichat, L., Glowinski, J. & Hamon, M. (1983): Identification of presynaptic serotonin autoreceptors using a new ligand: [^{3}H]PAT. *Nature* 305, 140-142.

Griebel, G., Misslin, R., Pawlowski, M., Guardiola-Lemaitre, B., Guillaumet, G. & Bizot-Espiard, J. (1992) Anxiolytic-like effects of a selective 5-HT$_{1A}$ agonist, S 20244, and its enantiomers in mice. *NeuroReport* 3, 84-86.

Guan, X.-M., Peroutka, S.J. & Kobilka, B.K. (1992): Identification of a single amino acid residue responsible for the binding of a class of ß-adrenergic receptor antagonists to 5-hydroxytryptamine$_{1A}$ receptors. *Mol. Pharmacol.* 41, 695-698.

Hamon, M. ed. (1992): Central and peripheral 5-HT$_3$ receptors, London: Academic Press, 314 p.

Hartig, P.R., Branchek, T.A. & Weinshank, R.L. (1992): A subfamily of 5-HT$_{1D}$ receptor genes. *Trends Pharmacol. Sci.* 13, 152-159.

Herrick-Davis, K. & Titeler, M. (1988): Detection and characterization of the serotonin 5-HT$_{1D}$ receptor in rat and human brain. *J. Neurochem.* 50, 1624-1631.

Hoyer, D. & Middlemiss, D.N. (1989): Species differences in the pharmacology of terminal 5-HT autoreceptors in mammalian brain. *Trends Pharmacol. Sci.* 10, 130-132.

Hoyer, D. & Schoeffter, P. (1988): 5-HT$_{1D}$ receptor-mediated inhibition of forskolin-stimulated adenylate cyclase activity in calf substantia nigra. *Eur. J. Pharmacol.* 147, 145-147.

Kilpatrick, G.J. & Tyers, M.B. (1992): Inter-species variants of the 5-HT$_3$ receptor. *Biochem. Soc. Trans.* 20, 118-121.

Kilpatrick, G.J., Jones, B.J. & Tyers, M.B. (1987): Identification and distribution of 5-HT$_3$ receptors in rat brain using radioligand binding. *Nature* 330, 746-748.

Koe, B.K., Lebel, L.A., Fox, C.B. & Macor, J.E. (1992): Characterization of [^{3}H]CP-96,501 as a selective radioligand for the serotonin 5-HT$_{1B}$ receptor: Binding studies in rat brain membranes. *J. Neurochem.* 58, 1268-1276.

Leonhardt, S., Herrick-Davis, K. & Titeler, M. (1989): Detection of a novel serotonin receptor subtype (5-HT$_{1E}$) in human brain: Interaction with a GTP-binding protein. *J. Neurochem.* 53, 465-471.

Leysen, J.E. (1990): Gaps and peculiarities in 5-HT$_2$ receptor studies. *Neuropsychopharmacology* 3, 361-369.

Mahle, C.D., Nowak, H.P., Mattson, R.J., Hurt, S.D. & Yocca, F.D. (1991): [^{3}H]5-carboxamidotryptamine labels multiple high affinity 5-HT$_{1D}$-like sites in guinea pig brain. *Eur. J. Pharmacol.* 205, 323-324.

Maricq, A.V., Peterson, A.S., Brake, A.J., Myers, R.M. & Julius, D. (1991): Primary structure and functional expression of the 5-HT$_3$ receptor, a serotonin-gated ion channel. *Science* 254, 432-437.

Matthes, H., Boschert, U., Amlaiky, N., Grailhe, R., Plassat, J.-L., Muscatelli, F., Mattei, M.-G. & Hen, R. (1993): Mouse 5-hydroxytryptamine$_{5A}$ and 5-hydroxytryptamine$_{5B}$ receptors define a new family of serotonin receptors: Cloning, functional expression, and chromosomal localization. *Mol. Pharmacol.* 43, 313-319.

McAllister, G., Charlesworth, A., Snodin, C., Beer, M.S., Noble, A.J., Middlemiss, D.N., Iversen, L.L. & Whiting, P. (1992): Molecular cloning of a serotonin receptor from human brain (5-HT$_{1E}$): A fith 5-HT$_1$-like subtype. *Proc. Natl. Acad. Sci. USA* 89, 5517-5521.

Meller, E., Goldstein, M. & Bohmaker, K. (1990): Receptor reserve for 5-hydroxytryptamine$_{1A}$-mediated inhibition of serotonin synthesis: Possible relationship to anxiolytic properties of 5-hydroxytryptamine$_{1A}$ agonists. *Mol. Pharmacol.* 37, 231-237.

Monsma, F.J.,Jr., Shen, Y., Ward, R.P., Hamblin, M.W. & Sibley, D.R. (1993): Cloning and expression of a novel serotonin receptor with high affinity for tricyclic psychotropic drugs. *Mol. Pharmacol.* 43, 320-327.

Oksenberg, D., Marsters, S.A., O'Dowd, B.F., Jin, H., Havlik, S., Peroutka, S.J. & Ashkenazi, A. (1992): A single amino-acid difference confers major pharmacological variation between human and rodent 5-HT$_{1B}$ receptors. *Nature* 360, 161-163.

Palacios, J.M., Waeber, C., Hoyer, D. & Mengod, G. (1990): Distribution of serotonin receptors. *Ann. N.Y. Acad. Sci.* 600, 36-52.

Preston, G.C., Milton, D.S., Ceuppens, P.R. & Warburton, D.M. (1992): Effects of the 5-HT$_3$ receptor antagonist GR 68755 on a scopolamine-induced cognitive deficit in healthy volunteers. *Brit. J. Clin. Pharmacol.* 70, 546.

Raymond, J.R., Albers, F.J. & Middleton, J.P. (1992): Functional expression of human 5-HT$_{1A}$ receptors and differential coupling to second messengers in CHO cells. *Naunyn-Schmiedeberg's Arch. Pharmacol.* 346, 127-137.

Sotelo, C., Cholley, B., El Mestikawy, S., Gozlan, H. & Hamon, M. (1990): Direct immunohistochemical evidence of the existence of 5-HT$_{1A}$ autoreceptors on serotoninergic neurons in the midbrain raphe nuclei. *Eur. J. Neurosci.* 2, 1144-1154.

Sprouse, J.S. & Aghajanian, G.K. (1987): Electrophysiological responses of serotonergic dorsal raphe neurons to 5-HT$_{1A}$ and 5-HT$_{1B}$ agonists. *Synapse* 1,3-9.

Vergé, D., Daval, G., Marcinkiewicz, M., El Mestikawy, S., Gozlan, H. & Hamon, M. (1986): Quantitative autoradiography of multiple 5-HT$_1$ receptor subtypes in the brain of control or 5,7-dihydroxytryptamine-treated rats. *J. Neurosci.* 6, 3474-3482.

Voigt, M.M., Laurie, D.J., Seeburg, P.H. & Bach, A. (1991): Molecular cloning and characterization of a rat brain cDNA encoding a 5-hydroxytryptamine$_{1B}$ receptor. *EMBO J.* 10, 4017-4023.

Waeber, C. & Palacios, J.M. (1990): 5-HT$_1$ receptor binding sites in the guinea pig superior colliculus are predominantly of the 5-HT$_{1D}$ class and are presynaptically located on primary retinal afferents. *Brain Res.* 528, 207-211.

Résumé

Les données récentes de la neurobiologie moléculaire confirment l'existence d'une multiplicité de récepteurs pour un même neuromédiateur, et ceci est particulièrement vrai dans le cas de la sérotonine. Quatre classes de récepteurs pour ce neuromédiateur, appelées 5-HT$_1$, 5-HT$_2$, 5-HT$_3$ et 5-HT$_4$, ont été définies sur la base de critères pharmacologiques. A l'exception du récepteur 5-HT$_3$ qui est en fait un canal ionique, tous les autres récepteurs de la sérotonine sont couplés à des protéines G et modulent positivement (5-HT$_4$) ou négativement (5-HT$_{1A}$, 5-HT$_{1B}$, 5-HT$_{1D}$, 5-HT$_{1E}$) l'adénylate cyclase, ou encore la phospholipase C (5-HT$_{1C}$, 5-HT$_2$) voire des canaux ioniques (5-HT$_{1A}$, 5-HT$_{1C}$, 5-HT$_2$). L'application des techniques de clonage a révélé l'existence d'autres récepteurs (5-HT$_5$, 5-HT$_6$) en plus de ceux qui ont été découverts par des approches pharmacologiques. Cependant, leur caractérisation est encore très incomplète, et il sera nécessaire de développer des ligands sélectifs pour en préciser les propriétés fonctionnelles.

IV. Potential anxiolytic drugs - therapeutic perspectives

IV. Anxiolytiques potentiels - perspectives thérapeutiques

Serotonin and anxiety: mixed 5-HT$_{1A}$ agonists - 5-HT$_{1C/2}$ antagonists as potential anxiolytic agents

Mark J. Millan and Mauricette Brocco

Institut de Recherches Servier (I.D.R.S.), 7, rue Ampère, 92800 Puteaux, France

SUMMARY

An overactivity of ascending serotoninergic pathways plays an important role in the pathogenesis of anxiety. In analogy to benzodiazepines, the activity of these projections is inhibited by 5-HT$_{1A}$ autoreceptors which mediate, correspondingly, anxiolytic actions. In addition, whereas postsynaptic 5-HT$_{1C/2}$ and, possibly, 5-HT$_3$ receptors may mediate the anxiogenic effects of 5-HT, postsynaptic 5-HT$_{1A}$ receptors may act oppositely; that is, like their presynaptic counterparts, to reduce anxiety. This paper provides a possible mechanistic basis for such actions and hypothesises that a synergistic 5-HT$_{1A}$ agonist - 5-HT$_{1C/2}$ antagonist action might be associated with a particularly efficacious anxiolytic action. This hypothesis was explored with the novel ligands, S 14506 and S 14671, which display such joint properties. Under certain conditions, their effects are, indeed, superior to those of 5-HT$_{1A}$ agonists, 5-HT$_{1C/2}$ antagonists or benzodiazepines. Nevertheless, this theory requires a more extensive evaluation before a final conclusion can be reached.

INTRODUCTION

The traditional treatment of anxiety with benzodiazepines (BZPs) presents several major problems (see Barrett, 1992; Barrett and Gleeson, 1991; Lader, 1991; Millan *et al.*, 1992a; Traber and Glaser, 1987; Treit, 1991). *First*, upon long-term treatment, tolerance may develop to their anxiolytic actions; that is, for a given dose, therapeutic efficacy progressively declines and an increase in dose is required to restore the original effect. *Second*, long-term exposure is associated with the development of dependence; that is, upon discontinuation of their administration, a withdrawal syndrome is seen. *Third*, BZPs exert highly disruptive side effects (e.g. sedation and amnesia). *Fourth*, BZPs are of limited utility in the management of anxiety-related diseases such as phobic anxiety, panic attacks and obsessive-convulsive disorders. These observations emphasize the need for novel approaches for the treatment of anxiety and the following sections discuss the significance of central serotoninergic pathways in this respect.

SEROTONIN AND ANXIETY

There exist major ascending serotoninergic projections from midbrain raphe nuclei to the cortex, limbic system (amygdala, hippocampus, nucleus accumbens and olfactory tubercule) and to the periaqueductal grey (PAG) (Törk, 1990); these target structures are intimately involved in the integration of the processes underlying anxiety and there is evidence that anxiety relates to an overactivity of these ascending serotoninergic pathways. Indeed, BZPs are thought to exert their anxiolytic actions (at least partially) by an inhibition of serotoninergic transmission to these regions (Barrett and Gleeson, 1991; Deakin, 1988; Lader, 1991; Schweizer and Rickels, 1991; Treit, 1991).

A key feature of the pharmacology of 5-HT is the existence of a *multiplicity* of receptor types via which it exerts its actions. These are currently defined as 5-HT$_1$, 5-HT$_2$, 5-HT$_3$ and 5-HT$_4$, though subclasses of these types as well as several other classes of 5-HT receptor also exist (Hoyer and Schoeffter, 1991; Glennon and Lucki, 1988). In the context of anxiety, 5-HT$_{1A}$ receptors have emerged as of especial pertinence. Indeed, the "partial" 5-HT$_{1A}$ agonist, buspirone, displays anxiolytic properties in man and it was the recognition that buspirone possesses substantial affinity for 5-HT$_{1A}$ receptors which originally suggested the possibility of treating anxiety via a specific action at this receptor type. Notably, 5-HT$_{1A}$ receptors are enriched in the PAG, cortex and the above-mentioned limbic system structures, all of which are implicated in the control of mood and in the processes underlying anxiety (Pazos et al., 1988). Further, 5-HT$_{1A}$ receptor agonists mimic BZPs in inhibiting ascending serotoninergic transmission (Aghajanian et al., 1978, Millan et al, 1992b). In addition, in a diversity of paradigms of anxiety involving both operant and exploratory end-points, 5-HT$_{1A}$ agonists manifest anxiolytic properties (Barrett and Gleeson, 1991; Treit, 1991) while buspirone and other 5-HT$_{1A}$ agonists display anxiolytic effects in man (see Lader, 1991; Millan et al., 1992a; Schweizer and Rickels, 1991).

PRE- AND POST-SYNAPTIC LOCALIZATION OF 5-HT$_{1A}$ RECEPTORS

5-HT$_{1A}$ receptors are localized not only *post*synaptically but also presynaptically as *inhibitory auto*receptors upon serotoninergic perikarya in raphe nuclei (Aghajanian et al., 1978; Bobker and Williams, 1990). These populations can exert contrasting functional roles in the control of certain parameters (see Glennon and Dukat, 1991; Glennon and Lucki, 1988). For example, 5-HT$_{1A}$ autoreceptors mediate hyperphagia while postsynaptic 5-HT$_{1A}$ receptors mediate corticosterone secretion. However, there is good evidence that *each* of these populations play a role in psychiatric disorders. In fact, both pre- *and* post-synaptic 5-HT$_{1A}$ receptors have been implicated in the anxiolytic (and antidepressant) actions of 5-HT$_{1A}$ agonists athough their respective contributions remain to be further defined (see above references). It may seem surprising that an agonist action at both presynaptic *and* postsynaptic 5-HT$_{1A}$ receptors can be involved in such therapeutic effects but a consideration of their mechanisms of action relative to *other* 5-HT receptor types explains how this might be possible.

NEURONAL MECHANISMS OF ACTION OF 5-HT$_{1A}$ RECEPTORS

As summarized in Figure 1, there is evidence that 5-HT$_{1C}$ receptors mediate the anxiogenic effects of 5-HT - as well as other deleterious effects upon mood (Kennett, 1992; Kennett et al., 1989; Glennon et al., 1991; Lucki, 1992; Murphy et al., 1991; Whitton and Curzon, 1990). Indeed, the 5-HT$_{1C}$ receptor agonist, mCPP, exerts anxiogenic actions in man and there is evidence that antagonism of 5-HT$_{1C}$ receptors is associated with an anxiolytic effect both in experimental models and, possibly, man (Brocco et al., 1990; Ceulemans et al., 1985; Hensman et al., 1991; Kennett, 1992) . There is also evidence that 5-HT$_2$ receptors mediate similar actions and that their antagonism may likewise be beneficial (Benjamin et al., 1992; Deakin, 1988; Motta et al., 1992; Stutzmann et al., 1991). In addition, the putative anxiolytic actions of 5-HT$_3$ antagonists (Barrett and Gleeson, 1991; Treit, 1991) implies that 5-HT$_3$ receptors might also be involved in the expression of anxiogenic actions. That is 5-HT$_{1C}$, 5-HT$_2$ and 5-HT$_3$ receptors mediate a generally negative influence (anxiogenic) which is opposite to that of 5-HT$_{1A}$ agonists (anxiolytic). There is a clear mechanistic basis to this difference in the functional properties of agonists at 5-HT$_{1A}$ as compared to 5-HT$_{1C/2}$ and 5-HT$_3$ receptors which may provide an explanation as to how both postsynaptic 5-HT$_{1A}$ receptors *and* 5-HT$_{1A}$ autoreceptors may mediate anxiolytic actions.

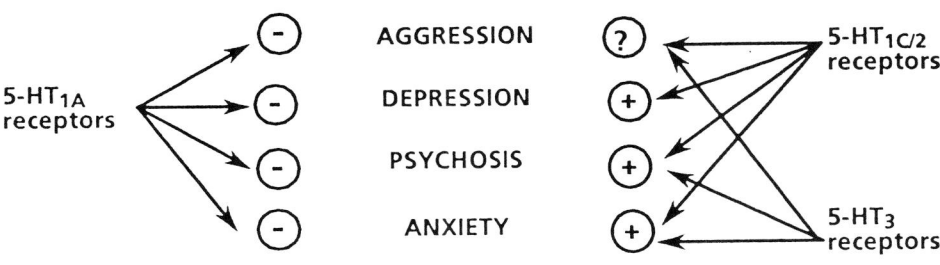

Fig. 1. 5-HT$_{1A}$ receptors may have opposite effects to 5-HT$_{1C/2}$ and 5-HT$_3$ receptors upon mood.

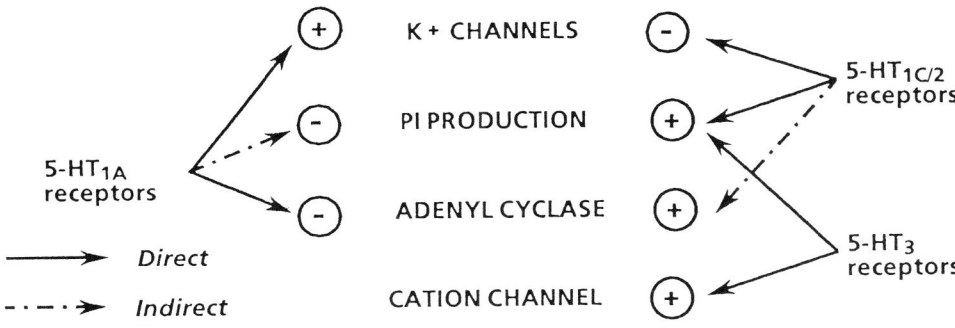

Fig. 2. Differential coupling of 5-HT$_{1A}$ as compared to 5-HT$_{1C/2}$ and 5-HT$_3$ receptors to intracellular transduction mechanisms. Indirect actions may also be expressed under certain conditions.

As indicated in Figure 2, 5-HT$_{1A}$ receptors are positively coupled to K$^+$-ion channels (Bobker and Williams, 1990). Correspondingly, 5-HT$_{1A}$ agonists lead to hyperpolarization and a reduction in cellular excitability (Goldfarb, 1990). That is, 5-HT$_{1A}$ agonists reduce neuronal firing. In addition to this action, 5-HT$_{1A}$ receptors inhibit the activity of adenylate cyclase and may *indirectly* inhibit phosphoinositide turnover under certain physiological conditions (Claustre et al., 1991 and 1988; Fan Liu and Albert, 1988 and 1991; Fargin et al., 1991; Fowler et al., 1991; Hill and Kendall, 1989 and 1992; Hoyer and Schoeffter, 1991; Raymond et al., 1989 and 1991). These second messenger actions are diametrically opposed to those mediated by 5-HT$_{1C/2}$ receptors which depolarize neurones by closing K$^+$-ion channels (Bobker and Williams, 1990; Goldfarb, 1990; Panicker et al., 1991). Further, 5-HT$_{1C/2}$ receptors enhance phosphoinositide turnover and may indirectly augment the activity of adenylate cyclase by increasing intracellular Ca^{2+} (Conn and Sanders-Bush, 1987; Hill and Kendall, 1989 and 1992; Paulssen et al., 1992). Similarly 5-HT$_3$ agonists depolarize neurones by opening cation channels and facilitate phosphoinositide turnover (Bobker and Williams, 1990; Edwards et al., 1991; Hoyer and Schoeffter, 1991). Overall, then, 5-HT$_{1A}$ receptors mediate a decrease in neuronal activity whereas 5-HT$_{1C/2}$ and 5-HT$_3$ receptors mediate an increase in neuronal activity. That is, 5-HT$_{1A}$ receptors and 5-HT$_{1C/2}$ (and 5-HT$_3$) receptors exert *opposite* effects at the cellular level. Now, there are many indications for functional interactions between 5-HT$_{1A}$ and 5-HT$_{1C/2}$ receptors (Bervoets et al., 1990; Glennon et al., 1991) and these have been shown to be co-localized (on the *same* neurones) in structures controlling mood, such the cortex, hippocampus and septum (Araneda et al., 1991; Brandão et al., 1991; Claustre et al., 1988 and 1991; Frances-Davies et al., 1987; Joëls et al., 1987; Stevens et al., 1992; Tan and Miletic, 1992; Van der hooff and Galvan, 1992). Figure 3 explains the relevance of these opposite effects. There are *two* ways in which 5-HT$_{1A}$ agonists can exercise anxiolytic actions. *First*, at 5-HT$_{1A}$ autoreceptors: by inhibiting serotoninergic transmission and thereby diminishing the release of 5-HT onto postsynaptic 5-HT$_{1C/2}$ and 5-HT$_3$ receptors. *Second*, at postsynaptic 5-HT$_{1A}$ receptors: by functionally interfering with actions mediated by postsynaptic 5-HT$_{1C/2}$ and 5-HT$_3$ receptors.

As concerns the therapeutic utility of a drug acting as an agonist at both 5-HT$_{1A}$ autoreceptors and postsynaptic 5-HT$_{1A}$ receptors, ligands displaying *high* efficacy (high intrinsic activity) should be the most effective. That is, a *full* rather than a partial agonist should logically be a better agent for the treatment of anxiety and other psychiatric disorders. In this context, one critical difference between 5-HT$_{1A}$ autoreceptors and postsynaptic 5-HT$_{1A}$ receptors should be mentioned. Owing to their *greater* receptor reserve, the efficacy required for full activation of 5-HT$_{1A}$ *auto*receptors is much *less* than that required for activation of their postsynaptic counterparts (Meller et al., 1990). Correspondingly, many drugs which act as full agonists at 5-HT$_{1A}$ autoreceptors act only as partial agonists at postsynaptic 5-HT$_{1A}$ receptors (Glennon and Dukat, 1991; Lucki, 1992). For example, buspirone. This implies that the therapeutic efficacy of buspirone is limited (Lader, 1991) and that a full agonist at both 5-HT$_{1A}$ autoreceptors and postsynaptic 5-HT$_{1A}$ receptors would be a more effective therapeutic agent.

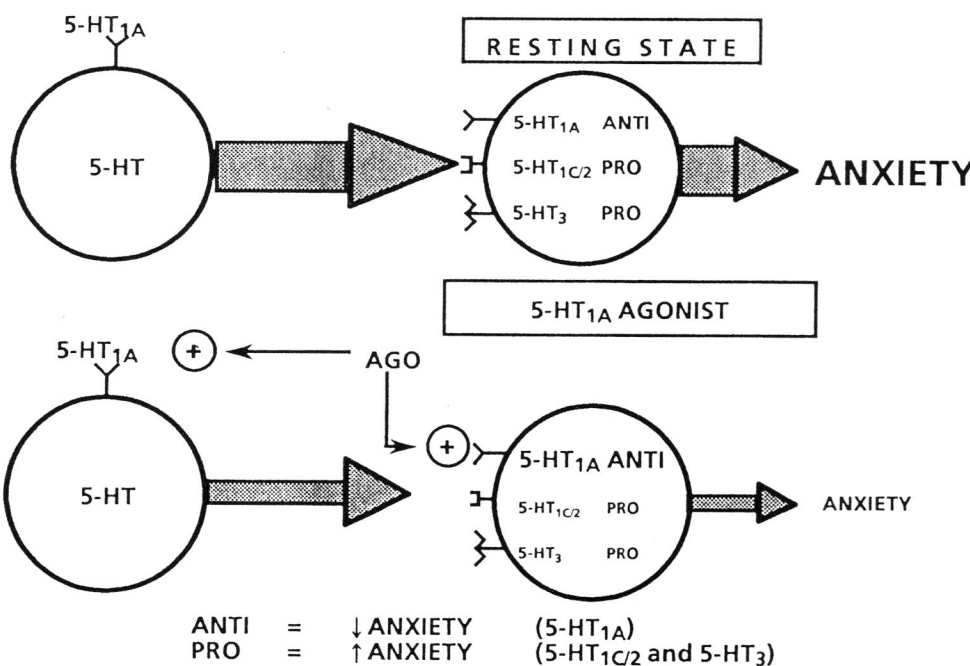

Fig. 3. 5-HT$_{1A}$ autoreceptors and postsynaptic 5-HT$_{1A}$ receptors express anxiolytic actions.

5-HT$_{1A}$ AGONISTS-5-HT$_{1C/2}$ ANTAGONISTS

In summary, there is evidence that ligands displaying high efficacy at both 5-HT$_{1A}$ autoreceptors and postsynaptic 5-HT$_{1A}$ receptors might be especially favourable in the treatment of anxiety - as well as depression and, possibly, other psychiatric disorders. In addition, ligands displaying antagonist actions at 5-HT$_{1C/2}$ and/or 5-HT$_3$ receptors may share such actions. Clearly, the combination of such properties in a single molecule would be of interest and the remainder of this article characterises the anxiolytic actions of two molecules, S 14506 and S 14671, which behave as (potent) high efficacy 5-HT$_{1A}$ agonists and also as (weak) 5-HT$_{1C/2}$ antagonists (Colpaert et al., 1992; Millan et al., 1992a and b). Their actions are compared to those of: the 5-HT$_{1A}$ agonist, 8-OH-DPAT; the 5-HT$_{1C/2}$ antagonist, ritanserin and the BZPs, clorazepate (CZP) and chlordiazepoxide (CDZ).

TESTS OF ANXIOLYTIC ACTIVITY EMPLOYED

Tests currently employed for the detection of anxiolytic activity are of essentially two types (see Barrett and Gleeson, 1991; Treit et al., 1991). In a first set of paradigms, disinhibition of anxiety-induced *suppression of natural behaviour* is analysed: for example, exploratory behaviour in the (+)-maze and the light-dark box or ultrasonic vocalizations in the infant rat separation test. In a second set of *response-suppression* paradigms, on the other hand, the ability of drugs to inhibit the anxiety-induced suppression of operant responding is examined; for example, the Vogel or Geller conflict tests in the rats. Although the evidence that 5-HT$_{1A}$ agonists possess anxiolytic properties in both types of models is convincing overall, their activity is particularly variable in models of natural behaviour (see above references). Further, the Geller conflict test in the rat fails to reliably detect anxiolytic properties of 5-HT$_{1A}$ agonists (Treit et al., 1991). In contrast, a conflict procedure has been described in the pigeon in which the anxiolytic properties of 5-HT$_{1A}$ agonists can be detected with great reliability (Barrett and Gleeson, 1991; Barrett and Zhang, 1991; Barrett et al., 1989; Brocco et al., 1990; Gleeson et al., 1989; Nanry et al., 1991). Further, this procedure allows for the precise quantification of their activity in terms of active dose-response ranges and the maximal effect obtained. For these reasons, the pigeon conflict test was chosen for an evaluation of the anxiolytic properties of S 14506 and S 14671. In addition, we undertook a comparison of behaviour in this test to that in the (+)-maze in the rat (Lister, 1987; Pellow et al., 1985).

METHODS

Pigeon conflict test.

Briefly, food-deprived pigeons were trained in operant chambers to peck an illuminated (green or red) key for food (Brocco et al., 1990). During green components, every 30th response produced access to food; during red components, every 30th response produced both food and electric shock to the groin. Sessions ended after the 5th cycle of alternating components and lasted 30 min in all. Saline, vehicle, or test compounds were injected intramuscularly (i.m., 1 ml/kg) 5 min prior to the session. Response rates during the unpunished (green) and punished (red) components of test sessions were expressed for each pigeon as a percentage of its own control rates observed during the previous (saline) session.

Rat (+)-maze test.

Naive, male Wistar rats were exposed to an elevated (+)-maze consisting of crossed open and closed arms subject to homogenous ambient light of equal intensity. The time spent on the open as compared to the closed arms as well as the number of entries into the open as compared to the closed arms was determined. In preliminary studies, about half (55 of 106) of control, vehicle-treated animals spent one-tenth (10 %) of their time on the open arms. This criteria was used for evaluation of drug effects such that, for each dose, the percentage of rats spending one-tenth (10 %) of time on the open arms was calculated.

RESULTS

Pigeon conflict test.

The BZPs, CZP and CDZ each elicited a robust and significant increase in punished but not non-punished responding (Fig. 4). Similarly, both the 5-HT_{1A} agonist, 8-OH-DPAT and the 5-$HT_{1C/2}$ antagonist, ritanserin, enhanced punished responding (Fig. 4). However, the former also markedly depressed unpunished responding at only 4-fold higher doses. In contrast to these two ligands, both S 14506 and S 14671 elicited an extremely pronounced increase in punished responding over a broad range of doses (Fig. 4). Their maximal effects were much more marked than for 8-OH-DPAT, ritanserin and CDZ. S 14506 and S 14671 also significantly depressed unpunished responding though, in the latter case, only at 16-fold higher doses. The 5-HT_{1A} antagonist, (-) alprenolol, at a dose of 10.0 mg/kg, abolished the anxiolytic action of S 14506 (not shown, seeColpaert et al., 1992).

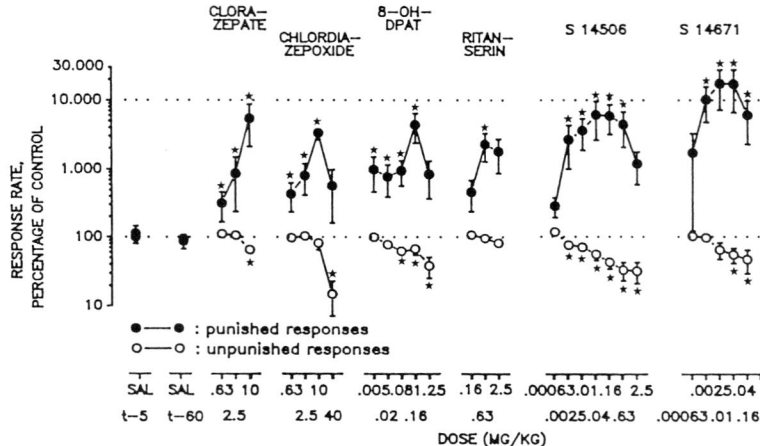

Fig. 4. Influence of drugs in the pigeon conflict test. Drugs were given i.m.. * p<0.05 to vehicle in the permutation test for paired replicates (Siegel and Castellan, 1988).

Rat (+)-maze test.

In the (+)-maze, both CZP and CDZ increased the percentage of time spent on the open vs the closed arms (Fig. 5). In addition, they selectively increased the number of entries into the former without changing the number of entries into the latter. 8-OH-DPAT elicited a mild increase in %time spent in open arms and in open arm entries only at a single low dose (Fig. 5). Indeed, it showed a biphasic pattern of activity with a loss of this increase at higher doses and a reduction in time in the open arms. Similarly, it biphasically enhanced total arm entries at lower doses and decreased these at high doses (Fig. 5). Ritanserin was ineffective in this model. S 14506 and S 14671 both tended to enhance presence in open arms at low doses (Fig. 6). However, it would probably have been necessary to test even lower doses in order to obtain significance. At high doses, % time in open arms as well as open arms entries was diminished. Both S 14506 and S 14671 also reduced total entries at high doses (Fig. 6).

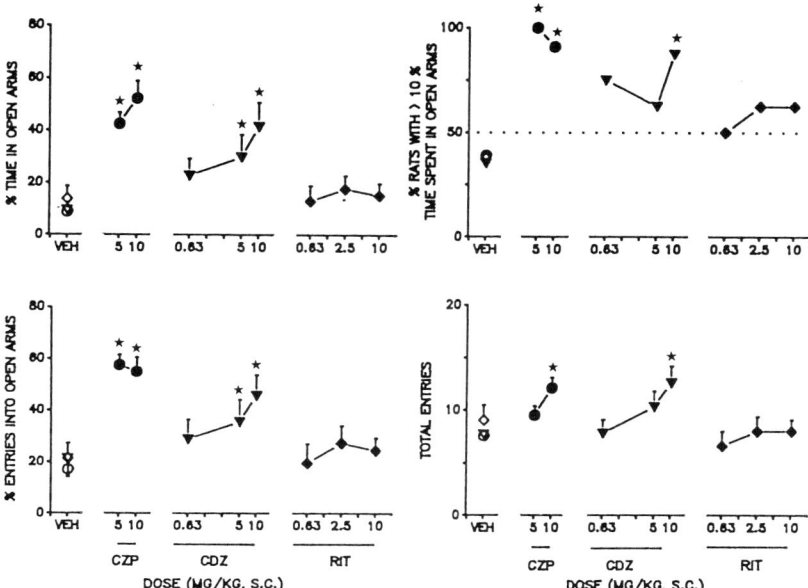

Fig. 5. Influence of the BZPs, clorazepate and chlordiazepoxide, and of the 5-HT$_{1C/2}$ antagonist, ritanserin, in the (+)-maze test. * p<0.05 to vehicle in Dunnetts' test or Fishers' test.

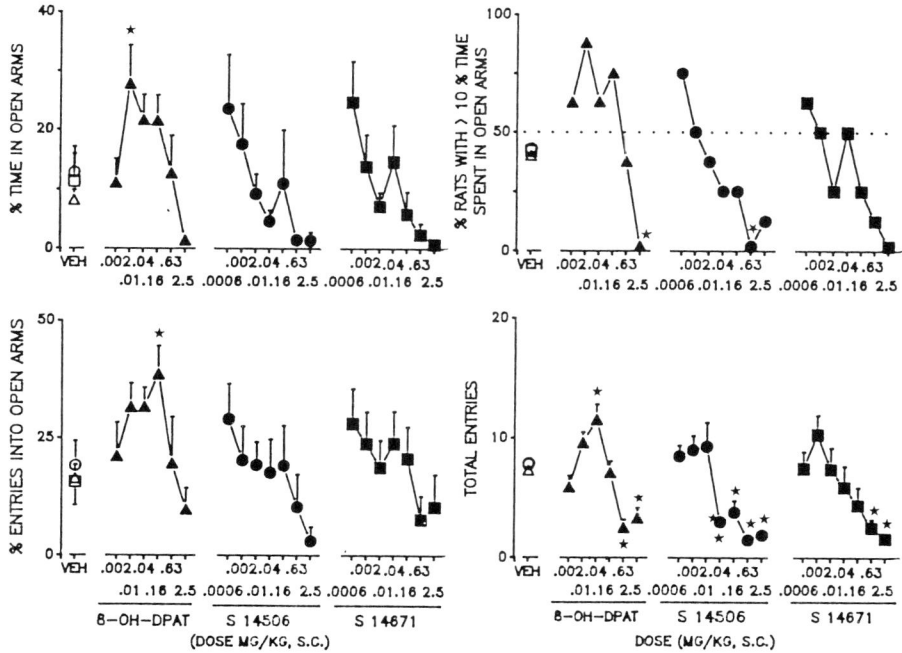

Fig. 6. Influence of 8-OH-DPAT, S 14506 and S 14671 in the (+)-maze test.* p<0.05 to vehicle in Dunnetts' test or Fishers' test.

DISCUSSION

A major observation which emerges from these studies is that the pattern of data acquired - as has also been suggested by previous investigators (Barrett et al., 1991) - is very different between the pigeon conflict test and the rat (+)-maze test.

In fact, in the pigeon conflict test, S 14506 and, most strikingly, S 14671, were exceptionally efficacious anxiolytic agents as judged by their maximal increase in punished responding. These were greater than for either ritanserin or 8-OH-DPAT. In addition, we have previously shown that their actions are more pronounced than those of buspirone (Millan et al., 1992a). One might argue that these effects may simply be attributed to their actions at 5-HT$_{1A}$ receptors. Indeed, S 14506 and S 14671 possess the (possibly unique) feature of positive Hill Coefficients at 5-HT$_{1A}$ receptors for which they display very high affinity (pKis = 9.0 and 9.3, respectively) (Colpaert et al., 1992; Millan et al., 1992b and unpublished data). These factors cannot, however, be easily related to their in vivo actions. Further, the efficacy of S 14506 and S 14671 as agonists at pre- and post-synaptic 5-HT$_{1A}$ receptors is not superior to that of 8-OH-DPAT (Colpaert et al., 1992; Millan et al., 1992b). Thus, an alternative explanation for this pattern of data may, indeed, be derived from the theory elaborated in the Introduction suggesting possible synergistic anxiolytic actions of 5-HT$_{1A}$ agonists and 5-HT$_{1C/2}$ antagonists. That is, whereas the anxiolytic action of 8-OH-DPAT falls off upon increasing the dose, the anxiolytic actions of S 14506 and S 14671 are maintained owing to their respective 5-HT$_{1C}$ and 5-HT$_{1C/2}$ antagonist properties (Millan et al., 1992a and b) which intervene at high doses. Nevertheless, one should be cautious in interpreting these data for several reasons. First, it remains to be demonstrated that co-administration of 8-OH-DPAT with ritanserin is as efficacious as S 14506 or S 14671. Second, S 14506 and S 14671 each possess antagonistic activity at D$_2$/D$_3$ dopamine receptors at doses around 10-fold higher than for their 5-HT$_{1A}$ effects, and these effects might also contribute to their functional actions in the conflict test (Rivet et al., in press). Third, and most obviously, their actions in the (+)-maze were very different to those in the pigeon conflict test.

Thus, in the (+)-maze, 8-OH-DPAT showed an anxiolytic action only at a low dose which was transformed into an *apparent* anxiogenic action at high doses, a profile mimicked by S 14506 and S 14671 which did *not* show any greater anxiolytic effect than 8-OH-DPAT. In addition, ritanserin was *not* active in this model. This absence of activity of ritanserin may help to explain the lack of the superior activity of S 14506 and S 14671 in the (+)-maze vs. the conflict test. A further difference between these two tests is that, in the pigeon conflict test, exclusively postsynaptic 5-HT$_{1A}$ receptors appear to be involved whereas, for the rat (+)-maze, the situation is less clear and both pre- (predominantly) and post-synaptic sites may be implicated (Barrett, 1992; Carli et al., 1989; Critchley et al., 1992; Fernández-Guasti et al., 1992; Higgins et al., 1992; Klint, 1991; Kostowski et al., 1989; Kshama et al., 1990; Przegalinski et al., 1992; Wright et al., 1992b). According to the above theory detailed, it is at the *post*synaptic level that one would expect the greatest degree of synergism between 5-HT$_{1A}$ agonists and 5-HT$_{1C/2}$ antagonists. In addition, the precise conditions of study of the (+)-maze may be important; for example, degree of familiarity and light exposure (Critchley et al., 1992; Pellow et al., 1985). It is possible that under other conditions, the findings may have differed. Indeed, there is a certain degree of divergence in the literature concerning various 5-HT$_{1A}$ agonists and partial agonists for which anxiolytic actions, no effect and anxiogenic actions have been reported (see Barrett and Gleeson, 1991; Treit, 1991).

Indeed, in the context of this latter point, it should be emphasized that the significance of apparent "anxiogenic" actions in the (+)-maze model has been questioned (Thiébot et al., 1988). That is, decreases in time spent in open arms and in entries therein may *not*, necessarily, reflect anxiogenic actions and their interpretation remains problematic. Indeed, several drugs not considered genuinely anxiogenic, such as mianserin and other antidepressants, reduce open arm presence (Pellow et al., 1985; Thiébot et al., 1988). In addition, we have found buspirone to elicit a very similar "anxiogenic" pattern as

S 14506, S 14671 and 8-OH-DPAT (not shown). Therefore, in view of the results in the pigeon, it is possible that the reduction in open arm presence for 8-OH-DPAT, S 14506 and S 14671 may *not* reflect an anxious state. This argument is supported by the observation that *closed* arm entries were reduced in parallel to the reduction in *open* arm entries. In other words, this was *not* a specific pattern of "anxiogenic" effect in contrast to, e.g. BZP inverse agonists (unpublished data). Finally, while the present experiments were performed acutely, several recent findings (Benjamin *et al.*, 1992; Schefke *et al.*, 1989; Wright *et al.*, 1992a) suggest that chronic schedules - allowing for adaptive mechanisms playing a key role in the development of drugs actions - may be more appropriate for the demonstration of the potential anxiolytic properties of serotoninergic ligands. Such studies remain to be performed for S 14506 and S 14671.

In conclusion, while the theory of 5-HT_{1A} agonist-5-$HT_{1C/2}$ antagonist synergism for obtention of optimal anxiolytic actions is intriguing, both this theory, as well as the precise roles of 5-HT_{1A}, 5-HT_{1C} and 5-HT_2 receptors in the control anxiety, require further investigation. Indeed, the 5-HT_{1A} actions of S 14506 and S 14671 *in vivo* appear to predominate on their 5-$HT_{1C/2}$ actions (Millan *et al.*, 1992a) and the discovery of novel ligands displaying more precisely equilibrated activity at 5-HT_{1A} and 5-$HT_{1C/2}$ sites will be a necessary step for a rigorous evaluation of this theory. Irrespective of the final outcome of such investigations, it is clear that a serotoninergic approach to the treatment represents a major avenue of research for the improved treatment of anxiety and the final testing of all such hypotheses can only be in the clinic.

AKNOWLEGMENTS

We would like to express our thanks to C. Le Roy for preparation of the manuscript and B. Lefèbvre de Ladonchamps and H. Gressier for technical assistance.

REFERENCES

Abdel-Latif, A.A., (1991): Biochemical and functional interactions between the inositol 1,4,5-trisphosphate-Ca^{2+} and cyclic amp signalling systems in smooth muscle. Cellular Signaling 5: 371-385.
Aghajanian, G.K., Wang, R.Y., and Baraban, J. (1978): Serotonergic and non-serotonergic neurons of the dorsal raphe: reciprocal changes in firing induced by peripheral nerve stimulation. Brain Res. 153: 169-175.
Araneda, R., and Andrade, R. (1991): 5-Hydroxytryptamine$_2$ and 5-Hydroxytryptamine$_{1A}$ receptors mediate opposing responses on membrane excitability in rat association cortex. Neuroscience. 40: 399-412.
Barrett, J.E. (1992): Studies on the effects of 5-HT_{1A} drugs in the pigeon. Drug Devel. Res. 26: 299-317.
Barrett. J.E., and Gleeson, S. (1991): Anxiolytic effects of 5-HT_{1A} agonists, 5-HT_3 antagonists and benzodiazepines: conflict and drug discrimination studies. In 5-HT_{1A} agonists, 5-HT_3 antagonists and benzodiazepines: their comparative behavioural pharmacology, eds. R.J. Rogers and S.J. Cooper, pp. 59-105. Chischester, Wiley & Sons Ltd.
Barrett. J.E., Gleeson, S., Nader, M.A., and Hoffmann, S.M. (1989): Anticonflict effects of the 5-HT_{1A} compound flesinoxan. J. Psychopharmacology 3: 64-69.
Barrett. J.E., and Zhang L. (1991): Anticonflict and discriminative stimulus effects of the 5-HT_{1A} compounds WY-47,846 and WY-48,723 and the mixed 5-HT_{1A} agonist/5-HT_2 antagonist WY-50,324 in pigeons. Drug Devel. Res. 24: 179-188.
Benjamin, D., Saiff, E.I., Nevins, T., and Lal, H. (1992): Mianserin-induced 5-HT_2 receptor. Down-regulation results in anxiolytic effects in the elevated plus-maze test. Drug Devel. Res. 26:287-297.
Bervoets, K., Millan, M.J., and Colpaert, F.C. (1990): Agonist action at 5-HT_{1C} receptors facilitates 5-HT_{1A} receptor-mediated spontaneous tail-flicks in the rat. Eur. J Pharmacol. 191: 185-195.
Bobker, D.H., and Williams, J.T. (1990): Ion conductances by 5-HT receptor subtypes in mammalian neurons. Trends Neurosci. 13: 169-173.
Brandão, M.L., Lopez-Garcia, J.A., Graeff, F.G., and Roberts, M.H.T. (1991): Electrophysiological evidence for exitatory 5-HT_2 and depressant 5-HT_{1A} receptors on neurones of the rat midbrain tectum. Brain Res. 556: 259-266.

Brocco, M.J., Koek, W., Degryse, A.-D., and Colpaert, F.C. (1990): Comparative studies on the anti-punishment effects of chlordiazepoxide, buspirone and ritanserin in the pigeon, Geller-Seifter and Vogel conflict procedures. Behav. Pharmacol. 1: 403-418.

Carli, M., Prontera, C., and Samanin, R. (1989): Evidence that central 5-hydroxytryptaminergic neurones are involved in the anxiolytic activity of buspirone. Br. J. Pharmacol. 96, 829-836.

Ceulemans, D.L.S., Hoppenbrouwers, M.L.J.A., Gelders, Y.G., Reyntjens, A.J.M. (1985): The influence of ritanserin, a serotonin antagonist, in anxiety disorders: A double-blind placebo-controlled study versus lorazepam. Pharmacopsychiatry 18: 303-305.

Claustre, Y., Bénavidès, J., and Scatton, B. (1991): Potential mechanisms involved in the negative coupling between serotonin 5-HT$_{1A}$ receptors and carbachol-stimulated phosphoinositide turnover in the rat hippocampus. J. Neurochem. 56: 1276-1285.

Claustre, Y., Bénavidès, J., and Scatton, B. (1988): 5-HT$_{1A}$ receptor agonists inibit carbachol-induced stimulation of phosphoinositide turnover in the rat hippocampus. Eur. J. Pharmacol. 149: 149-153.

Colpaert, F.C., Koek, W., Lehmann, J., Rivet, J.-M., Lejeune, F., Canton, H., Bervoets, K., Millan, M.J., Laubie, M., and Lavielle, G. (1992): S 14506: a novel, potent, high-efficacy 5-HT$_{1A}$ agonist and potential anxiolytic agent. Drug Dev. Res. 26: 21-48.

Conn, P.J., and Sanders-Bush, E. (1987): Relative efficacies of piperazines at the phosphoinositide hydrolysis-linked serotoninergic (5-HT$_2$ and 5-HT$_{1C}$) receptors. J. Pharmacol. Exp. Ther. 242: 552.

Critchley, M.A.E., Njung'e, K., and Handley, S.L. (1992): Actions and some interactions of 5-HT$_{1A}$ ligands in the elevated X-maze and effects of dorsal raphe lesions. Psychopharmacology 106: 484-490.

Deakin, J.F.W. (1988): 5-HT$_2$ receptors, depression and anxiety. Pharmacol. Biochem. Behav. 29: 819-820.

Di Marzo, V., Galadari, S.H.I., Tippins, J.R., and Morris, H.R. (1991): Interactions between second messengers: cyclic amp and phospholipase A$_2$- and phospholipase C-metabolites. Life Sci. 49: 247-259.

Edwards, E., Harkins, K., Ashby, C.R., and Wang, R.Y. (1991): Effect of 5-hydroxytryptamine$_3$ receptor agonists on phosphoinositide hydrolysis in the rat fronto-cingulate and entorhinal cortices. J. Pharmacol. Exp. Ther. 256: 1025-1032.

Fan Liu, Y., and Albert, P.R. (1991): Cell-specific signaling of 5-HT$_{1A}$ receptors. J. Biol. Chem. 266: 23689-23697.

Fargin, A., Raymond, J.R., Regan, J.W., Cotecchia, S., Lefkowitz, M.G., and Caron, M.G. (1989): Effector coupling mechanisms of the cloned 5-HT$_{1A}$ receptor. J. Biol. Chem. 264: 14848-14852.

Fargin, A., Yamamoto, K., Cotecchia, S., Goldsmith, P.K., Spiegel, A.M., Lapetina, E.G., Caron, M.G,. and Lefkowitz, M.G. (1991): Dual coupling of the cloned 5-HT$_{1A}$ receptor to both adenylyl cyclase and phospholipase C is mediated via the same G$_i$ protein. Cellular Signaling 3: 547-557.

Fernández-Guasti, A., López-Rubalcava, C., Pérez-Urizar, J., and Catañeda-Hernández, G. (1992): Evidence for a postsynaptic action of the serotonergic anxiolytics: ipsapirone, indorenate and buspirone. Brain Res. Bull. 28: 497-501.

Fowler, C.J., Ahlgren, P.C., and O'Neill, C. (1991): Antagonism by 8-hydroxy-2(di-N-propylamino)tetralin and other serotonin agonists of muscarinic M1-type receptors coupled to inositol phospholipid breakdown in human IMR-32 and SK-N-MC neuroblastoma cells. Life Sci. 48: 959-967.

Frances Davies, M., Deisz, R.A., Prince, D.A., and Peroutka, S.J. (1987): Two distinct effects of 5-hydroxytryptamine on single cortical neurons. Brain Res. 423: 347-352.

Gleeson, S., Ahlers, S.T., Mansbach, R.S., Foust, J.M., and Barrett, J.E. (1989): Behavioural studies with anxiolytic drugs. VI., Effects on punished responding of drugs interacting with serotonin receptor subtypes. J. Pharmacol. Exp.Ther. 250: 809-817.

Glennon, R.A., and Dukat, M. (1991): Serotonin receptors and their ligands: a lack of selective agents. Pharmacol. Biochem. Behav. 40: 1009-1017.

Glennon, R.A., and Lucki, I (1988): Behavioural models of serotonin receptor activation. In The serotonin receptors, eds by E. Sanders-Bush, pp. 253-292. Clifton, Humana Press.

Glennon, R.A., Darmani, N.A., and Martin, B.R. (1991): Multiple populations of serotonin receptors may modulate the behavioral effects of serotoninergic agents. Life Sci. 48: 2493-2498.

Goldfarb, J. (1990): Electrophysiologic studies of serotonin receptor activation. Neuropsychopharmacology 3: 435-446.

Handley, S.L., and Mithani, S. (1984): Effects of alpha-adrenoceptor agonists and antagonists in a maze-exploration model of 'fear'-motivated behaviour. Naunyn-Schmiedeberg's Arch. Pharmacol. 327: 1-5.

Hensman, R., Guimarães, F.S., Wang, M., and Deakin, J.F.W. (1991): Effects of ritanserin on aversive classical conditioning in humans. Psychopharmacology 104: 220-224.

Higgins, G.A., Jones, B.J., and Oakley, N.R. (1992): Effect of 5-HT$_{1A}$ receptor agonists in two models of anxiety after dorsal raphe injection. Psychopharmacology 106: 261-267.

Hill, S.J., and Kendall, D.A. (1989): Cross-talk between different receptor-effector systems in the mammalian CNS. Cellular Signalling 1: 135-141.

Hill, S.J., and Kendall, D.A. (1992): Cross-talk between intracellular second messenger transduction systems. Drugs, News, & Perspectives 5: 39-48.

Hoyer, D., and Schoeffter, P. (1991): 5-HT receptors: subtypes and second messengers. J. Receptor Res. 11: 197-214.

Joëls, M., Shinnick-Gallagher, P., and Gallagher, J.P. (1987): Effect of serotonin and serotonin analogues on passive membrane properties of lateral septal neurons in vitro. Brain Res. 417: 99-107.

Kennett, G.A. (1992): 5-HT$_{1C}$ receptor antagonists have anxiolytic-like actions in the rat social interaction model. Psychopharmacology 107, 379-384.

Kennett, G.A., Whitton, P., Shah, K., and Curzon, G. (1989): Anxiogenic-like of mCPP and TFMPP in animal models are opposed by 5-HT$_{1C}$ receptor antagonists. Eur. J. Pharmacol. 164: 445-454.

Klint, T. (1991): Effect of 8-OH-DPAT and buspirone in a passive avoidance test and in the elevated plus-maze test in rats. Behavioural Pharmacol. 2: 481-489.

Kostowski, W., Plaznik, A., and Stefanski, R. (1989): Intra-hippocampal buspirone in animal models of anxiety. Eur. J. Pharmacol. 168: 393-396.

Kshama, D., Hrishikeshavan, H.J., Shanbhogue, R., and Munonyedi, U.S. (1990): Modulation of baseline behavior in rats by putative serotonergic agents in three ethoexperimental paradigms. Behavioral & Neural Biol. 54: 234-253.

Lader, M.H. (1991): Benzodiazepines and novel anxiolytics: clinical pharmacology, dependence and withdrawal. In 5-HT$_{1A}$ agonists, 5-HT$_3$ antagonists and benzodiazepines: their comparative behavioural pharmacology, eds R.J. Rodgers and S.J. Cooper, pp. 343-363. Chichester, Wiley & Son.

Lister, R.G. (1987): The use of a plus-maze to measure anxiety in the mouse. Psychopharmacology 92: 180-185.

Lucki, I. (1992): 5-HT$_1$ receptors and behavior. Neuroscience & Behavioral Rev. 16: 83-93.

Meller, E., Goldstein, M., and Bohmaker, K. (1990): Receptor reserve for 5-hydroxytryptamine$_{1A}$-mediated inhibition of serotonin synthesis: possible relationship to anxiolytic properties of 5-hydroxytryptamine$_{1A}$ agonists. Molec. Pharmacol. 37: 231-237.

Millan, M.J., Canton, H and G. Lavielle (1992a): Targetting multiple serotonin receptor types: mixed 5-HT$_{1A}$ agonists - 5-HT$_{1C/2}$ antagonists as therapeutic agents. Drug News & Perspectives 5: 397-406.

Millan, M.J., Rivet, J.-M., Canton, H., Lejeune, F., Bervoets, K., Brocco, M., Gobert, A., Lefèbvre De Ladonchamps, B., Le Marouille-Girardon, S., Verrièle, L., Laubie, M., and Lavielle, G. (1992b): S 14671: A naphtylpiperazine 5-HT$_{1A}$ agonist of exceptional potency and high efficacy possessing antagonist activity at 5-HT$_{1C/2}$ receptors. J. Pharmacol. Exp. Ther. 262:451-463.

Moser, P.C. (1989): An evaluation of the elevated plus-maze test using the novel anxiolytic buspirone. Psychopharmacology 99: 48-53.

Moser, P.C., Tricklebank, M.D., Middlemiss, D.N., Mir, A.K., Hibert, M.F., and Fozard, J.R. (1990): Characterization of MDL 73005EF as a 5-HT$_{1A}$ selective ligand and its effects in animal models of anxiety: comparison with buspirone, 8-OH-DPAT and diazepam. Br. J. Pharmacol. 99: 343-349.

Motta, V., Maisonnette, S., Morato, S., Castrechini, P., and Brandão, M.L. (1992): Effects of blockade of 5-HT$_2$ receptors and activation of 5-HT$_{1A}$ receptors on the exploratory activity of rats in the elevated plus-maze. Psychopharmacology 107: 135-139.

Murphy, D.L., Lesch, K.P., Aulakh, C.S., and Pigott, T.A. (1991): Serotonin-selective arylpiperazines with neuroendocrine, behavioral, temperature, and cardiovascular effects in humans. Pharmacol. Rev. 43: 527-552.

Nanry, K.P., Howard, J.L., and Pollard, G.T. (1991): Effects of buspirone and other anxiolytics on punished key-pecking in the pigeon. Drug Development Res. 24: 269-276.

Panicker, M.M., Parker, I., and Miledi, R. (1991): Receptors of the serotonin 1C subtype expressed from cloned DNA mediate the closing of K$^+$ membrane channels encoded by brain mRNA. Proc. Natl. Acad. Sci. 88: 2560-2562.

Paulssen, E.J., Paulssen, R.H., Gautvik, K.M., and Gordeladze, J.O. (1992): 'Cross-talk' between phospholipase C and adenylyl cyclase involves regulation of G-protein levels in GH$_3$ rat pituitary cells. Cellular Signalling 4: 747-755.

Pazos, A., Hoyer, D., Dietl, M and Palacios, J.M. (1988): Autoradiography of serotonin receptors. In Neuronal Serotonin, eds by N.N. Osborne and M. Hamon, pp. 507-544. London, Wiley and Sons.

Pellow, S., Chopin, P., File, S.E., and Briley, M. (1985): Validation of open: closed arm entries in an elevated plus-maze as a measure of anxiety in the rat. J. Neurosci. Methods 14: 149-167.

Przegalinski, E., Chojnacka-Wójcik, E., and Filip, M. (1992): Stimulation of postsynaptic 5-HT$_{1A}$ receptors is responsible for the anticonflict effect of ipsapirone in rats. J. Pharm. Pharmacol. 44: 780-782.

Raymond, J.R., Albers, F.J., Middleton, J.P., Lefkowitz, R.J., Caron, M.G., Obeid, L.M., and Dennis, V.W. (1991): 5-HT$_{1A}$ and histamine H$_1$ receptors in HeLa cells stimulate phosphonositide hydrolysis and phosphate uptake via distinct G protein pools. J. Biol. Chem. 266: 372-379.

Raymond, J.R., Fargins, A., Middleton, J.P., Graff, J.M., McNeill Haupt, D., Caron, M.G., Lefkowitz, R.J., and Dennis, V.W. (1989): The human 5-HT$_{1A}$ receptor expressed in HeLa cells stimulates sodium-dependent phosphate uptake via protein kinase C. J. Biol. Chem. 264: 21943-21950.

Rivet, J.-M., Audinot, V., Gobert, A., Cistarelli, L., Chaput, C., Brocco, M., Lavielle, G., and Millan, M.J., (1993): Actions of the potent, methoxynaphthylpiperazine 5-HT$_{1A}$ receptor agonists, S 14506 and S 14671, at dopamine D$_1$, D$_2$ and D$_3$ receptors in vitro/in vivo. Neuroscience, Abst., in press.

Rodgers, R.J., Cole, J.C., Cobain, M.R., Daly, P., Doran, P.J., Eells, J.R., and Wallis, P. (1992): Anxiogenic-like effects of fluprazine and eltoprazine in the mouse elevated plus-maze: profile comparisons with 8-OH-DPAT, CGS 12066B, TFMPP and mCPP. Behavioural Pharmacology 3: 621-634.

Schefke, D.M., Fontana, D.J., and Commissaris, R.L. (1989): Anti-conflict efficacy of buspirone following acute versus chronic treatment. Psychopharmacology 99: 427-429.

Schweizer, E., and Rickels, K. (1991): Serotonergic anxiolytics: a review of their clinical efficacy. In 5-HT$_{1A}$ agonists, 5-HT$_3$ antagonists and benzodiazepines: their comparative behavioural pharmacology, eds R.J. Rodgers and S.J. Cooper, pp. 365-376. Chichester, Wiley & Son Ltd.

Shimizu, H., Tatsuno, T., Tanaka, H., Hirose, A., Araki, Y., and Nakamura, M. (1992): Serotonergic mechanisms in anxiolytic effect of tandospirone in the vogel conflict test. Japan. J. Pharmacol. 59: 105-112.

Siegel, S., and Castellan, N.J. (1988): Non-parametric statistics for the behavioral sciences. New-York, McGrawHill.

Stevens, D.R., McCarley, R.W., and Greene, R.W. (1992): Serotonin$_1$ and serotonin$_2$ receptors hyperpolarize and depolarize separate populations of medial pontine reticular formation neurons in vitro. Neurosci. 47: 545-553.

Stutzmann, J.M., Eon, B., Darche F., Lucas, M., Rataud, J., Piot, O., Blanchard, J.C., and Laduron, P.M. (1991): Are 5-HT$_2$ antagonists endowed with anxiolytic properties in rodents? Neurosci. Lett. 128: 4-8.

Tan, H., and Miletic, V. (1992): Diverse actions of 5-hydroxytryptamine on frog spinal dorsal horn neurons in vitro. Neurosci. 49: 913-923.

Thiébot, M.-H., Soubrié, P., and Sanger, D. (1988): Anxiogenic properties of beta-CCE and FG 7142: a review of promises and pitfalls. Psychopharmacology 94: 452-463.

Törk, I. (1990): Anatomy of the serotonergic system. N.Y. Acad. Science 38: 9-35.

Traber, J., and Glaser, T. (1987): 5-HT$_{1A}$ receptor related anxiolytics. Trends Pharm. 8: 432-437.

Treit, D. (1991): Anxiolytic effects of benzodiazepines and 5-HT$_{1A}$ agonists: animal models. In 5-HT$_{1A}$ agonists, 5-HT$_3$ antagonists and benzodiazepines: their comparative behavioural pharmacology, eds R.J. Rodgers and S.J. Cooper, pp. 107-131. Chichester, Wiley & Son Ltd.

Van den Hooff, P., and Galvan, M. (1992): Actions of 5-hydroxytryptamine and 5-HT$_{1A}$ receptor ligands on rat dorso-lateral septal neurones in vitro. Br. J. Pharmacol. 106: 893-899.

Whitton, P., and Curzon, G. (1990): Anxiogenic-like effect of infusing 1-(3-chlorophenyl) piperazine (mCPP) into the hippocampus. Psychopharmacology 100: 138-140.

Wright, I.A., Heaton, M., Upton, N., and Marsden, C.A. (1992a): Comparison of acute and chronic treatment of various serotonergic agents with those of diazepan and idazoxan in the rat elevated X-maze. Psychopharmacology 107: 405-414.

Wright, I.A., Upton, N., and Marsden, C.A. (1992b): Effect of established and putative anxiolytics on extracellular 5-HT and 5-HIAA in the ventral hippocampus of rats during behaviour on the elevated X-maze. Psychopharmacology 109: 338-346.

Résumé

Le rôle du système sérotoninergique dans les phénomènes d'anxiété a été particulièrement étudié, depuis la mise en évidence des propriétés agonistes vis-à-vis des récepteurs sérotoninergiques 5-HT$_{1A}$, de la buspirone, anxiolytique non-benzodiazépinique, actif chez l'Homme. L'activation des récepteurs 5-HT$_{1A}$ (pré- et post-synaptiques) par des produits agonistes résulte en un effet anxiolytique : une action de ces agonistes (au niveau présynaptique) réduirait l'hyperactivité anormale des voies sérotoninergiques ascendantes limbiques et corticales, liée au phénomène d'anxiété. Les autres récepteurs sérotoninergiques (postsynaptiques) 5-HT$_{1C}$, 5-HT$_2$, 5-HT$_3$, seraient impliqués de façon inverse dans le phénomène d'anxiété ; ainsi, l'agoniste 5-HT$_{1C}$, le mCPP, exerce un effet anxiogène chez l'Homme, alors que les antagonistes 5-HT$_{1C/2}$ et 5-HT$_3$ semblent posséder des propriétés anxiolytiques. En raison de l'antagonisme apparent entre récepteurs 5-HT$_{1A}$ et 5-HT$_{1C/2}$ dans les mécanismes intervenant dans l'anxiété, il semble intéressant d'évaluer les propriétés anxiolytiques de molécules, telles que le S 14506 et le S 14671, qui possèdent à la fois des propriétés agonistes 5-HT$_{1A}$ et antagonistes 5-HT$_{1C/2}$. Les effets anxiolytiques de ces produits ont été évalués chez le Pigeon (test de conflit) et chez le Rat (test d'exploration : labyrinthe en croix) et comparés à ceux des benzodiazépines, clorazépate (CZP) et chlordiazepoxide (CDZ), de l'agoniste 5-HT$_{1A}$, 8-OH-DPAT, et de l'antagoniste 5-HT$_{1C/2}$, ritansérine. Dans le test de conflit chez le Pigeon, les S 14506 et S 14671 exercent une activité anxiolytique (augmentation des réponses punies) plus marquée que celle obtenue avec les autres produits. Par contre, dans le test d'exploration chez le Rat, les S 14506 et S 14671 ont une activité anxiolytique très faible, voisine de celle du 8-OH-DPAT ; la ritansérine se révèle inactive dans ce test. Bien que l'explication de la différence entre ces deux tests n'est pas aujourd'hui évidente, ces résultats servent à renforcer l'intérêt d'une approche sérotoninergique pour le traitement de l'anxiété. La découverte de produits plus équilibrés 5-HT$_{1A}$ agonistes/5-HT$_{1C/2}$ antagonistes sera nécessaire par une évaluation plus approfondie de l'hypothèse de leur potentialité thérapeutique dans le traitement de l'anxiété.

Potential therapeutic applications of CCK antagonists in anxiety and panic disorders

Valérie Daugé, Nathalie Ladurelle, Muriel Derrien, Christiane Durieux and Bernard-P. Roques

Département de Pharmacochimie Moléculaire et Structurale, INSERM U.266 - CNRS URA D1500, Université René Descartes, 4, avenue de l'Observatoire, 75270 Paris Cedex 06, France

Summary

Numerous pharmacological studies performed in humans, monkeys and rodents are in favor of the participation of CCKergic system in some adaptative behaviors. Some of them could occur by counteraction of the endogenous enkephalins acting on ∂ opioid receptors as shown in emotional stressfull situations, showing a possible antidepressant-like effects for CCK-B antagonists. A dysfunctioning of CCKergic system could lead to psychiatric disorders such as panic attacks in humans and monkeys. Peripheral and central CCK-B receptors and CCK-A receptors of particular brain structures (nucleus tractus solitarius, hippocampus, mesocorticolimbic system) seem to be involved in the behavioral expression of the anxiogenic-like effects and the associated neurovegetative and neuroendocrine changes induced by CCK compounds. In several animal models of fear and anxiety (black and white box, elevated plus maze, social interaction..), peripheral administration of CCK-B agonists (BC264, BC197) and antagonists (L365,260, CI988, RB211) support the role of CCK as an endogenous anxiogenic factor. The CCK-B antagonists could have therapeutic applications in treating panic attacks and anxiety. In the posterior nucleus accumbens, CCK_8 through interaction with CCK-A receptors increases extracellular DA levels in freely moving rats and induces anxiogenic-like effects suppressed by 6-OHDA lesions of DAergic mesoaccumbens pathways and D_2 antagonists. Biochemical and behavioral data suggest that several CCK-B receptor subtypes could be involved in CCK_8-induced modifications of emotional and cognitive processes.

Introduction

CCK was first recognized as a gastrointestinal hormone, mediating digestive function and feeding behavior. Nevertheless numerous physiological processes such as respiratory functions (Morin-Surun et al., 1983) and cardiovascular tonus (Koyama et al., 1990), vigilance states (St Hilaire et al., 1991), memory processes (Itoh and Lai, 1990 ; Lemaire et al., 1992), nociception (Faris et al., 1983 ; Wiertelak et al., 1992 ; Noble et al., 1993 ; Derrien et al., 1993b ; Maldonado et al., 1993) and emotional and /or motivational states (Daugé et al., 1989a,b ; Singh et al., 1991) were also shown to be modulated by CCK. The sulfated octapeptide fragment of cholecystokinin (CCK_8) which interacts with the same affinity with CCK-A and CCK-B receptors (Table 1) is the most abundant form found in the brain. Low amounts of shorter fragments such as the C-terminal tetrapeptide CCK_4, which exhibits a better selectivity for CCK-B than for CCK-A receptors (Table 1) were also shown to occur in the brain (Rehfeld and Hansen, 1986).

The distribution of the two types of CCK receptors in the organism is quite different. The A type is abundant in the peripheral system but is also found in a few discrete regions of the rat brain i.e. area postrema, interpeduncular nucleus, posterior hypothalamus and the nucleus tractus solitarius (NTS).

In contrast the B type is the predominent form found in the brain, particularly in the cerebral cortex and in limbic structures such as olfactory tubercles, hippocampus, amygdala and the nucleus accumbens (N.Acc.) (Moran et al., 1986 ; Hill et al., 1987), raising interesting questions as to its possible role in psychiatric disorders including schizophrenia, depressive syndromes, anxiety. The recent purification and molecular cloning of the CCK receptors from rat pancreas (CCK-A) and brain (CCK-B) have shown that these two distinct receptors contain seven putative transmembrane domains, suggesting that they belong to the guanine nucleotide-binding regulatory protein-coupled receptor superfamily (Wank et al., 1992 ; Beinborn et al., 1993). Furthermore, the stomach gastrin receptor and the CCK-B receptor appear to be identical (Bienborn et al., 1993).

Extensive pharmacological studies have shown that CCK_4 and the related molecule pentagastrin, can produce panic attacks after i.v. administration in humans (Bradwjen et al., 1990 ; Abelson and Nesse, 1990). Indeed, CCK_4 was found to induce various symptoms; anxiety, apprehension, tension and fear in addition to somatic and cognitive symptoms characteristic of panic attacks. These effects were suppressed by the CCK-B antagonist, L365,260 (Bradwjen et al., 1992). Interestingly patients with panic disorders were found to be more sensitive to the effects of CCK_4 than healthy volunteers (Bradwjen et al., 1991). Furthermore the CCK concentration detected in the cerebrospinal fluid of these patients was decreased (Lydiard et al., 1992). Nevertheless, the efficiency of CCK antagonists to treat panic attacks not induced by CCK_4 remains to be demonstrated and the mechanism and site of action of CCK_4 and CCK-B antagonists have not yet been determined.

It is interesting to note that a communication between peripheral and central nervous systems has been demonstrated for the satiety reflex, in which CCK released during feeding binds to CCK-A receptors localized on the vagus nerve to send information to the NTS (Smith et al., 1981 ; Smith and Gibbs, 1992). A CCK_4 interaction with receptors at the peripheral level to trigger panic attacks cannot therefore be excluded. The involvement of CCK in behavior related to anxiety requires selective agonists and antagonists for CCK-A and CCK-B binding sites, able or not to cross the blood brain barrier. The affinities and selectivities for the rat pancreas (CCK-A) and the mouse brain (CCK-B) binding sites of currently available CCK agonists and antagonists, are shown in Table1. Furthermore behavioral studies performed after peripheral injection or local administration in brain will give information on the role of CCK and its functional pathways.

Table 1 : Affinities of CCK analogs on rat pancreas (CCK-A) and mouse brain (CCK-B) binding sites.

COMPOUNDS		CCK-A K_i nM $^3HpCCK_8$	CCK-B K_i nM $^3HpBC\ 264$	CCK-A / CCK-B
CCK-B agonists				
CCK_8	Asp-Tyr(SO_3H)-Met-Gly-Trp-Met-Asp-PheNH$_2$	0.87 ±0.16	0.48 ± 0.07	1.8
CCK_4	Trp-Nle-Asp-PheNH$_2$	5113 ±1802	16.4± 3.4	311
BC 197	Boc-(D).Asp-Tyr(SO_3H)-Nle-(D).Lys-Trp-Nle-Asp-PheNH$_2$	1845 ± 402	26.8 ± 2.7	69
BC 264	Boc-Tyr(SO_3H)-gNle-mGly-Trp-(NMe)Nle-Asp-PheNH$_2$	355 ± 98	0.32 ± 0.02	1109
CCK-A agonist				
	Boc-Tyr-Lys(CO-NH-o-tol)-Asp-PheNH$_2$	1.17 ±0.17	37.6± 4.3	0.031
CCK-B antagonists				
RB 211	N-(2-adamantyloxycarbonyl)-(D)-α-methyl-tryptophanyl-[N-{2-(4-chlorophenyl)ethyl}]glycine	1232 ± 130	13.6± 1.6	90
CI 988	[R-(R*, R*)]-4-[[2-[[3-(1H-Indol-3-yl)-2-methyl-1-oxo-2-[[(tricyclo[3.3.1.1.",7]dec-2-yloxy)carbonyl]amino]propyl]-amino]-1-phenylethyl]amino]-4-oxobutanoic acid	2382 ± 514	1.2 ± 0.2	1985
L-365,260	(3R)-N-(2,3-dihydro-1-methyl-2-oxo-5-phenyl-1H-1,4-benzodiazepin-3-yl)-N'-(3-methylphenyl)urea	1170 ± 330	5.2 ± 0.6	225
CCK-A antagonist				
L-364,718 or MK 329	(3S)-N-(2,3-dihydro-1-methyl-2-oxo-5-phenyl-1H-1,4-benzodiazepin-3-yl)-1H-indole-2-carboxamide	1.55 ±0.15	62.7± 7.6	0.025

I Evidence for the involvement of CCK in panic attacks and anxiety in monkeys and rodents

Recent interesting results from Ervin and coll., show anxiogenic effects of CCK agonists in a non human primate model. CCK_4 given i.v. to African green monkeys has strong and dose related effects on behaviors thought to reflect anxiety and panic. It is interesting that other CCK analogues, notably BC264, a highly selective CCK-B agonist (table1) synthesized in our laboratory (Charpentier et al., 1988) also produce behavioral change, but the profile of behavior is somewhat different. Vigilance and stereotypy are prominent after administration of BC264 which is known to penetrate the brain efficiently (Durieux et al., 1991). While CCK_4 effects are potently and dose-responsively blocked by various CCK-B antagonists (LY262691, LY247348, CI988 (Table1)), but not by CCK-A antagonist (LY219057), there is no attenuation of stereotypy or vigilance produced by BC264 or CCK_4 when a CCK-B antagonist, which does not effectively cross the blood brain barrier, RP71483, is injected (Palmour et al., 1993). These data are therefore consistent with the hypothesis that some of the behavioral effects of CCK_4 are mediated centrally, while others may follow the interaction of the peptide with peripheral receptors (Branchereau et al., 1992). They also suggest the existence of CCK receptor subtypes since BC264 does not produce the same behavioral profile as CCK_4 after peripheral administration.

Furthermore CCK-B antagonists such as CI988 produce anxiolytic effects in a marmoset "human threat" model accounting for a physiological involvement of the CCKergic system in anxiety (Hughes et al., 1990).

While there is no data in rodents, due to the lack of a specific animal model of panic attack, several studies indicate that CCK may also act as an endogenous anxiogenic peptide. Thus, various CCK-B antagonists (L365,260, CI988 (Table1)) were able to produce anxiolytic effects in several models of fear and/or anxiety in rodents, such as the black and white box in mice (Singh et al., 1991) the elevated plus maze in mice and rats (Rataud et al., 1991 ; Singh et al., 1991) an ethological model for measuring behavioral responses to predation (Hendrie and Neill, 1992), and the social interaction and conflict (alternations of footshock punished and unpunished periods) tests in rats (Singh et al., 1991). Moreover, the involvement of CCK-B receptors was emphasized by the anxiogenic-like effects produced by BC264 or BC197 (selective CCK-B agonists, Charpentier et al.,1988) and their suppression by CCK-B antagonists (CI988, L365,260) in the black and white box test in mice (Fig.1A). Furthermore a new selective CCK-B antagonist, RB211, synthesized in the laboratory (Blommaert et al., submitted) (Table1) produced anxiolytic effects after i.p. injection in mice, supporting a physiological regulation of emotional states by CCK, (Fig.1B).

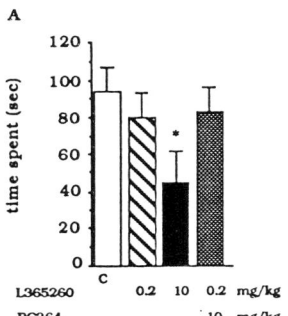 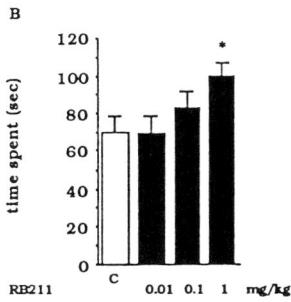

Fig. 1 A : Antagonism of the anxiogenic-like effects of BC 264 (CCK-B agonist) by L-365,260 (CCK-B antagonist) in the black and white box test in mice. L-365,260 was injected i.p. 15 min before BC 264 i.p. injected 30 min before the 5 min test. **B** : Anxiolytic-like effect induced by RB 211 (CCK-B antagonist) in the black and white box test in mice. RB 211 was i.p. injected 30 min before the 5 min test. C = control. *$p<0.05$; Newman-Keuls test.

In contrast to CCK-B, CCK-A receptor stimulation induced sedative effects when a CCK-A agonist (tetrapeptide modified, Table1) was i.p. administered in the black and white box test and in animex studies (Daugé et al., submitted). Nevertheless CCK-A receptor activation have been claimed by some authors to produce anxiolytic effects (review in Ravard and Dourish, 1990 ; Hendrie and Neill, 1992). The often observed lack of dose-response curves following administration of non selective compounds in behavioral studies could result from successive activation of CCK-B and CCK-A receptors (review in Ravard and Dourish, 1990). Furthermore, the effects of CCK compounds could vary considerably in regard to the studied animals due to differences in the distribution and binding characteristics of CCK receptor types among species (Sekiguchi and Moroji 1986; Durieux et al., 1988, Beinborn et al., 1993) or subtypes (Durieux et al., 1986, 1992 ; Knapp et al., 1990), (Table 2).

Table 2 : Inhibitory potencies of CCK analogues on the specific binding of 0.2 nM [^{3}H]pBC 264, at CCK-B sites in different species *(from Durieux et al., 1992).*

	Guinea pig cortex		Rat cortex		Mouse brain	
	K_I nM	n_H	K_I nM	n_H	K_I nM	n_H
CCK$_8$	0.23 ± 0.03	0.94 ± 0.08	1.01 ± 0.05	0.82 ± 0.07	0.48 ± 0.07	0.95 ± 0.09
pCCK$_8$	0.13 ± 0.01	0.96 ± 0.06	0.55 ± 0.15	0.90 ± 0.07	0.33 ± 0.04	0.91 ± 0.05
pBC 264	0.13 ± 0.01	0.90 ± 0.08	0.17 ± 0.03	0.92 ± 0.03	0.17 ± 0.04	0.97 ± 0.03
CCK$_8$NS	6.0 ± 1.1	0.89 ± 0.03	10.2 ± 3.1	0.71 ± 0.08	4.6 ± 0.1	0.76 ± 0.04
CCK$_5$	11.0 ± 2.0	0.78 ± 0.03	19.7 ± 2.8	0.63 ± 0.03	13.2 ± 2.4	0.84 ± 0.03
CCK$_4$	49.9 ± 9.9	0.81 ± 0.12	55.7 ± 10.2	0.65 ± 0.04	16.4 ± 3.4	0.78 ± 0.05
BC 254	0.76 ± 0.09	0.83 ± 0.04	43.9 ± 6.7	0.88 ± 0.08	23.3 ± 1.0	0.95 ± 0.01
L-364,718	132.0 ± 18.3	1.02 ± 0.04	549 ± 69	0.93 ± 0.08	62.4 ± 7.6	0.80 ± 0.05
L-365,260	2.32 ± 0.27	0.92 ± 0.06	10.9 ± 2.0	0.87 ± 0.01	5.2 ± 0.6	0.88 ± 0.07
PD134308	0.28 ± 0.01	1.02 ± 0.01	6.1 ± 0.5	0.97 ± 0.08	1.2 ± 0.2	0.83 ± 0.07

Results are mean ± S.E.M. from three to four experiments performed in triplicate. Each determination was obtained from the analysis of Hill plots using eight to ten concentrations of analogues.

II Anatomical substrate of CCK-inducing anxiogenic-like effects

There is some evidence for the participation of several brain structures in the behavioral expression of the anxiogenic-like effects and the associated neurovegetative and neuroendocrine changes induced by CCK agonists.

The solitary complex (SC) which is composed of dorsal motor nucleus of the vagus (DVMN) and the NTS, plays a major role in translating peripheral information to the brain. This was clearly demonstrated in the case of the satiety reflex which involves initial peripheral CCK-A receptor activation (Smith et al., 1981 ; Crawley et al., 1991 ; Smith and Gibbs, 1992). The involvement of the NTS has been recently visualized using immunohistochemical techniques to map C-fos expression. The i.p. administration of CCK$_8$ (low dose) induced C-fos expression in the rostral and the caudal part of the NTS and in the paraventricular nuclei of the hypothalamus. The suppression of CCK$_8$ effects by MK329 is in favor of a CCK interaction with the CCK-A receptors (Chen et al., 1993). These experiments are in agreement with electrophysiological data showing that CCK-A-mediated inhibition of preganglionic DVMN neurons in coronal brainstem slices could be in keeping with a relaxation of the digestive tract by CCK which occurs during the satiety reflex. The NTS was postulated to directly or indirectly participate in some components of panic attacks (Branchereau et al., 1992) triggerred by stimulation of CCK-B binding sites. Indeed CCK-B receptor stimulation by BC264 induces postsynaptic excitation. Moreover the proper action of the CCK-B antagonists L365,260 and CI988 on neurons of the SC suggest that tonically released endogenous CCK8 acts on CCK-B receptors to control presynaptic inhibition induced by GABAergic interneurons (Branchereau et al., 1992). The resulting postsynaptic neuronal stimulation could produce local excitation of neurons involved in cardiorespiratory control and in emotional responses through activation of direct or indirect ascending pathways projecting to the N.Acc. (Wang et al., 1992), amygdala, periaqueductal grey matter and the locus coeruleus (review in Jean, 1991).

Other brain regions linked or not to the NTS seem to be involved in CCK-induced anxiogenic effects. Thus, CCK_8 has been shown to activate rat hippocampal neurons, an effect suppressed by activation of the neuronal type of benzodiazepine receptor (Bradwejn and De Montigny, 1984). The authors have suggested that this electrophysiological link between CCK and benzodiazepine might be related to the anxiolytic properties of benzodiazepine. Moreover local administration of CCK_8 in the dorsal periaqueductal grey matter which contains neurons where CCK and enkephalins are colocalized, induced a selective decrease in exploration of the aversive part (open arms) of the elevated plus maze in rats (Guimaraès et al., 1992). Besides microinjection of CCK_8 and unsulfated CCK_8 into the central amygdaloid nucleus delayed the extinction of active avoidance and increased the retention of passive avoidance behavior which have been possibly related to an enhancement of behavioral arousal and/or fear-motivation of the animals (Fekete et al., 1984).

More complex results have been described after local injection of CCK_8 into the N.Acc., that may be due to the anatomical and biochemical heterogeneity of the CCKergic system in this brain structure. While neuroleptic-like effects have been found with CCK_8 (Fekete et al., 1984 ; Heidbreder et al., 1992), a hypoexploration in the four hole box and in the open-field (only observed in a novel environment) and an anxiogenic-like effect in the elevated plus maze were observed after stimulation of CCK-A receptors in the postero-median part of the N.Acc., but not into the anterior part (Daugé et al., 1989a,b, 1990). Interestingly this part of the nucleus receives DA-CCK colocalized fibers issuing from the ventral tegmental area (Hökfelt et al., 1980) but also CCK fibers from the NTS (Wang et al., 1992). In agreement with this neuroanatomical organization, CCK_8 inducing effects were suppressed by 6-hydroxydopamine lesions of the DA mesoaccumbens fibers and by D_2 but not D_1 antagonists (Derrien et al., 1993a). Moreover, several studies have described CCK effects on extracellular DA levels in the N.Acc.. In agreement with the neuroanatomical heterogeneity of this structure, different effects have been found after injection into the anterior or the posterior N.Acc., but some discrepancies remain. For instance, CCK_8 has been found to decrease and increase DA release from rostral and caudal slices of N.Acc. respectively (Marshall et al., 1991), while it has been shown to increase this release only in the anterior N.Acc. after microdialysis in anesthetized rats (Ruggeri et al., 1987). This latter method seems to be the best approach to study the regional release of various transmitters in brain. However, it is essential to respect a delay between the probe insertion and the beginning of the perfusion (Santiago and Westerink, 1990) and to avoid anesthesia which has been shown to modify neuronal responsiveness (Stähle et al., 1990). Under these conditions, we have recently studied the effects of CCKergic stimulation on DA release in the N.Acc. of freely moving rats (Ladurelle et al., 1993). The animals were implanted with a probe the day before perfusion and housed in individual boxes. The treatment consisted of a 40 min perfusion of CCK compounds directly through the microdialysis probes. Under these conditions, the perfusion of CCK_8 (25pmol) in the posterior N.Acc. induced a 64% increase of DA release in this region. It also increased, but on a lower scale, the extracellular levels of DA catabolites (DOPAC, HVA). In contrast, the selective CCK-B agonist BC264, perfused in the anterior N.Acc. (350pmol) had no effect on the metabolites but reduced DA release to approximately 55% of basal levels (Fig.2). These data suggest that the CCK modulation of DA involves two different mechanisms in the rostral and the caudal regions of the N.Acc. which could be related to the heterogeneity of responses obtained in CCK behavioral studies (Daugé et al., 1989b, 1992 ; review in Crawley, 1991). This is in agreement with anatomical data which indicate that the predominant organizational pattern of the N.Acc. appears to be one in which the core, shell and rostral pole engage different forebrain systems, that possibly subserve entirely different functions mediated by distantly related mechanisms (review by Zahm and Brog, 1992).

The different interactions obtained between CCK and DA in these two parts of the N.Acc., suggest an important regulatory role of this peptide in limbic DA function which could be disturbed in several psychiatric disorders (schizophrenia, depressive syndroms, anxiety...). In line with this, it is of particular interest to note that BC264 peripherally injected in African green monkeys produced vigilance and stereotypy (Palmour et al., 1993) and CCK-B antagonists a decrease of the firing of the DA neurones of the ventral tegmental area in the mesencephalon which project to the N.Acc. (Rasmussen et al.,1993).

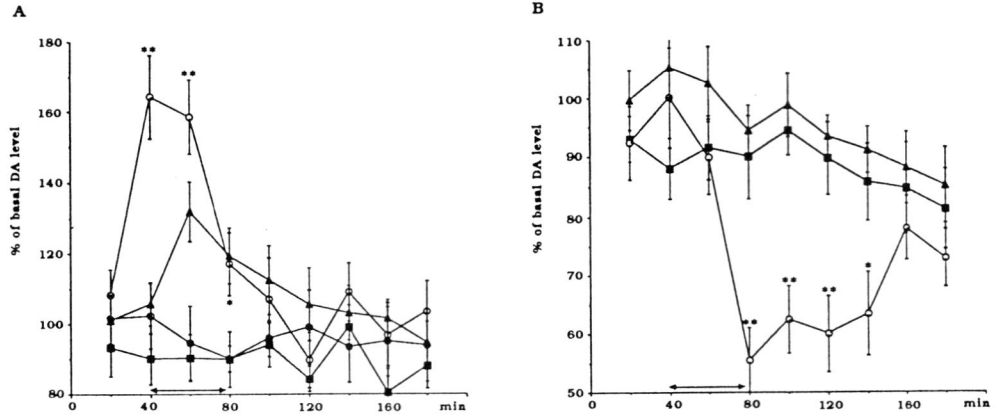

Fig. 2 A : Effect of the 40 min perfusion of CCK_8 on the extracellular DA level in the postero-median nucleus accumbens. ■ : Saline ; ● : CCK_8 10^{-9}M ; ▲ : CCK_8 10^{-7}M ; O : CCK_8 10^{-5}M. B : Effect of the 40 min perfusion of BC 264 on the extracellular DA level in the anterior nucleus accumbens. ■ : Saline ; ▲ : BC 264 10^{-5}M ; O : BC 264 10^{-4}M. *, $p<0.05$; **, $p<0.01$; Dunnett's test.

Conclusion

Experiments using CCK antagonists and agonists showed that the CCKergic system was activated in several stressfull and conflicting situations in humans, monkeys and rodents. Thus CCK was shown to produce a hypoexploration only in rats not habituated to their environment (Daugé et al., 1989a). Moreover CCK antagonists potentiated the analgesia induced by morphine only in non acclimatized rats exposed to a novel environment (Lavigne et al., 1992 ; see also references in section I). The phasic release of CCK could lead to various behavioral responses such as antinociception (by the interaction of CCK with CCK-A receptors and consequently an increase of endogenous enkephalin release) or nociception (by the interaction of CCK with CCK-B receptors leading to a decrease in endogenous enkephalin release) (Noble et al., 1993), anorexia, anxiety (by the interaction of CCK on CCK-B receptors)... and could participate in the coordinated control of some adaptative behaviors. In line with this, the recent work showing that CCK is markedly elevated in plasma before (and after) competitive marathon runs compared to controls (non competitive marathon runs) suggests that CCK could be an important factor in responses to anticipatory stress (Philipp et al., 1992). Moreover, endogenous CCK, through CCK-B receptors, will re-establish the nociceptive threshold increased by endogenous opioids when the stimuli that signal the occurence of aversive or dangerous events is no longer present or when a safety stimuli occurs (Wiertelack et al., 1992). It has been proposed that CCKergic and opioidergic systems could be functional antagonists. Thus it has been shown that the release of endogenous enkephalins leading to nociception, was decreased by the activation of CCK-B receptors and increased by the blockade of CCK-B but not CCK-A receptors (Noble et al., 1993 ; Maldonado et al., 1993). Conversely activation of the opioidergic system can in turn regulate the extracellular levels of CCK (Benoliel et al., 1992 ; Ruiz-Gayo et al., 1992). Peripheral administration of BC264 or BC197 accentuated the suppression of motor activity in the conditioned suppression of motility paradigm, in shocked mice but not in non-shocked animal. This effect was suppressed by L365,260 and the CCK-B antagonist induced a reduction in stress-induced immobilization. This first demonstration of antidepressant-like effects resulting from CCK-B receptor blockade seems to result from a functional antagonism between CCK and enkephalins acting on ∂ sites (Durieux et al., 1993).

In conclusion several experimental studies are in favor of the participation of the CCKergic system as an endogenous anxiogenic factor required for some adaptative behaviors. A dysfunctioning of this system could lead to psychiatric disorders, as reported for panic attacks. It seems that CCK could interact with its receptors at the peripheral level to participate in the satiety reflex (CCK-A) but also in anxiety and panic disorders (CCK-B/gastrin). Although, the role of CCK receptors in the brain is not yet well understood, several experiments support their participation in emotional and cognitive processes. Several structures of the brain are involved: N.Acc. amygdala, hippocampus, periaqueductal gray matter. The NTS could play a major role in translating peripheral information to the brain. CCK-B antagonists could therefore have interesting therapeutic implications. Indeed, unlike classical neuroleptics, they could act at the mesocorticolimbic level, minimizing the extrapyramidal effects observed with DA antagonists. Likewise the anxiolytic effects produced by CCK-B antagonists could be restricted to situations perceived as aversive, thus avoiding the side effects generated by tranquilisers as benzodiazepines.

REFERENCES

Abelson, J.L. and Nesse, R.M. (1990) : Cholecystokinin-4 and panic. Arch. Gen. Psychiat. 47, 395.

Beinborn, M., Lee, Y.-M., McBride, E.W., Quinn, M. and Kopin, A.S. (1993) : A single amino acid of the cholecystokinin-B/gastrin receptor determines specificity for non-peptide antagonists. *Nature* 362, 348-350.

Benoliel, J.J., Mauborgne, A., Bourgoin, S., Legrand, J.C., Hamon, M. and Cesselin, F. (1992) : Opioid control of the in vitro release of CCK-like material from the rat substantia nigra. *J. Neurochem.* 58, 916-922.

Blommaert, A.G.S., Weng, J.H., Dorville, A., McCort, I., Ducos, B., Durieux, C. and Roques, B.P. (1993) : Cholecystokinin peptidomimetics as selective CCK-B antagonists : Design, synthesis and in vitro and in vivo biochemical properties. J. Med. Chem., submitted.

Bradwejn, J. and De Montigny, C. (1984) : Benzodiazepines antagonize cholecystokinin-induced activation of rat hippocampal neurons. *Nature* 312, 363-364.

Bradwejn, J., Koszycki, D. and Meterissian, G. (1990) : Cholecystokinin-tetrapeptide induces panic attack in patients with panic disorder. *Can. J. Psychiat.* 35, 83-85.

Bradwejn, J., Koszycki, D. and Shriqui, C. (1991) : Enhanced sensitivity to cholecystokinin tetrapeptide in panic disorder clinical and behavioral findings. *Arch. Gen. Psychiatry* 48, 603-610.

Bradwejn, J., Koszycki, D., Dutertre, A.C., Megen, H.V., Boer, J.D., Westenberg, H., Karkanias, C. and Haigh, J. (1992) : L-365,260, a CCK-B antagonist, blocks CCK_4-panic in panic disorder. *Clin. Pharmacol.* 15suppl. 1, 5.

Branchereau, P., Böhme, G.A., Champagnat, J., Morin-Surun, M.P., Durieux, C., Roques, B.P. and Denavit-Saubié, M. (1992) : Cholecystokinin and cholecystokinin receptors in neurons of the brainstem solitary complex of the rat : pharmacological identification. *J. Pharmacol. Exp. Ther.* 260, 1433-1440.

Charpentier, B., Durieux, C., Pélaprat, D., Dor, A., Reibaud, M., Blanchard, J.C. and Roques, B.P. (1988) : Enzyme resistant CCK analogs with high affinities for central receptors. *Peptides* 9, 835-841.

Chen, D.Y., Deutsch, J.A., Gonzalez, M.F. and Gu, Y. (1993) : The induction and suppression of c-fos expression in the rat brain by cholecystokinin and its antagonist L-365,718. *Neurosci. Lett.* 149, 91-94.

Crawley, J.N. (1991) : Cholecystokinin-dopamine interactions. *Trends Pharmacol. Sci.* 12, 232-236.

Crawley, J.N., Fiske, S.M., Durieux, C., Derrien, M. and Roques, B.P. (1991) : Centrally administered cholecystokinin suppresses feeding through a peripheral type receptor mechanism. *J. Pharmacol. Exp. Ther.* 257, 1076-1080.

Daugé, V., Dor, A., Féger, J. and Roques, B.P. (1989a) : The behavioral effects of CCK_8 injected into the medial nucleus accumbens are dependent on the motivational state of rat. *Eur. J. Pharmacol.* 163, 25-32.

Daugé, V., Steimes, P., Derrien, M., Beau, N., Roques, B.P. and Féger, J. (1989b) : CCK_8 effects on motivational, and emotional states of rats involve CCK-A receptors of the postero-median part of the nucleus accumbens. *Pharmacol. Biochem. Behav.* 34, 157-163.

Daugé, V., Böhme, G.A., Crawley, J.N., Durieux, C., Stutzmann, J.M., Féger, J., Blanchard, J.C. and Roques, B.P. (1990) : Investigation of behavioral and electrophysiological responses induced by selective stimulation of CCK-B receptors by using a new highly potent CCK analog BC 264. *Synapse* 6, 73-80.

Daugé, V., Derrien, M., Blanchard, J.C. and Roques, B.P. (1992) : The selective CCK-B agonist, BC 264 injected in the antero-lateral part of the nucleus accumbens, reduces the spontaneous alternation behavior of rats. *Neuropharmacol.* **31**, 67, 75.

Daugé, V., Corringer, P.J. and Roques, B.P. (1993) : Peripheral administration of selective CCK-B but not CCK-A agonists produced anxiogenic-like effects in the black and white box test in mice. *Brit. J. Pharmacol.*, Submitted.

Derrien, M., Durieux, C., Daugé, V. and Roques, B.P. (1993a) : Involvement of D_2 dopamine receptors in the emotional and motivational responses induced by injection of CCK_8 in the posterior part of the nucleus accumbens. *Brain Res.*, in press.

Derrien, M., Noble, F., Maldonado, R. and Roques, B.P. (1993b) : Cholecystokinin-A but not cholecystokinin-B receptor stimulation induces endogenous opioid dependent antinociceptive effect in the hot plate test in mice. *Neurosci. Lett.*, in press.

Durieux, C., Coppey, M., Zajac, J.M. and Roques, B.P. (1986) : Occurence of two cholecystokinin binding sites in guinea-pig brain cortex. *Biochem. Biophys. Res. Commun.* **137**, 1167-1173.

Durieux, C., Pham, H., Charpentier, B. and Roques, B.P. (1988) : Discrimination between CCK receptors of guinea-pig and rat brain by cyclic CCK_8 analogues. *Biochem. Biophys. Res. Commun.* **154**, 1301-1307.

Durieux, C., Ruiz-Gayo, M. and Roques, B.P. (1991) : In vivo binding affinities of cholecystokinin agonists and antagonists determined using the selective CCK-B agonist [^{3}H]pBC 264. *Eur. J. Pharmacol.* **209**, 185-193.

Durieux, C., Ruiz-Gayo, M., Corringer, P.J., Bergeron, F., Ducos, B. and Roques, B.P. (1992) : [^{3}H]pBC 264, a suitable probe for studying cholecystokinin-B-receptors : binding characteristics in rodent brains and comparison with [^{3}H]SNF 8702. *Mol. Pharmacol.* **41**, 1089-1095.

Durieux, C., Derrien, M., Maldonado, R., Valverde, O., Fournié-Zaluski, M.C. and Roques, B.P. (1993) : Pharmacological investigation of CCK-B receptors using systemically active selective agonists and antagonists. *CCK 93, May 19-22, 1993, Chatham, Cape Cod, Ma. p13.*

Faris, P.L., McLaughlin, C.L., Baile, C.A., Olney, J.W. and Komisaruk, B.R. (1983) : Morphine analgesia potentiated but tolerance not affected by active immunization against cholecystokinin. *Science* **226**, 1215-1217.

Fekete, M., Lengyel, A., Hegedüs, B., Penke, B., Zarandy, M., Toth, G.K. and Telegdy, G. (1984) : Further analysis of the effects of cholecystokinin octapeptides on avoidance behaviour in rats. *Eur. J. Pharmacol.* **98**, 79-91.

Guimaraès, F.S., Russo, A.S., De Aguiar, J.C., Ballejo, G. and Graeff, F.G. (1992) : Anxiogenic-like effect of CCK8 micro-injected into the dorsal periaqueductal grey of rats in the elevated plus maze. *In Multiple Cholecystokinin Receptors in the CNS*, ed. C.T. Dourish, S.J. Cooper, S.V. Iversen & L.L. Iversen, pp. 149-154. Oxford Science Publications.

Heidbreder, C., Gewiss, M., De Mot, B., Mertens, I. and De Witte, P. (1992) : Balance of glutamate and dopamine in the nucleus accumbens modulates self-stimulation behavior after injection of cholecystokinin and neurotensin in the rat brain. *Peptides* **13**, 441-449.

Hendrie, C.A. and Neill, J.C. (1992) : Ethological analysis of the role of CCK in anxiety. *In Multiple Cholecystokinin Receptors in the CNS*, ed. C.T. Dourish, S.J. Cooper, S.D. Iversen & L.L. Iversen, pp. 132-142. Oxford Science Publications.

Hill, R.G., Hughes, J. and Pittaway, K.M. (1987) : Antinociceptive action of cholecystokinin octapeptide (CCK_8) and related peptides in rats and mice : effects of naloxone and peptidase inhibitors. *Neuropharmacol.* **26**, 289-300.

Hökfelt, T., Rehfeld, J.F., Skirboll, L., Ivemark, M. and Markey, K. (1980) : Evidence for coexistence of dopamine and cholecystokinin in mesolimbic neurons. *Nature* (Lond.) **285**, 476-478.

Hughes, J., Boden, P., Costall, B., Domeney, A., Kelly, E., Horwell, D.C., Hunter, J.C., Pinnock, R.D. and Woodruff, G.N. (1990) : Development of a class of selective cholecystokinin type B receptor antagonists having potent anxiolytic activity. *Proc. Natl. Acad. Sci. USA* **87**, 6728-6732.

Itoh, S. and Lai, H. (1990) : Influences of cholecystokinin and analogues on memory processes. *Drug. Dev. Res.* **21**, 257-276.

Jean, A. (1991) : Le noyau du faisceau solitaire : aspects neuroanatomiques, neurochimiques et fonctionnels. *Arch. Int. Physiol. Bioch. Biophys.* **99**(5), A3-A52.

Knapp, RJ., Vaughn, L.K., Fang, S.N., Bogert, C.L., Yamamura, M.S., Hruby, V.J. and Yamamura, H.I. (1990) : A new, highly selective CCK-B receptor radioligand ([^{3}H] [N.methyl-

Nle^{28,31}]CCK$_{26-33}$) : evidence for CCK-B receptor heterogeneity. *J. Pharmacol. Exp. Ther.* 255, 1278-1283.

Koyama, S., Fujita, T., Shibamoto, T., Matsuda, Y., Uematsu, H. and Jones, R.O. (1990) : Contribution of baroreceptor reflexes to blood pressure and sympathetic responses to cholecystokinin and vasoactive intestinal peptide in anaesthesized dogs. *Eur. J. Pharmacol.* 175, 245-251.

Ladurelle, N., Keller, G., Roques, B.P. and Daugé, V. (1993) : Effects of CCK$_8$ and of the CCK-B selective agonist BC 264 on extracellular dopamine content in the anterior and posterior nucleus accumbens : A microdialysis study in freely moving rats. *Brain Res.*, in press.

Lavigne, G.J., Millington, W.R. and Mueller, G.P. (1992) : The CCK-A and CCK-B receptors antagonists devazepide and L-365,260, enhance morphine antinociception only in non-acclimated rats exposed to a novel environment. *Neuropeptides* 21, 119-129.

Lemaire, M., Piot, O., Roques, B.P., Böhme, G.A. and Blanchard, J.C. (1992) : Evidence for an endogenous cholecystokininergic balance in social memory. *Neuroreport* 3, 929-932.

Ley, R. (1988) : Panick attacks during sleep : a hyperventilation-probably model. *J. Behav. Ther. & Exp. Psychiat.* 19, 181-192.

Lydiard, R.B., Ballenger, J.C., Laraia, M.T., Fossey, M.D. and Beinfeld, M.C. (1992) : CSF cholecystokinin concentrations in patients with panic disorders and in normal comparison subjects. *Am. J. Psychiatry* 149, 691-693.

Maldonado, R., Derrien, M;, Noble, F. and Roques, B.P. (1993) : Association of the peptidase inhibitor RB 101 and a CCK-B antagonist strongly enhances antinociceptive responses. *NeuroReport*, in press.

Marshall, F.H., Barnes, S., Hughes, J., Woodruff, G.N. and Hunter, J.C. (1991) : Cholecystokinin modulates the release of dopamine from the anterior and posterior nucleus accumbens by two different mechanisms. *J. Neurochem.* 56, 917-922.

Moran, T.H., Robinson, P.H., Goldrich, M.S. and McHugh, P.R. (1986) : Two brain cholecystokinin receptors : implication for behavioral actions. *Brain Res.* 362, 175-179.

Morin-Surun, M.P., De Marchi, J., Vanderhaeghen, J.J., Rossier, J. and Denavit-Saubié, M. (1983) : Inhibitory effect of cholecystokinin octapeptide on neurons in the nucleus tractus solitarius. *Brain Res.* 265, 333-338.

Noble, F., Derrien, M. and Roques, B.P. (1993) : Modulation of opioid analgesia by CCK : evidence of regulatory mechanisms between CCK and enkephalin systems in the supraspinal control of pain. *Brit. J. Pharmacol.*, in press.

Palmour, R.M., Durieux, C., Roques, B.P., Bertrand, P., Capet, M., Dubroeucq, M.-C., Howbert, J.J., Woodruff, G., Bradwejn, J. and Ervin, F.R. (1993) : Anxiogenic effects of CCK agonists in a non-human primate model : central or peripheral ? *CCK 93, May 19-22, 1993, Chatham, Cape Cod, Ma. p52.*

Philipp, E., Wilckens, T., Friess, E., Platte, P. and Pirke, K.-M. (1992) : Cholecystokinin, gastrin and stress hormone responses in marathon runners. *Peptides* 13, 125-128.

Rasmussen, K., Czachura, J.F., Stockton, M.E. and Howbert, J.J. (1993) : Electrophysiological effects of diphenylpyrazolidine cholecystokinin B and cholecystokinin A antagonists on midbrain dopamine neurons. *J. Pharmacol. Exp. Ther.* 264, 480-488.

Rataud, J., Darche, F., Piot, O., Stutzmann, J.M., Böhme, G.A. and Blanchard, J.C. (1991) : "Anxiolytic" effect of CCK-antagonists on plus maze behavior in mice. *Brain Res.* 548, 315-317.

Ravard, S. and Dourish, C.T. (1990) : Cholecystokinin and anxiety. *Trends Pharmacol. Sci.* 11, 271-273.

Rehfeld, J.F. and Hansen, H.F. (1986) : Characterization of preprocholecystokinin products in the porcine cerebral cortex : evidence of different processing pathways. *J. Biol. Chem.* 261, 5832-5840.

Ruggeri, M., Ungerstedt, U., Agnati, F., Mutt, V., Härfstrand, A. and Fuxe, K. (1987) : Effects of cholecystokinin peptides and neurotensin on dopamine release and metabolism in the rostral and caudal part of the nucleus accumbens using intracerebral dialysis in the anaesthesized rat. *Neurochem. Int.* 10(4), 509-520.

Ruiz-Gayo, M., Durieux, C., Fournié-Zaluski, M.C. and Roques, B.P. (1992) : Stimulation of δ opioid receptors reduces the in vivo binding of the cholecystokinin CCK-B selective agonist

[³H]pBC 264 : evidence for a physiological regulation of CCKergic systems by endogenous enkephalins. *J. Neurochem.* **59**, 1805-1811.

Saint-Hilaire, Z., Roques, B.P. and Nicolaidis, S. (1991) : Effect of a highly selective central CCK-B receptor agonist : BC 264 on rat sleep. *Pharmacol. Biochem. Behav.* **38**, 545-548.

Santiago, M. and Westerink, B.H.C. (1990) : Characterization of the in vivo release of dopamine as recorded by different types of intracerebral microdialysis probes. *Naunyn-Schmied. Arch. Pharmacol.* **342**, 407-414.

Sekiguchi, R. and Moroji, T. (1986) : A comparative study on characterization and distribution of cholecystokinin binding sites among the rat, mouse and guinea-pig brain. *Brain Res.* **399**, 271-281.

Singh, L., Lewis, A.S., Field, M.J., Hugues, J. and Woodruff, G.N. (1991) : Evidence for an involvement of the brain cholecystokinin B receptor in anxiety. *Proc. Natl. Acad. Sci. USA* **88**, 1130-1133.

Smith, G.P., Jerome, C., Cushin, B.J., Eterno, R. and Smasky, K.J. (1981) : Abdominal vagotomy blocks the satiety effects of cholecystokinin in rats. *Science* **213**, 1036-1037.

Smith, G.P. and Gibbs, J. (1992) : Development and proof of the CCK hypothesis of satiety. *In Multiple Cholecystokinin Receptors in the CNS*, ed. C.J. Dourish, S.J. Cooper, S.D. Iversen & L.L. Iversen, pp. 166-182. Oxford Science Publications.

Stähle, L., Collin, A.K. and Ungerstedt, U. (1990) : Effect of halothane anaesthesia on extracellular levels of dopamine, dihydroxyphenylacetic acid, homovanillic acid and 5-hydroxyindolacetic acid in rat striatum : a microdialysis study. *Naunyn-Schmied. Arch. Pharmacol.* **342**, 136-140.

Wang, Z.-J., Rao, Z.-R. and Shi, J.-W. (1992) : Tyrosine hydroxylase, neurotensin, or cholecystokinin-containing neurons in the nucleus tractus solitari send projection fibers to the nucleus accumbens in the rat. *Brain Res.* **578**, 347-350.

Wank, S.A., Harkins, R., Jensen, R.T., Shapira, H., De Weerth, A. and Slattery, T. (1992) : Purification, molecular cloning, and functional expression of the cholecystokinin receptor from rat pancreas. *Proc. Natl. Acad. Sci. USA* **89**, 3125-3129.

Wiertelak, E.P., Maier, S.F. and Watkins, L.R. (1992) : Cholecystokinin antianalgesia : safety cues abolish morphine analgesia. *Science* **256**, 830-833.

Zahm, D.S. and Brog, J.S. (1992) : On the significance of subterritories in the "accumbens" part of the rat ventral striatum. *Neurosci.* **50**, 751-767.

Résumé

Un certain nombre d'études pharmacologiques effectuées chez l'homme, le singe et les rongeurs sont en faveur de la participation du système CCKergique dans certains comportements adaptatifs. Il pourrait dans certains cas intervenir en s'opposant aux effets des enképhalines endogènes interagissant avec les récepteurs δ, comme ceci est démontré dans une situation de stress émotionnel chez l'animal, montrant des effets de type antidépresseur des antagonistes CCK-B. Un dysfonctionnement du système CCKergique pourrait conduire à des désordres psychiatriques comme il est postulé, lors d'attaques de panique chez l'homme et chez le singe. Les récepteurs périphériques (CCK-B/gastrine) ainsi que les récepteurs CCK-B et CCK-A centraux (noyau du tractus solitaire, hippocampe, système mésolimbique) semblent être impliqués dans les effets de type anxiogène et dans les changements neurovégétatifs et neuroendocriniens associés. Dans plusieurs modèles animaux de peur ou d'anxiété (boîte noire et blanche, labyrinthe en croix surélevé, interaction sociale...) l'administration périphérique d'agonistes CCK-B (BC264, BC197) et d'antagonistes (L365,260, CI988, RB211) sont en faveur du rôle de la CCK comme facteur endogène d'anxiété. Les antagonistes CCK-B pourraient donc avoir des applications thérapeutiques dans le traitement des attaques de panique et de l'anxiété. Dans le noyau accumbens postérieur, le CCK_8 en interagissant avec les récepteurs CCK-A augmente les taux extracellulaires de dopamine chez l'animal éveillé et induit un effet de type anxiogène qui est supprimé par une lésion des voies dopaminergiques mésoaccumbens ou par un antagoniste D_2. Des études biochimiques et comportementales suggèrent que plusieurs sous-types de récepteurs CCK-B pourraient être impliqués dans les modifications induites par le CCK_8 au niveau des processus émotionnels et cognitifs.

NMDA antagonists: a novel class of anxiolytics?

Jenny L. Wiley and Robert L. Balster

Medical College of Virginia, Department of Pharmacology and Toxicology, MCV Station, Box 613, Richmond, Virginia 23298-0613, USA

SUMMARY

Competitive NMDA antagonists produce reliable anxiolytic effects in punishment and nonpunishment procedures with rats, pigeons and mice. In squirrel monkeys, neither competitive nor PCP-like NMDA antagonists are active in punishment procedures. Other types of NMDA antagonists have not been tested in this species. In rats, pigeons, and mice, PCP-like antagonists show variable effects in punishment procedures as do other types of noncompetitive NMDA antagonists, although the latter types of drugs have not been extensively studied. In nonpunishment procedures, MK-801, the only known PCP-like drug investigated, is active in all models. Glycine-site antagonists show similar activity in nonpunishment procedures whereas the polyamine-site antagonist, ifenprodil, is active, but nonselective. Thus, all types of NMDA antagonists tested exhibit anxiolytic activity in both punishment and nonpunishment procedures in many studies. The antipunishment effect of competitive and PCP-like NMDA antagonists appears to be species specific, occurring in rodents and pigeons but not in squirrel monkeys. Overall, the anxiolytic effects of competitive NMDA antagonists are the most consistent, which is encouraging for the continued evaluation of these drugs as potential antianxiety agents.

The benzodiazepines, the most frequently prescribed class of antianxiety medication, are believed to produce their anxiolytic effect via facilitation of inhibitory pathways in the central nervous system. Specifically, benzodiazepines bind to specific sites associated with the α-subunit of the γ-aminobutyric acid (GABA) receptor complex. Agonist binding to the GABA receptor produces channel opening and an influx of chloride ions, resulting in cellular inhibition. Benzodiazepine binding increases the frequency of channel opening (Study & Barker, 1981). In addition to their anxiolytic effects, the benzodiazepines have a number of other therapeutic effects in humans and behavioral effects in animals, including muscle relaxation, sedation, and anticonvulsant effects (Sanger, 1985).

One class of drug that has a preclinical behavioral profile which resembles that of GABA agonists is N-methyl-D-aspartate (NMDA) antagonists. NMDA antagonists have been shown to have anticonvulsant (Croucher et al., 1982) and muscle relaxant effects (Turski et al., 1985). Preclinical evaluation suggests that they may also have anxiolytic effects (Wiley & Balster, 1992).

The NMDA receptor is one of a subclass of receptors that bind excitatory amino acids. The NMDA receptor is actually a receptor complex that is comprised of at least six different binding sites: a NMDA site, strychnine-insensitive glycine site, phencyclidine (PCP) site, magnesium site, polyamine site, and zinc site. Agonist binding to the NMDA site opens a channel and allows influx of calcium and sodium ions, resulting in cellular excitation (Lodge & Johnson, 1990; Watkins, 1989). Competitive NMDA antagonists compete with agonists for binding at the NMDA site (Olverman & Watkins, 1989). Glycine is required as a co-transmitter; hence, glycine binding is facilitory and glycine blockers function as NMDA antagonists. The PCP and magnesium sites are located within the channel and binding at these sites results in inhibition of channel opening (Lodge et al., 1989). Ligands at the zinc site are also inhibitory modulators of NMDA function; ligands at the polyamine site are facilatory. The present review examines preclinical research on potential anxiolytic effects of antagonists acting at various sites within the NMDA receptor complex.

The methods used to study anxiolytic effects of drugs in animals can be classified as punishment procedures, nonpunishment procedures, or drug discrimination. Studies using drug discrimination as an anxiolytic screening procedure and studies of drug discrimination with NMDA antagonists are reviewed elsewhere (Andrews & Stephens, 1990; Willetts et al., 1990) and will not be covered in this chapter. The results of tests with the other two types of procedures are presented separately.

PUNISHMENT PROCEDURES

Punishment can be defined as suppression of behavior that occurs subsequent to the presentation of an aversive stimulus such as electric shock. Punishment procedures used to screen for the anxiolytic effects of drugs typically involve delivery of an electric shock when a hungry or thirsty animal performs a specific response (e.g., lever press or licking response) in order to obtain food or water. Alternatively, exploratory behavior of the animal may be curtailed through the use of punishment (e.g., in the four-plate test). Punishment procedures usually consist of a multi-component operant schedule in which behavior in one or more components is punished and behavior in the other components is unpunished.

Benzodiazepines and barbiturates, known antianxiety agents, selectively disinhibit behavior suppressed by punishment; hence, animals exhibit increased rates of responding during punished components without showing changes in unpunished responding. Other drug classes, such as stimulants, analgesics, and antidepressants, generally do not increase rates of punished responding (Cook & Davidson, 1973; Cook & Sepinwall, 1975; Geller & Seifter, 1960).

NMDA antagonists have been tested in several types of punishment procedures, including conflict tests as well as tests of the conditioned emotional response and the four-plate test (for a review of methods, see File, 1987). Species tested include rats, pigeons, mice, and squirrel monkeys. In rats, all of the competitive NMDA antagonists tested to date produced antipunishment effects. AP7 (Bennett & Amrick, 1986, 1987), CGS 19755 (Bennett et al., 1989, 1990; Liebman & Bennett, 1988), (+)-CPP (Corbett & Dunn, 1991; Dunn et al., 1990; Liebman & Bennett, 1988), NPC 12626 (Wiley et al., 1992; Willetts et al., 1993), and NPC 17742 (Willetts et al., 1993) increased punished responding, usually without affecting unpunished responding. In some studies, the magnitude of the antipunishment effect was comparable to that produced by the benzodiazepines (Liebman & Bennett, 1988; Willetts et al., 1993); in other cases, the magnitude of the antipunishment effect was smaller than that of the benzodiazepines (Bennett & Amrick, 1986; Wiley et al., 1992). Tolerance to the antipunishment effect of two of these compounds, NPC 12626 and NPC 17742, did not develop with repeated dosing over a period of 5-6 days (Wiley et al., 1992; Willetts et al., 1993). When administered orally, some of the competitive NMDA antagonists have shown activity in anticonvulsant screening tests (Chapman et al., 1990, 1991); however, CGS 19755 did not show oral activity in a punishment procedure (Bennett et al., 1990).

In contrast to the consistent antipunishment effect seen with competitive NMDA antagonists in rats, noncompetitive NMDA antagonists produce more variable results across studies. PCP-like antagonists have received the majority of research attention. In most rat studies, PCP-like antagonists increase punished responding (Corbett & Dunn, 1991; Dunn et al., 1990; Hoehn-Saric et al., 1991; Lerner et al., 1986; McMillan et al., 1991; Porter et al., 1989; Snell & Harris, 1982); in a few rat studies, the results are negative (Liebman & Bennett, 1988; Sanger & Jackson, 1989). These variable results cannot be readily explained by differences in drug or training schedules or by other procedural variations. Indeed, in the context of a single study, Sanger & Jackson (1989) found that, whereas MK-801 was active in a punishment procedure, PCP and both isomers of NANM were inactive. When active, PCP-like drugs also produce a variable magnitude of antipunishment effects, similar to the situation with competitive NMDA antagonists. MK-801 has been the most frequently studied drug of this class. The effect of MK-801 appears to be time-dependent (Clineschmidt et al., 1982; Xie & Commissaris, 1992), requiring long pre-treatment intervals (up to 24 hours). This drug has been shown to have oral activity in rats (Clineschmidt et al., 1982; Goldberg et al., 1983) and to be stereoselective with activity in the (+)-isomer (Xie and Commissaris, 1992). MK-801's antipunishment effect is not mediated by benzodiazepine receptors as the benzodiazepine receptor antagonist, flumazenil, does not block activity (Clineschmidt, 1982).

Noncompetitive NMDA antagonists acting at sites other than the PCP site have received very little testing in punishment procedures in rats. Riluzole, a noncompetitive glutamate antagonist, was shown to be inactive in a punishment procedure (Stutzman et al., 1989), as was ifenprodil, an antagonist at the polyamine site (Sanger & Jackson, 1989). On the other hand, results of punishment tests with antagonists of the strychnine-insensitive glycine site seem more promising. Dunn et al. (1992) have shown that (+)-HA-966, a glycine antagonist, increased punished responding, as did the racemate (Corbett & Dunn, 1991). Further, this drug's antipunishment effect was stereoselective with the (-)-isomer being inactive (Dunn et al., 1992). The same group has reported that two new noncompetitive NMDA antagonists, 7189 and 8319, exhibit antipunishment effects in rats (Dunn et al., 1990). Based on results from binding studies, these drugs are believed to act at the PCP receptor.

The profile of antipunishment effects of NMDA antagonists in pigeons and in mice is similar to the profile in rats, although fewer studies have been done with these species. Competitive NMDA antagonists produce increases in punished responding in pigeons (Koek & Colpaert, 1991) and in mice (Stephens & Andrews, 1988; Stephens et al., 1986). The effect of PCP-like antagonists is variable in both species. Some studies report activity in punishment procedures (Brandao et al., 1980: Chait et al., 1981; Kuribara et al., 1990; Wenger, 1980); other studies report that these drugs are inactive (Koek & Colpaert, 1991; Stephens & Andrews, 1988). Other types of noncompetitive NMDA antagonists have been tested in a single study with pigeons. Koek and Colpaert (1991) found that riluzole, ifenprodil, and several glycine-site antagonists were inactive in a punishment procedure.

Finally, tests of NMDA antagonists in punishment procedures with squirrel monkeys have shown that the competitive NMDA antagonists, CPP and NPC 12626, and the PCP-like antagonists, PCP and MK-801, do not produce increases in punished responding in this species (Clineschmidt et al., 1982; Goldberg et al., 1983; Mansbach et al., 1991). Interestingly, buspirone, the prototypic 5-HT$_{1A}$ anxiolytic, produces antipunishment effects in rats and pigeons but not in squirrel monkeys (Barrett & Witkin, 1991).

In summary, studies with rats, pigeons and mice reveal that competitive NMDA antagonists reliably increase punished responding in all three species. PCP-like antagonists show variable effects in punishment procedures as do other types of noncompetitive NMDA antagonists, although the latter types of drugs have not been extensively studied. In squirrel monkeys, neither competitive nor PCP-like NMDA antagonists increase punished responding. Other types of NMDA antagonists have not been tested in this species.

NONPUNISHMENT PROCEDURES

Nonpunishment procedures involve investigation of drug effects on behaviors that naturally occur in rodents, including exploratory behavior, social interaction, and separation-induced ultrasonic vocalizations in rat pups. In the elevated plus-maze test, exploratory behavior is suppressed through elevation and introduction of a novel environment. This test involves placing a mouse or rat in the center of an elevated 4-arm maze shaped like a plus sign. Two of the arms are open and two are enclosed. Upon initial exposure to this apparatus, rodents typically spend a significantly greater amount of time in the closed arms. Administration of a benzodiazepine or other known anxiolytic agent increases the number of entries and amount of time spent in the open arms (Pellow & File, 1986; Pellow et al., 1985).

The social interaction test also involves suppression of behavior through the introduction of novelty. In this test, a rodent is placed in a novel environment with an unfamilar conspecific. Drugs with anxiolytic effects increase social interaction without increasing general motor activity (File 1980, 1988).

A third nonpunishment procedure that has been used to screen for anxiolytic effects of drugs is the separation-induced ultrasonic vocalization test (Gardner, 1985). This test involves recording the ultrasonic vocalizations emitted by rat pups when they are removed from the dam. Benzodiazepines suppress these vocalizations without producing overt signs of sedation (Kehne et al., 1991).

Competitive NMDA antagonists are active in all three screening procedures. In rats, AP5 (Dunn et al., 1989) and (+)-CPP (Corbett & Dunn, 1991; Dunn et al., 1989, 1990) increase the number of open arm entries and amount of time spent in the open arms of an elevated plus-maze. AP7 shows only weak activity in this model in rats and mice (Dunn et al., 1989; Stephens et al., 1986); however, the lower efficacy of this compound may be due to its poor CNS penetrability. When injected directly into the dorsal periaqueductal grey (DPAG) area of the midbrain of rats, AP7 increased number of open arm entries, as do the other competitive NMDA antagonists (Guimaraes et al., 1991). AP5, AP7, and (+)-CPP also selectively increased social interaction in rats (Dunn et al., 1989, 1990) and decreased separation-induced ultrasonic vocalizations in rat pups (Kehne et al., 1991; Winslow & Insel, 1991; Winslow et al., 1990). In rat pups, these drugs were 10-fold more potent in the separation-induced ultrasonic vocalization procedure than in antipunishment and anticonvulsant procedures (Winslow & Insel, 1991), perhaps reflecting the immaturity of the blood-brain barrier in rat pups or differences in the number and distribution of NMDA receptors in infant animals. In contrast with competitive antagonists, NMDA itself decreases open arm exploration and social interaction time (Dunn et al., 1989).

MK-801 is the only traditional PCP-like NMDA antagonist which has been tested in nonpunishment procedures. In rats, this drug is potent in increasing open arm exploration in the elevated plus-maze procedure (Corbett & Dunn, 1991; Dunn et al., 1989, 1990) and in increasing social interaction time in the social interaction test (Corbett & Dunn, 1991; Dunn et al., 1989, 1990). Overall motor activity remained unchanged in both types of tests. MK-801 has also been found to reduce signs of anxiety/fear in an antipredator defensiveness test in rats (Blanchard et al., 1992). In tests of separation-induced ultrasonic vocalizations in rat pups, MK-801 decreases ultrasonic vocalizations (Kehne et al., 1991; Winslow & Insel, 1991; Winslow et al., 1990), although this decrease is sometimes accompanied by a general decrease in motor activity (Winslow & Insel, 1991; Winslow et al., 1990). In general, MK-801 shows activity in all three nonpunishment models as well as in an antipredator defensiveness test. Two newer noncompetitive NMDA antagonists, 7189 and 8319, show similar anxiolytic activity in the elevated plus-maze and the social interaction test (Dunn et al., 1990).

Other types of noncompetitive NMDA antagonists are active in nonpunishment procedures. Glycine-site antagonists such as KYN, 7-Cl-KYN, and 5,7-DCKA increase open arm exploration in mice (Trullas et al., 1989) and decrease separation-induced ultrasonic vocalizations in rat pups (Kehne et al., 1991; Winslow et al., 1990). The partial glycine-site agonist, ACPC, produces similar results in both types of tests (Trullas et al., 1989; Winslow & Insel, 1991; Winslow et al., 1990). Dunn et al. (1992) found that the effect of HA-966, a glycine-site antagonist, was stereoselective. The (+)-isomer and the racemate (Corbett & Dunn, 1991) increased open arm exploration and social interaction time with an efficacy similar to that of diazepam; the (-)-isomer was inactive in both procedures. Finally, ifenprodil, an antagonist at the polyamine site, has been tested in the separation-induced ultrasonic vocalization procedure with rat pups. Although the drug decreased ultrasonic vocalizations, the decrease was accompanied by disturbances in motor activity (Winslow & Insel, 1991; Winslow et al., 1990).

In conclusion, although results of anxiolytic screening procedures with NMDA antagonists are not as consistently positive as results with benzodiazepines, it should be remembered that most of these tests were developed using benzodiazepines as positive controls. Buspirone also produces a mixed pattern of results in these clinical tests (Barrett & Witkin, 1991). Overall, the anxiolytic effects of competitive NMDA antagonists are the most consistent, which is encouraging for the continued evaluation of these drugs as potential anxiolytic agents.

ABBREVIATIONS

ACPC = 1-aminocyclopropanecarboxylic acid
AP5 = 2-amino-5-phosphonopentanoate
AP7 = 2-amino-7-phosphonoheptanoate
CGS 19755 = cis-4-phosphonomethyl-2-piperidinecarboxylic acid

CPP = (+)-2-carboxypiperazine-4-yl-propyl-1-phosphonic acid
5,7-DCKA = 5,7-dichlorokynurenic acid
HA-966 = (+)-3-(2-carboxypiperazin-4yl)-propyl-1-phosphonic acid
KYN = kynurenic acid
MK-801 = (+)-5-methyl-10,11-dihydro-5H-dibenzo[a,d]cyclohepten-5,
  10-imine maleate
NANM = (+)-N-allylnormetazocine
NPC 12626 = 2-amino-4,5-(1,2-cyclohexyl)-7-phosphonoheptanoate
NPC 17742 = 2R,4R,5S-2-amino-4,5-(1,2-cyclohexyl)-7-phosphonoheptanoate
PCP = phencyclidine
7-CL-KYN = 7-chlorokynurenic acid

ACKNOWLEDGEMENTS

Support for the preparation of this review was provided by the National Institute on Drug Abuse Grant DA-01442. J.L. Wiley is a postdoctoral fellow supported by training grant DA-07027.

REFERENCES

Andrews, J.S. & Stephens, D.N. (1990): Drug discrimination models in anxiety and depression. Pharmacol. Ther. 47, 267-280.
Barrett, J.E. & Witkin, J.M. (1991): Buspirone in animal models of anxiety. In Buspirone: Mechanisms and clinical aspects, ed. G. Tunnicliff, A.S. Eison, & D.P. Taylor, pp. 37-79. San Diego, CA: Academic Press.
Bennett, D.A. & Amrick, C.L. (1987): Antagonists at the N-methyl-D-aspartate receptor produce anticonflict effects. In Excitatory amino acid transmission, ed. T.P. Hicks, D. Lodge, & H. McLennan, pp. 213-216. New York: Alan R. Liss, Inc.
Bennett, D.A. & Amrick, C.L. (1986): 2-amino-7-phosphono-heptanoic acid (AP7) produces discriminative stimuli and anticonflict effects similar to diazepam. Life Sci. 39, 2455-2461.
Bennett, D.A., Bernard, P.S., Amrick, C.L., Wilson, D.E., Liebman, J.M., & Hutchinson, A.J. (1989): Behavioral pharmacological profile of CGS 19755, a competitive antagonist at N-methyl-D-aspartate receptors. J. Pharmacol. Exp. Ther. 250, 454-460.
Bennett, D.A., Lehmann, J., Bernard, P.S., Liebman, J.M., Williams, M., Wood, P.L., Boast, C.A., & Hutchison, A.J. (1990): CGS 19755: A novel competitive N-methyl-D-aspartate (NMDA) receptor antagonist with anticonvulsant, anxiolytic and anti-ischemic properties. In Current and Future Trends in Anticonvulsant, Anxiety, and Stroke Therapy, ed. B.S. Meldrum & M. Williams, pp. 519-524. New York: Wiley-Liss, Inc.
Blanchard, D.C., Blanchard, R.J., Corobrez, A.D.P., Veniegas, R., Rodgers, R.J., & Shepherd, J.K. (1992): MK-801 produces a reduction in anxiety-related antipredator defensiveness in male and female rats and a gender-dependent increase in locomotor behavior. Psychopharmacology 108, 352-362.
Brandao, M.L., Fontes, J.C.S., & Graeff, F.G. (1980): Facilitatory effect of ketamine on punished behavior. Pharmacol. Biochem. Behav. 13, 1-4.
Chait, L.D., Wenger, G.R., & McMillan, D.E. (1981): Effects of phencyclidine and ketamine on punished and unpunished responding by pigeons. Pharmacol. Biochem. Behav. 15, 145-148.
Chapman, A.G., Graham, J., & Meldrum, B.S. (1990): Potent oral anticonvulsant action of CPP and CPPene in DBA/2 mice. Eur. J. Pharmacol. 178, 97-99.
Chapman, A.G., Graham, J.L., Patel, S. & Meldrum, B.S. (1991): Anticonvulsant activity of two orally active competitive N-methyl-D-aspartate antagonists, CGP 37849 and CGP 39551, against sound-induced seizures in DBA/2 mice and photically induced myoclonus in Papio papio. Epilepsia 32, 578-587.
Clineschmidt, B.V. (1982): Effect of the benzodiazepine receptor antagonist Ro 15-1788 on the anticonvulsant and anticonflict actions of MK-801. Eur. J. Pharmacol. 84, 119-121.
Clineschmidt, B.V., Williams, M., Witoslawski, J.J., Bunting, P.R., Risley, E.A., & Totaro, J.A. (1982): Restoration of shock-suppressed behavior by treatment with (+)-5-methyl-10,11-dihydro-5H-dibenzo[a,d]cyclohepten-5,10-imine (MK-801), a substance with potent anticonvulsant, central sympathomimetic, and apparent anxiolytic properties. Drug Dev. Res. 2, 147-163.
Cook, L. & Davidson, A.B. (1973): Effects of behaviorally active drugs in a conflict-punishment procedure in rats. In The benzodiazepines, ed. S. Garattini, E. Mussini, and L.O. Randall, pp. 327-345. New York: Raven Press.
Cook, L. & Sepinwall, J. (1975): Behavioral analysis of the effects and

mechanisms of action of benzodiazepines. In <u>Mechanism of action of benzodiazepines</u>, ed. E. Costa & P. Greengard, pp. 1-28. New York: Raven Press.

Corbett, R. & Dunn, R.W. (1991): Effects of HA-966 on conflict, social interaction, and plus maze behaviors. <u>Drug Dev. Res.</u> **24**, 201-205.

Croucher, M.J., Collins, J.F., & Meldrum, B.S. (1982): Anticonvulsant action of excitatory amino acid antagonists. <u>Science</u> **216**, 899-901.

Dunn, R.W., Corbett, R., & Fielding, S. (1989): Effects of 5-HT1A receptor agonists and NMDA receptor antagonists in the social interaction test and the elevated plus maze. <u>Eur. J. Pharmacol.</u> **169**, 1-10.

Dunn, R.W., Corbett, R., Martin, L.L., Payack, J.F., Laws-Ricker, L., Wilmot, C.A., Rush, D.K., Cornfeldt, M.L., & Fielding, S. (1990): Preclinical anxiolytic profiles of 7189 and 8319, novel non-competitive NMDA antagonists. In <u>Current and Future Trends in Anticonvulsant, Anxiety, and Stroke Therapy</u>, ed. B.S. Meldrum & M. Williams, pp. 495-512. New York: Wiley-Liss, Inc.

File, S.E. (1988): How good is social interaction as a test of anxiety. In <u>Selected models of anxiety, depression and psychosis</u>, ed. P. Simon, P. Soubrie, & D. Wildlocher, pp. 151-166. Basel: Karger.

File, S.E. (1987): The contribution of behavioural studies to the neuropharmacology of anxiety. <u>Neuropharmacol.</u> **26**, 877-886.

File, S.E. (1980): The use of social interaction as a method for detecting anxiolytic activity of chlordiazepoxide-like drugs. <u>J. Neurosci. Meth.</u> **2**, 219-238.

Gardner, C.R. (1985): Distress vocalization in rat pups: A simple screening method for anxiolytic drugs. <u>J. Pharmacol. Meth.</u> **14**, 181-187.

Geller, I. & Seifter, J. (1960): The effects of meprobamate, barbiturates, d-amphetamine and promazine on experimentally induced conflict in the rat. <u>Psychopharmacologia</u> **1**, 482-492.

Goldberg, M.E., Salama, A.I., Patel, J.B., & Malick, J.B. (1983): Novel non-benzodiazepine anxiolytics. <u>Neuropharmacol.</u> **22**, 1499-1504.

Guimaraes, F.S., Carobrez, A.P., DeAguiar, J.C., & Graeff, F.G. (1991): Anxiolytic effect in the elevated plus-maze of the NMDA receptor antagonist AP7 microinjected into the dorsal periaqueductal grey. <u>Psychopharmacology</u> **103**, 91-94.

Hoehn-Saric, R., McLeod, D.R., & Glowa, J.R. (1991): The effects of NMDA receptor blockade on the acquisition of a conditioned emotional response. <u>Biol. Psychia.</u> **30**, 170-176.

Kehne, J.H., McCloskey, T.C., Baron, B.M., Chi, E.M., Harrison, B.L., Whitten, J.P., & Palfreyman, M.G. (1991): NMDA receptor complex antagonists have potential anxiolytic effects as measured with separation-induced ultrasonic vocalizations. <u>Eur. J. Pharmacol.</u> **193**, 283-292.

Koek, W. & Colpaert, F.C. (1991): Use of conflict procedure in pigeons to characterize anxiolytic drug activity: Evaluation of N-methyl-D-aspartate antagonists. <u>Life Sci.</u> **49**, PL37-PL42.

Kuribara, H., Fujiwara, S., Yasuda, H., & Tadokoro, S. (1990): The anticonflict effect of MK-801, an NMDA antagonist: Investigation by punishment procedure in mice. <u>Japan. J. Pharmacol.</u> **54**, 250-252.

Lerner, T., Feldon, J., & Myslobodsky, M.S. (1986): Amphetamine potentiation of anticonflict action of chlordiazepoxide. <u>Pharmacol. Biochem. Behav.</u> **24**, 241-246.

Liebman, J.M. & Bennett, D.A. (1988): Anxiolytic actions of competitive N-methyl-D-aspartate receptor antagonists: A comparison with benzodiazepine modulators and dissociative anesthetics. In <u>Frontiers in excitatory amino acid research</u>, ed. E.A. Cavalheiro, J. Lehmann, & L. Turski, pp. 301-308. New York: Alan R. Liss, Inc.

Lodge, D. & Johnson, K.M. (1990): Noncompetitive excitatory amino acid receptor antagonists. <u>Tr. Pharmacol. Sci.</u> **11**, 81-86.

Lodge, D., Jones, M., & Fletcher, E. (1989): Non-competitive antagonists of N-methyl-D-aspartate. In <u>The NMDA receptor</u>, ed. J.C. Watkins & G.L. Collingridge, pp. 37-51. Oxford: IRL Press.

Mansbach, R.S., Willetts, J., Jortani, S.A., & Balster, R.L. (1991): NMDA antagonists: Lack of antipunishment effect in squirrel monkeys. <u>Pharmacol. Biochem. Behav.</u> **39**, 977-981.

McMillan, D.E., Hardwick, W.C., DeCosta, B.R., & Rice, K.C. (1991): Effects of drugs that bind to PCP and sigma receptors on punished responding. <u>J. Pharmacol. Exp. Ther.</u> **258**, 1015-1018.

Olverman, H.J. & Watkins, J.C. (1989): NMDA agonists and competitive antagonists. In <u>The NMDA receptor</u>, ed. J.C. Watkins & G.L. Collingridge, pp. 19-36. Oxford: IRL Press.

Pellow, S. & File, S.E. (1986): Anxiolytic and anxiogenic drug effects on exploratory activity in an elevated plus-maze: A novel test of anxiety in the rat. Pharmacol. Biochem. Behav. **24**, 525-529.

Pellow, S., Chopin, P., File, S.E., & Briley, M. (1985): Validation of open: closed arm entries in an elevated plus-maze as a measure of anxiety in the rat. J. Neurosci. Meth. **14**, 149-167.

Porter, J.H., Wiley, J.L., & Balster, R.L. (1989): Effects of phencyclidine-like drugs on punished behavior in rats. J. Pharmacol. Exp. Ther. **248**, 991-1002.

Sanger, D.J. (1985): GABA and the behavioral effects of anxiolytic drugs. Life Sci. **36**, 1503-1513.

Sanger, D.J. & Jackson, A. (1989): Effects of phencyclidine and other N-methyl-D-aspartate antagonists on the schedule-controlled behavior of rats. J. Pharmacol. Exp. Ther. **248**, 1215-1221.

Snell, D. & Harris, R.A. (1982): Interactions between narcotic agonists, partial agonists and antagonists on punished and unpunished behavior in the rat. Psychopharmacology **76**, 177-181.

Stephens, D.N. & Andrews, J.S. (1988): N-methyl-D-aspartate antagonists in animal models of anxiety. In Frontiers in excitatory amino acid research, ed. E.A. Cavalheiro, J. Lehmann, & L. Turski, pp. 309-316. New York: Alan R. Liss, Inc.

Stephens, D.N., Meldrum, B.S., Weidmann, R., Schneider, C., & Grutzner, M. (1986): Does the excitatory amino acid receptor antagonist 2-APH exhibit anxiolytic activity. Psychopharmacology **90**, 166-169.

Study, R.E. & Barker, J.L. (1981): Diazepam and (-)-pentobarbital: fluctuation analysis reveals different mechanisms for potentiation of gamma-aminobutyric acid responses in cultured central neurons. Proc. Nat. Acad. Sci. **78**, 7180-7184.

Stutzmann, J.M., Cintrat, P., Laduron, P.M., & Blanchard, J.C. (1989): Riluzole antagonizes the anxiogenic properties of the B-carboline FG7142 in rats. Psychopharmacology **99**, 515-519.

Trullas, R., Jackson, B., & Skolnick, P. (1989): Anxiolytic properties of 1-aminocyclopropanecarboxylic acid, a ligand at strychnine-insensitive glycine receptors. Pharmacol. Biochem. Behav. **34**, 313-316.

Turski, L., Schwarz, M., Turski, W.A., Klockgether, T., Sontag, K.H., & Collins, J.F. (1985): Muscle relaxant action of excitatory amino acid antagonists. Neurosci. Let. **53**, 321-326.

Watkins, J.C. (1989): The NMDA receptor concept: Origins and development. In The NMDA receptor, ed. J.C. Watkins & G.L. Collingridge, pp. 1-17. Oxford: IRL Press.

Wenger, G.R. (1980): Effects of phencyclidine and ketamine in pigeons on behavior suppressed by brief electrical shocks. Pharmacol. Biochem. Behav. **12**, 865-870.

Wiley, J.L. & Balster, R.L. (1992): Preclinical evaluation of N-methyl-D-aspartate antagonists for antianxiety effects: a review. In Multiple Sigma and PCP Receptor Ligands: Mechanisms for Neuromodulation and Neuroprotection?, ed. J.M. Kamenka & E.F. Domino, pp. 801-815. Ann Arbor, MI: NPP Books.

Wiley, J.L., Compton, A.D., Porter, J.H., & Balster, R.L. (1992): Antipunishment effects of NPC 12626 during acute and repeated dosing in rats. Life Sci. **50**, 1519-1528.

Willetts, J., Clissold, D.B., Hartman, T.L., Brandsgaard, R.R., Hamilton, G.S., & Ferkany, J.W. (1993): Behavioral pharmacology of NPC 17742, a competitive N-methyl-D-aspartate (NMDA) antagonist. J. Pharmacol. Exp. Ther. **264**, 256-264.

Willetts, J., Balster, R.L., & Leander, J.D. (1990): The behavioral pharmacology of NMDA receptor antagonists. Tr. Pharmacol. Sci. **11**, 423-428.

Winslow, J.T. & Insel, T.R. (1991): Infant rat separation is a sensitive test for novel anxiolytics. Prog. Neuro-Psychopharmacol. Biol. Psychia. **15**, 745-757.

Winslow, J.T., Insel, T.R., Trullas, R., & Skolnick, P. (1990): Rat pup isolation calls are reduced by functional antagonists of the NMDA receptor complex. Eur. J. Pharmacol. **190**, 11-21.

Xie, Z. & Commissaris, R.L. (1992): Anxiolytic-like effects of the noncompetitive NMDA antagonist MK-801. Pharmacol. Biochem. Behav. **43**, 471-477.

Résumé

Les antagonistes compétitifs des récepteurs NMDA exercent des effets de type anxiolytique dans des situations expérimentales appropriées chez le rat, le pigeon et la souris. En revanche, chez le singe écureuil, ces composés, de même que les antagonistes de type PCP, ne sont pas anxiolytiques dans des tests impliquant une punition. Ces mêmes tests chez le rat, le pigeon et la souris, révèlent des effets inconstants avec les antagonistes de type PCP ou d'autres types d'antagonistes non-compétitifs des récepteurs NMDA. En revanche, dans des tests sans punition, le MK-801 (le seul agent de type PCP qui ait été étudié jusqu'à présent) est clairement anxiolytique, de même que les antagonistes agissant sur le site "glycine" et un antagoniste du site "polyamine", l'ifenprodil. D'une manière générale, les antagonistes des récepteurs NMDA exercent donc une activité anxiolytique dans les tests appropriés chez l'animal. Cependant, il existe des différences d'espèces puisque les antagonistes compétitifs et les composés de type PCP ont des potentialités anxiolytiques chez les rongeurs et le pigeon, mais pas chez le singe écureuil. A ce jour, les données les plus convaincantes ont été obtenues avec les antagonistes compétitifs des récepteurs NMDA ce qui justifie les études en cours en vue de leur développement éventuel comme anxiolytiques chez l'homme.

Poster presentations

Communications affichées

Plasma cortisol and ACTH responses to o-CRF stimulation in patients with obsessive compulsive disorder

D. Bailly, D. Servant, D. Dewailly, R. Beuscart and P.-J. Parquet

Centre d'Information et de Traitement des Dépendances, C.H.R.U., 57, boulevard de Metz, 59037 Lille Cedex, France

According to some clinical data, obsessive-compulsive disorder (OCD) and endogenous depression may share common biological mechanisms. Patients with endogenous depression show a blunted ACTH response to corticotropin-releasing factor (CRF) stimulation. This result is consistent with the view that central hyperactivity of CRF secreting neurons may be involved in mediating several endocrine and behavioral characteristics of endogenous depression (Gold & Chrousos, 1985 ; Holsboer et al., 1987). Recently, Altemus et al (1992) showed that concentrations of cerebrospinal fluid CRF were significantly elevated in patients with OCD compared with controls. Same results were previously reported in depressed patients (Nemeroff et al., 1984). These data suggest hyperactivity of the hypothalamic-pituitary-adrenal (HPA) axis resulting from an increase of CRF secretion in OCD as well as in endogenous depression. In order to check this hypothesis, we have studied plasma cortisol and ACTH responses to the stimulation by ovine CRF (o-CRF) in patients with OCD.

Ten non-depressed patients (5 men and 5 women) with OCD (according to the DSM III-R criteria) were studied. They were aged 20-44 years (mean age : 35.3 ± 7 years). None had other clinically detectable psychiatric or organic disease and none took medication at least two weeks before the study. Mean scores on the Hamilton Rating Scales were 17.1 ± 4.4 for Anxiety and 8.2 ± 2.6 for Depression. For a comparison group we used ten normal control subjects (5 men and 5 women) matched on age (mean age : 32.4 ± 5.8 years). Mean scores on the Hamilton Rating Scales were 6.4 ± 4.7 for Anxiety and 6.4 ± 5 for Depression.

The o-CRF stimulation test was conducting according to the method previously reported (Bailly et al., 1989). Ovine CRF was injected as an intravenous bolus at 12:00. Blood was collected every 15 min. for 1 h., then every 30 min. for 1 h. Plasma ACTH was determined using a radioimmunoassay. The sensitivity was 10 pg/ml of plasma. The intra-assay and inter-assay coefficients of variation averaged 6.2 % and 8.3 %, respectively. In that assay beta and delta endorphins did not significantly cross-react and cross-reactivity of beta lipotropin was o.1 %. Plasma cortisol was assayed by a fluorimetric method. The sensitivity was 1 µg/dl of plasma. Statistical comparisons were performed by variance analysis with repeated measures and by Fisher's multiple comparison test. The net area under the curve (AUC) and the ratio of the AUC ACTH to AUC cortisol were studied in complement of absolute values.

Results showed a significantly lower ACTH response to o-CRF in patients with OCD compared to controls ($F = 13.56$, $p<0.01$), with significant differences in all the time points measures. The mean basal ACTH level was significantly lower in patients than in controls (11.8 ± 44 vs 22.3 ± 12.1 pg/ml ; $F = 6.72$, $p<0.01$). The AUC for ACTH was 1857 ± 595.2 pg/ml per hour in patients vs 4185.7 ± 1891.2 pg/ml per hour in controls (Z = -2.8, p<0.01). In contrast, the cortisol response did not significantly differ between OCD patients and controls. As expected according to these data, the ratio of ACTH to cortisol responses was found significantly lower in patients than in controls (0.9 ± 0.4 vs 2.5 ± 1.4 ; Z = -2.8, p<0.01).

These results are consistent with the hypothesis of HPA axis hyperactivity resulting from an increase of CRF secretion in OCD that might explain some clinical similarities observed between OCD and endogenous depression.

References
Altemus, M., Pigott, T., Kalogeras, K.T., Demitrack, M., Dubbert, B., Murphy, D.L. & Gold, P.W. (1992) : Abnormalities in the regulation of vasopressin and corticotropin-releasing factor secretion in obsessive compulsive disorder. *Arch. Gen. Psychiatry* 49 : 9-20.
Bailly, D., Dewailly, D., Beuscart, R., Couplet, G., Dumont, P., Racadot, A., Fossati, P. & Parquet, P.J. (1989) : adrenocorticotropin and cortisol responses to ovine corticotropin-releasing factor in alcohol dependence discrder. *Horm. Res.* 31 : 72-75.
Gold, P.W. & Chrousos, G.P. (1985) : Clinical studies with corticotropin-releasing factor : implications for the diagnosis and pathophysiology of depression, Cushing's disease and adrenal insufficiency. *Psychoneuroendocrinology* 10 : 401-419.
Holsboer, F., Von Bardeleben, U., Buller, R. Heuser, I. & Steiger, A. (1987) : Stimulation response to corticotropin-releasing hormone (CRH) in patients with depression, alcoholism, and panic disorder. *Horm Metab. Res.* 16 : 80-88.
Nemeroff, C.B., Widerlov, E., Bissette, G., Walleus, H., Karlsson, I., Eklund, K., Kilts, C.S., Loosen, P.T. & Vale, W. (1984) : Elevated concentrations of CSF corticotropin-releasing factor-like immunoreactivity in depressed patients. *Science* 226 : 1342-1344.

Effects of specific modulation of neurotransmitter systems in the septal region on anxiety level and working memory performance in C57BL/6

Muriel Belotti, Marie-Pierre Mano and Daniel Galey

Laboratoire de Neurosciences Comportementales et Cognitives, URA CNRS 339, Université de Bordeaux 1, avenue des Facultés, 33405 Talence Cedex, France

Substantial literature provides convergent evidence that the septal region is involved in the regulation of anxiety-related behaviors. However, the septal region is anatomically and chemically complex and the role of its different components in anxiety is not presently established.

The aim of this study was to investigate, by using selective pharmacological approach, the possible differential effects of intraseptal modulation of neurotransmitter systems (i.e. gabaergic/cholinergic or noradrenergic) in the anxiety phenomenon and spatial working memory. The anxiety level was evaluated in an elevated-plus maze, using the activity and time ratios.

In this task, the more elevated is the time ratio, the less "anxious" are the subjects. In addition, under the same treatments, exploratory behavior was assessed in a four hole board in order to control exploratory abilities.

The results (Table 1) showed that injection of diazepam (0,5 mg/kg, i.p.) or intraseptal infusion of scopolamine (2,5 µg/0,2 µl) in medial septal region (MS) resulted in level of anxiety, as well as exploratory abilities, that were comparable to those displayed by saline group animals. However, the animals which received both treatments exhibited decreased level of anxiety, thus showing that septal gabaergic-cholinergic interaction can modulate this phenomenon. This result supports Gray hypothesis (Gray, 1982) which postulates that septo-hippocampal cholinergic activation produces anxiety. Furthermore spatial working memory performance evaluated in a sequential alternation procedure was impaired after the same combined treatment ($P < 0.01$ as compared to the other groups).

	Four hole board			Elevated-plus maze	
	Exploration number	Exploration time (s)	Locomotor activity	Activity ratio	Time ratio
Control	39.8 ± 4.0	26.0 ± 3.4	26.3 ± 2.4	0.149 ± 0.03	0.135 ± 0.04
Saline	37.8 ± 5.5	24.4 ± 6.7	23.2 ± 2.0	0.298 ± 0.07	0.298 ± 0.07
Scopol.	27.8 ± 4.2	13.0 ± 2.1	17.0 ± 2.8	0.278 ± 0.08	0.354 ± 0.11
Diazepam	40.7 ± 3.3	26.8 ± 4.8	24.7 ± 3.9	0.237 ± 0.05	0.238 ± 0.07
Scop + Diaz	42.7 ± 7.4	23.1 ± 4.5	20.7 ± 3.5	0.33 ± 0.05	0.605 ± 0.09*

Table 1 : * $P < 0.05$ as compared to the other groups.

On the other hand, an improvement of the anxiety level is showed after the infusion of a selective α_1 antagonist, the BE 2254 (500 ng/0.2 µl) in each lateral septal nucleus (LS), but this phenomenon is also observable in the saline group animals, thus suggesting a non specific effect induced by non identified LS component lesion (Table 2)..

In addition, the spatial working memory investigation was achieved in a radial-maze during the acquisition of a delayed non-matching to place rule. In these conditions, selective blockade of noradrenergic activation did not induce changes on working memory performance evaluated in two different conditions. However, when the treatment was applied before the habituation session, when animals were initially exposed to the context they were impaired in subsequent acquisition of the rule ($P < 0.01$ as compared to the other groups) thus suggesting that noradrenergic activation is essential when animals process new environmental features.

	Four hole board			Elevated-plus maze	
	Exploration number	Exploration time (s)	Locomotor activity	Activity ratio	Time ratio
Control	30.3 ± 2.8	16.4 ± 2.4	16.9 ± 1.4	0.313 ± 0.01	0.205 ± 0.02
Saline	31.1 ± 4.0	14.8 ± 1.6	15.4 ± 2.2	0.269 ± 0.02	0.106 ± 0.02*
BE 2254	32.2 ± 4.4	18.4 ± 1.8	13.6 ± 1.8	0.212 ± 0.03	0.06 ± 0.01*

Table 2 : * $P < 0.05$ as compared to the other groups.

Taken together, these results suggest that these two divisions (MS and LS) of the septal region may intervene in an opposite manner in the control of anxiety and spatial working memory since we have previously showed an improvement of this last paradigm after the infusion of 6-hydroxydopamine in each LS nucleus (Jaffard et al., 1985; Galey et al., 1989).

References

Galey, D., Toumane, A., Durkin, T., & Jaffard, R. (1989) : *In vivo* modulation of septo-hippocampal cholinergic activity in mice : relationships with spatial reference and working memory performance. *Behav. Brain Res.* 32, 163-172.

Gray, J. (1982) : The neuropsychology of anxiety : an enquiry into the functions of the septo-hippocampal system. Oxford University Press, Oxford.

Jaffard, R., Galey, D., Micheau, J., & Durkin, T. (1985) : The cholinergic septo-hippocampal pathway, learning and memory. In *Brain Plasticity, learning and memory.* ed. B.E. Will, P. Schmitt & J.C. Dalrymple-Alford, Plenum Press, N.Y., 167-181.

Effects of methyl-beta-carboline-3-carboxylate (βCCM) on emotional and memory disorders resulting from experimental mamillary bodies lesions and chronic alcohol consumption in Balb/c mice

Daniel J. Béracochéa, Bruno Bontempi, Ali Krazem, Claude Destrade and Robert Jaffard

Laboratoire de Neurosciences Cognitives et Comportementales, URA CNRS 339, Université de Bordeaux 1, avenue des Facultés, 33405 Talence Cedex, France

We attempted here to determine the effects of the lesion of the mamillary bodies (MB) or chronic alcohol consumption (CAC) on emotional and memory processes, and the effects of the administration of βCCM, a benzodiazepine inverse agonist, on these processes using Balb/c mice as subjects.

Chronic ethanol administration (12-months) and surgical procedures for MB-lesions have been described in full elsewhere (see Béracochéa et al., 1987; Beracochéa & Jaffard,1987). βCCM was dissolved in a saline solution and administered subcutaneously 30 min before behavioral testing. Independant group of mice was used in each condition and received either βCCM or Saline. Memory was measured according to the evolution of alternation rate across trials in a sequential alternation task. Emotional effects of treatments were assessed in an elevated-plus maze, using the activity and latency ratios. In this task, the more elevated are these ratios, the less "anxious" are the subjects. In addition, the cerebral metabolic activity using the 2-DG relative method (Destrade et al., 1992) was studied in alcohol-treated and control mice performing a sequential alternation task following saline or βCCM administration.

In the elevated-plus maze, CAC and MB lesions increased both activity and latency ratios as compared to controls ($P<0.01$ in all comparisons); the administration of βCCM significantly reduced these ratios as indicated in Table 1.

Table 1	Control			MB			Alcohol	
	Saline	βCCM 0.5	βCCM 1.0	Saline	βCCM 0.5	βCCM 1.0	Saline	βCCM 0.5
Activity Ratio	35.2	19.6*	14.1*	52.0	40.3*	14.2*	48.4	35.0*
Latency Ratio	28.3	46.2**	15.3*	61.2	50	12.1**	43.4	23.5*
* $p < 0.05$; ** $p < 0.01$ as compared to the saline condition								

CAC and MB-lesions induced a significant alternation deficit on the three last but not on the two first trials of the series, as compared to controls ($P<0.01$ in all comparisons). The administration of βCCM totally suppressed the behavioral deficit in alcohol-treated and MB-lesioned mice (Table 2).

Table 2	Control			MB			Alcohol	
	Saline	βCCM 0.5	βCCM 1.0	Saline	βCCM 0.5	βCCM 1.0	Saline	βCCM 0.5
4 Th - 6 Th TRIALS (% Alternation)	71*	92*	68	47	56	82**	51	84**
* $p < 0.05$; ** $p < 0.01$ as compared to the saline condition								

The 2-DG study showed that CAC reduced significantly ($P<0.01$) the metabolic activity into the MB and anterior thalamic nucleï; the administration of βCCM (0.5mg/kg) significantly ($P<0.01$) increased the metabolic activity into these two brain areas, so that experimental subjects did not significantly differed from controls. No significant changes in metabolic activity was found in other brain areas, whatever the groups and drug administrations. Sequential alternation performances and MB metabolic activity were highly correlated in the alcohol group ($r=0.80$), the lower the metabolic activity, the lower the alternation rate.

In conclusion, MB-lesions and CAC reduced anxiety and induced memory deficits. βCCM administration at doses inducing anxiogenic effects alleviated the memory impairments in both groups. The effect of the drug is in part related to the activity of the mamillo-thalamic pathway. Indeed, i) the improvement of performance required, to be observed, a dose twice more important in MB-lesioned subjects than in alcohol ones; in alcohol-treated subjects, performances in the SA task were highly correlated with the MB metabolic activity .

References

Béracochéa, D.J., Lescaudron, L., Tako,A., Verna,A., & Jaffard,R (1987): Build-up and release from proactive interference during chronic ethanol consumption in mice: a behavioral and neuroanatomical study. Behav. Brain Res. 25, 63-74.

Beracochéa, D.J.& Jaffard,R (1987): Impairment of spontaneous alternation behavior in sequential test procedures folllowing mammillary bodies lesions in mice: evidence for time-dependent-interference-related memory deficits. Behav.Neurosci. 2, 187-197).

Destrade, C., Messier, C., Bontempi, B., Sif,J., & Jaffard, R: (1992): Investigations into time-dependent metabolic changes during memory processes in the mouse brain using the (14C) deoxyglucose and (14C)-glucose in *Advances in metabolic mappingtechniques for brain imaging of behavioral and learning function.* Kluver Academic Pub, 389-407.

Link between anxiety and memory: behavioural and pharmacological study in the mouse

A. Beuzen, C. Belzung, N. Pineau and E. Bouhou

Laboratoire d'Éthologie et de Psychophysiologie, parc de Grandmont, 37200 Tours, France

Several theories about the neural substrate of anxiety imply different cerebral structure that are also involved in learning and memory. Moreover, some pharmacological compounds such as benzodiazepine receptor agonists have both anxiolytics and amnesics effects (Thiebot,1985) while benzodiazepine inverse agonists have opposite action (Izquierdo et al., 1990). However, it is to be noticed that the benzodiazepine amnesic activity is obvious in testing paradigm including aversive components (Izquiedo et Medina, 1992) so that one cannot decide if the amnesic effect is due to a direct effect of the drug on memory processes or to an indirect anti-aversive activity. Moreover, the question is so the more controversal that "anxiety" is a concept and not an entity grouping together several different phenomenons. Indeed, two types of anxiety have been dissociated : state anxiety and trait anxiety (Misslin et al, 1993).The purpose of this study was to further clarify the link between anxiety and memory using first a behavioural approach and second a pharmacological study.

Three different behavioural situations were used in mice : the free exploration test was used to assess state anxiety , the light dark box to measure trait anxiety (Belzung C.,1992) and the passive avoidance test to evaluate memory of aversive events (emotional memory). Following parameters were presented : time in the lit box (TLB, Light/dark box), number of avoidance behaviour of the novel area (free exploration test), latency of entry in the dark compartment on the learning day (lat1) and on the retention day (lat2) (passive avoidance test).

First a correlational approach was employed. Fifty four animals from 9 isogenics groups were submitted to the three tests cited upper. Pearson correlation coeficients were computed. The results show that there is no link between the TLB in the light dark box and the avoidance in the free exploration test ($r=-0.089$, NS). In the passive avoidance test,the pearson correlation coefficient between the entry latency on the first day and the entry latency on the second day reach the significance $r=-.265$ (for $p=0.05$ the criterion value is 0.275). Moreover there is no link between parramaters recorded in the free exploration test and the retention latency to enter in the passive avoidance apparatus ($r=-0.182$,NS). On the contrary there is a negative correlation between the time spent in the lit box and the retention latency in passive avoidance ($r=-0.315$, $p<0.05$). The TLB is also correlated with the entry latency on the learning day (lat1) in the passive avoidance paradigm ($r=-0.485$, $p<0.01$). These results suggest that state and trait anxiety are two different phenomenons. Moreover there is a link between trait anxiety and emotional memory but we must qualify our remark because lat1 and lat2 are correlated.

Another approach was used to clarify this point. The effect of several pharmacological compounds were study in this three situations. Chlordiazepoxide (5 mg/kg) or CCK-B receptor antagonist PD-135158 (1 mg/kg) were administred to mice confronted to these various situations.

These two drugs enhance the TLB (PD-135158 : $U=27$, $p=0.008$; CDZ : $U=66$, $p=0.053$, Table 1).
In the free exploration test, chlordiazepoxide alone is efficient (CDZ : $U=82.5$, $p=0.001$; PD-135158 : $U=40.5$, $p=0.472$ NS, Table 1).

	CDZ DOSES		PD-135168	
	0 mg/kg	5 mg/kg	0 mg/kg	1 mg/kg
Light dark box (TLB)	39 (4/77)	56 * (45/79)	0 (0/69)	129 ** (64/158.5)
Free exploration test (avoidance)	4 (2/7)	0 ** (0/0)	29.5 (4/39)	39 (21/36)

TABLE 1 : Effects of chlordiazepoxide (CDZ) and PD-135158 in two different tests (median, first and third quartile (parentheses)). * : $p<0.05$, ** : $p<0.01$ compared with the control group (Mann-Withney test).

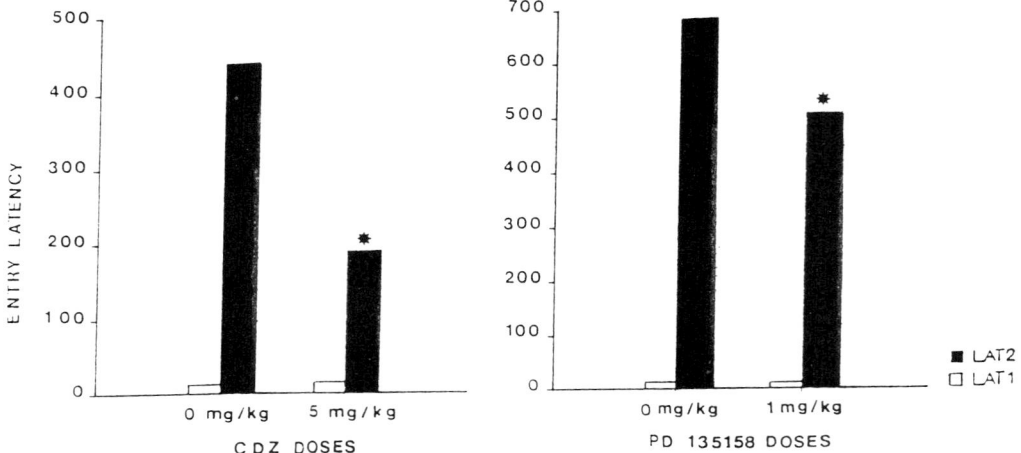

Fig 1 : Effects of chlordiazepoxide and PD-135158 on passive avoidance response. (Median values, lat1: training latency, Lat2: retention latency. * : $p<0.05$ compared with the control group (Mann-Withney test).

As regard with the passive avoidance paradigm these two drugs produce an amnesic effect, but the cholecystokinine agonist seems to be less efficient (PD-155158 : U=185, p=0.032; CDZ : U=698, p=0.024).

The key point to be emphazised about the results of this study is that the distinction between state and trait anxiety is very relevant as we show that these two entity are independant. Moreover, it allows to clarify the question of the link between anxiety and memory as we show that emotional memory is only related to trait anxiety.

References
Belzung C. (1992): Hippocampal mossy fibres: implication in novelty reactions or in anxiety behaviours? Behav. Brain Res., 51, 149-155.
Izquierdo,I.,Medina,J.H. (1991): GABA-A receptor modulation of memory : the role of endogenous benzodiazepines. TIPS,12, 260-265.
Izquierdo I., Pereira M.E. and Medina J.H.(1990): Benzodiazepine receptor ligand influences on acquisition: suggestion of an endogenous modulatory mechanism mediated by benzodiazepine receptors. Behav. Neural Biol.,54,27-41.
Misslin R., Belzung C., Neibel L. and Vogel E.(1993): The free exploratory paradigm : an effective method for measuring neophobie behaviour in mice and testing potential neophobia reducing drugs. Behav. Pharmacol.(in press).
Thiebot M.H. (1985): Some evidence for amnesic-like effects of benzodiazepines in animals. Neurosci. Biobehav. Rev., 9, 95-100.

Role of serotonin 1 receptors in hippocampal functions: a psychopharmacological study in the rat

M.-C. Buhot, S.K. Patra* and S. Naïli

*CNRS, Laboratoire de Neurobiologie, E6, B.P. 71, 31, chemin Joseph-Aiguier, 13402 Marseille Cedex 20, France and * Centre for Advanced Study in Psychology, UTKAL University, Bhubaneswar 751 004, Orissa, India*

The hippocampus has been repeatedly demonstrated as the key cerebral structure involved in memory, spatial orientation, and emotional states (O'Keefe & Nadel, 1978; Gray, 1984). A large number of studies suggests that these functions are mainly controlled by the septo-hippocampal cholinergic system. It is well-documented that this system receives modulatory influences of other neurotransmission systems, such as the serotonergic (5-HT) system, in particular through type 1 receptors. Consistent data also show that the 5-HT system is involved in the modulation of sensory and locomotor functions, memory, arousal and emotional states.

The aim of the present study was to define the role of hippocampal $5-HT_{1A}$ and $5-HT_{1B}$ receptors, using rats equipped with intracerebral cannulae for the injection of drugs in the CA_1 field of the dorsal hippocampus. Two behavioural tasks were used: object exploration in an open-field (for analyses of locomotor and exploratory activities, habituation and response to change), and spatial learning in a radial maze (for the evaluation of performance in spatial memory). We used scopolamine as a muscarinic antagonist (10 µg/µl), the 8-hydroxy-2-(di-n-propylamino)-tetralin (8-OH-DPAT) as a $5-HT_{1A}$ agonist (5µg/µl), the 3-(1,2,5,6-tetrahydropyrid-4-yl)pyrrolo[3,2-b]pyrid-5-one or CP 93,129 (Macor et al., 1990) as a $5-HT_{1B}$ agonist (5, 10 and 16 µg/µl), and a control, 9 °/∞ NaCl (saline) solution.

The local activation of $5-HT_1$ receptors affected behaviour differentially.
The 8-OH-DPAT did not modify locomotor activity (Fig. 1), while it reduced object exploration and habituation (as compared to saline injections: Student's $t_{[14]}= 2.43$, $p<0.05$), a result in contrast with previous observations where systemic injections were used (Buhot et al., 1989). A spatial change (by displacing a familiar object in the open-field) induced a selective increase of exploration, which suggests that attentional capacities were not affected. Nevertheless, the introduction of a novel object did not induce any particular reaction. Performance in the radial maze did not differ from that following saline injections suggesting that spatial memory was not affected (Fig. 2).

The CP-93,129 induced decreased locomotor activity in the open-field, especially during the first minutes of testing (Fig. 1), while no change in object exploration was observed. A lack of exploratory habituation did not impair the subsequent positive response to the spatial change. However, a novel object induced avoidance reactions and increased interest in a familiar object, a behaviour which differed significantly from that following saline injection (Student's t test: $t_{[14]}= 2.52$, $p<0.05$), and suggests a neophobic reaction. Spatial performance in the radial maze was significantly impaired at the higher concentration of the drug (Student's t test: $t_{[14]}= 4.13$, $p<0.01$), and was dose-dependent (Fig. 2).

Intrahippocampal treatment with scopolamine, a drug aimed at blocking the cholinergic septo-hippocampal pathway, resulted in the following main effects. First, an increased locomotor pattern (differing from that induced by CP-93,129: [$F_{(1,14)}=7.7$, $p<0.02$], Fig. 1), a well known effect previously observed using systemic injections or following hippocampal lesions (Save et al., 1992). Secondly, a lack of response to the spatial change was observed, which is in agreement with previous work, and relevant to the specificity of the cholinergic hippocampal system (Brito et al., 1983). The impairment in spatial memory observed in the radial maze (Student's t test: $t_{[14]}= 3.28$, $p<0.01$) agrees with this finding (Fig. 2).

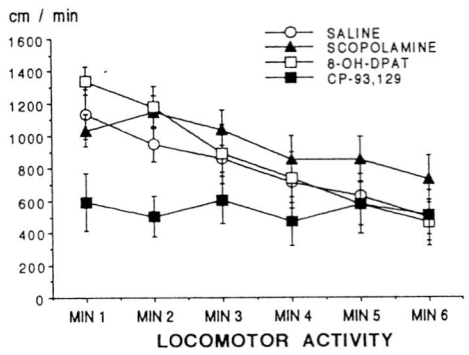

Fig. 1. Time course of locomotor activity displayed by rats during the first 6 min (MIN 1 to MIN 6) of the test (the CP-93,129 was used at 16 µg/µl).

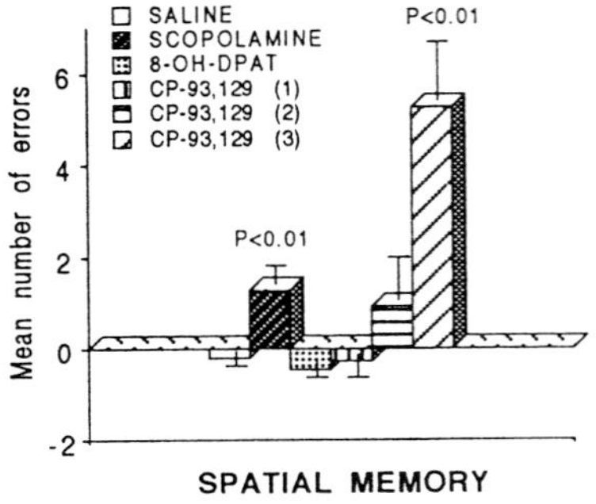

Fig. 2. Mean number of errors per trial as compared with non-injection trials [(1)= 5 µg/µl; (2)= 10 µg/µl; (3)= 16 µg/µl].

These results demonstrate that 5-HT$_{1A}$ and 5-HT$_{1B}$ do not play the same role in influencing hippocampal function. Furthermore, for the same receptor, the agonist effect is linked to the behavioural situation, showing thus a state-dependent effect. Part of these results may be attributed to the influence of 5-HT$_{1B}$ heteroreceptors located on the septal terminals (Maura & Raiteri, 1986), and/or to those 5-HT$_{1A/B}$ receptors located on the CA$_1$ neurons which project to the subiculum, one of the main hippocampal efferents to cortical areas. Finally, this study defines the role played by serotonine 1 receptors in spatial behavior, memory and emotion, related to the hippocampal functions.

Acknowledgements
The generous gift of CP-93,129 from Drs. Macor and Koe (Pfizer Inc., Groton, CT, USA).

References
Brito, G.N.O., Davis, B.J., Stopp, L.C. & Stanton, M.E. (1983): Memory and the septo-hippocampal cholinergic system in the rat. *Psychopharmacology* 81, 315-320.
Buhot, M.-C., Rage, P. & Segu, L. (1989): Changes in exploratory behaviour of hamsters following treatment with 8-hydroxy-2(di-n-propylamino)tetralin. *Behav. Brain Res.* 35, 163-179.
Gray, J.A. (1984): The hippocampus as an interface between cognition and emotion. In *Animal Cognition*, ed.H.L. Roitblat, T.G. Bever, & H.S. Terrace, H.S., vol 33, pp. 607-625. N.J.: LEA-Hillsdale.
Macor, J.E., Burkhart, C.A., Heym, J.H., Ives, J.L., Lebel, L.A., Newman, M.E., Nielsen, J.A., Ryan, K., Schulz, D.W., Torgersen, L.K. & Koe, B.K. (1990): 3-(1,2,5,6-Tetrahydropyrid-4-yl)pyrrolo[3,2-*b*]pyrid-5-one : a potent and selective serotonin (5-HT$_{1B}$) agonist and rotationally restricted phenolic analogue of 5-methoxy-3-(1,2,5,6-tetrahydropyrid-4-yl)indole. *J. Med. Chem.* 33, 2087-2093.
Maura, G. & Raiteri, M. (1986): Cholinergic terminals in rat hippocampus possess 5-HT$_{1B}$ receptors mediating inhibition of acetylcholine release. *Eur. J. Pharmacol.* 129, 333-337.
O'Keefe, J. et Nadel, L. (1978). *The hippocampus as a cognitive map*. Oxford: Oxford Clarendon Press.
Save, E., Poucet, B., Foreman, N. & Buhot, M.-C. (1992): Object exploration and reactions to spatial and nonspatial changes in hooded rats following damage to parietal cortex or hippocampal formation. *Behav. Neurosci.* 106, 447-456.

Implication of an autosomal locus in the activity in open-field by the analysis of two inbred strains of mice and their segregating populations

Yan Clément, Benoît Martin, Christine Adelbrecht, Patrice Venault and Georges Chapouthier

Génétique, Neurogénétique et Comportement, URA CNRS 1294, UFR Biomédicale, Université Paris V-René-Descartes, 45, rue des Saints-Pères, 75270 Paris Cedex 06, France

The open-field test measures the reactivity of animals placed in a new environment. In addition to other variables, grooming activity is considered as a specific behavior of rodents in response to stress. Grooming activity increases in a new environment and decreases after benzodiazepine administration. We can make the hypothesis that grooming could be modulated by a genetic determinism. We crossed a traditional inbred strain, C57BL/6ByJ (B) with the inbred strain, ABP/Le (P) known to carry five easily identifiable markers: *non agouti* (*a*, chromosome 2), *brown coat color* (*b*, chromosome 4), *pink-eyed dilution* (*p*, chromosome 7), *short-ear* (*se*, chromosome 9) and *belted* (*bt*, chromosome 15). From the two reciprocal F1's, PBF1 and BPF1, we made the two reciprocal F2 populations PB.PBF2 and BP.BPF2 and explored the possible role of four of the five segregating loci associated with these markers. We demonstrated that the two parental strains show different grooming measures, suggesting that genes belonging to P and B are implicated in grooming activity. Since data obtained in the reciprocal F1's can account for an effect of the maternal environment, we analysed the results in each F2 population. We compared the homozygous groups for one given marker z/z, and the groups $?/+$ for this marker. In both F2 populations, we show that on the chromosome 9, close to the *se* locus, there is one or more gene(s), which are associated with an increase in grooming activity. We suggest that on this chromosomal fragment exist one or more gene(s) that modulate the physiological processes associated with the anxiety of animals when there are placed in an open-field.

Effects of alpha-2 adrenoceptor agonist and antagonists in the safety signal withdrawal paradigm

Anne Dekeyne, Martine Guernier and Claude Oberlander

Centre de Recherches Roussel-Uclaf, Pharmacologie-Neurobiologie, 111, route de Noisy, 93230 Romainville, France

Safety signal withdrawal is a new method that seems sensitive to both anxiolytic and anxiogenic effects of drugs under identical procedural conditions (Thiébot et al., 1991). The aim of the present study was to investigate using this paradigm the effects of the alpha-2 adrenoceptor agonist clonidine, and antagonists yohimbine, idazoxan, and RU 52 583[1]. Rats were trained under a standard conflict procedure during which periods of nonpunished lever pressing for food alternated with punished periods. The nonpunished components were conducted under a FR8 schedule and signalled by a cue light above the lever (safety signal). Punished periods were conducted under a FR1 schedule with shocks randomly delivered with 50 ± 15 per cent of the presses, and were signalled by a cue light above and to the left of the lever (punishment signal). On tests sessions (safety signal withdrawal), the safety signal was turned off at the end of the first non punished period, but the punishment signal was not present. During this period (4 min), each lever press was food rewarded and no shocks were delivered. Typically, control rats exhibited a strong blockade of responding during the first minute, that lessened over the remaining three. As for the anxiolytic compound diazepam (1, 2 and 4 mg/kg i.p.), this behavioural blockade was reduced by clonidine (0.05 and 0.1 mg/kg p.o.). While 0.5 mg/kg i.p. of d-amphetamine enhanced the

---

[1] (-) (3α) - 11 - methyl - 20, 21 - dinoreburnamenine, maleate

behavioural blockade without reducing responding during the nonpunished periods of the test session. Such an anxiogenic-like effect was not found with RU 52 583 (from 5 to 100 mg/kg p.o.), but was seen with yohimbine (0.1 mg/kg p.o.) and idazoxan (0.5 mg/kg p.o.). Therefore, the safety signal withdrawal paradigm also appears to be sensitive to some molecules acting on alpha-2 adrenoceptors.

REFERENCES

Thiébot, M.H., Dangoumau, L., Richard, G. and Puech, A.J. (1991): Safety signal withdrawal: a behavioural paradigm sensitive to both "anxiolytic" and "anxiogenic" drugs under identical experimental conditions. *Psychopharmacology 103*, 415-424.

The free exploratory paradigm: an effective method for measuring neophobia behavior in mice and testing potential neophobia reducing drugs

G. Griebel, R. Misslin, L. Weibel and E. Vogel

Laboratoire de Psychophysiologie, 7, rue de l'Université, 67000 Strasbourg, France

When given the opportunity to choose between a novel and a familiar compartment, BALB/c mice exhibited a neotic preference for familiar places and a marked number of avoidance responses towards novelty. When novelty was reduced by two familiar odors, fresh sawdust or urine of conspecifics, neotic reactions of BALB/c mice were reversed and animals clearly showed a preference for the novel compartment. These latter results tended to demonstrate the specific role of novelty in revealing defensive reactions of BALB/c mice in this paradigm which is devoid of constraining components.

Chlordiazepoxide (2.5-10 mg/kg, IP, 30 min), diazepam (1-4 mg/kg, IP, 30 min) and the nonbenzodiazepine partial agonist Ro 19-8022 (0.5-2 mg/kg, IP, 30 min), strongly reduced neophobia. Alpidem (2.5-10 mg/kg, IP, 30 min) another partial agonist at these sites, 8-OH-DPAT (0.016-1 mg/kg, IP, 20 min) a full agonist at $5-HT_{1A}$ receptor, and zacopride (0.0001-1 mg/kg, IP, 30 min), a selective $5-HT_3$ receptor antagonist, were unable to conteract neophobia.

Taken together, these results show that:
1) this paradigm can be proposed as an effective animal model for exploring potential drugs able to reduce neophobia;
2) in this model, which is concerned with a particular type of anxiety termed as "trait" anxiety (Lister, 1990), serotoninergic drugs failed to present the same pharmacolo-gical profile as benzodiazepines.

References

Lister, R.G. (1990): Ethologically-based animal models of anxiety disorders. *Pharmac. Ther.* 46, 321-340.

Brain neurosteroids: dehydroepiandrosterone reduces aggression in mice

Marc Haug*, Fabrice Perche*, Jacques Young**, Etienne-E. Baulieu** and Paul Robel**

* Université Louis Pasteur, Laboratoire de Psychophysiologie, CNRS URA 1295, 7, rue de l'Université, 67000 Strasbourg, France and ** INSERM U.33, Laboratoire des Hormones, 94275 Bicêtre Cedex, France

Dehydroepiandrosterone (DHA) and Pregnenolone (Δ5P) are present in the rat and mouse brain at concentrations superior to those found in the blood. Brain DHA is not affected by adrenal stimulation with ACTH or adrenal inhibition by dexamethasone. Cerebral Δ5-P and DHA are subject to circadian fluctuations not in phase with those of adrenal steroids in the plasma. An indirectly related but nevertheless important finding to support the cerebral synthesis of neurosteroids is obtained after castration and adrenalectomy : cerebral DHA and Δ5-P persist in the brain despite several weeks of peripheral hormone deficit, in contrast with testosterone (T) of testicular origin, which rapidly disappears after castration. DHA and Δ5-P are present in the brain in the form of nonconjugated steroids, sulfate esters and fatty acid esters and their concentrations are on the order of 10^{-7}-10^{-8} M, identical in males and females.

Several experiments have indicated the potential of DHA to interfere with behavioral phenomena. An antiaggressive effect of DHA has been demonstrated in castrated male mice that become aggressive in presence of lactating females (Haug et al., 1983). This form of attack, strongly reduced in intact males, occurs in castrated animals and is suppressed by administration of either T or estradiol (Haug and Brain, 1979). Because DHA can be metabolically transformed into T, although the quantities of this steroid found at the brain level were quite small (Schlegel et al., 1985), we used (Haug et al., 1988) a derivative of DHA, 3β-methyl-Δ5-androstene-17-one (CH3-DHA), lacking hormonal action, to avoid any transformation into sex hormones. This compound had an inhibitory action on the attack at least equal to that of DHA, increasing brain DHA without concomitantly rising brain T levels (Young et al., 1991), and, thus reinforcing the hypothesis that the anti-aggressive action of DHA is probably unrelated to its conversion into sex steroid hormones.

Attack on lactating females is also displayed by intact or ovariectomized female mice, and can be suppressed by administration of T (but not E2). Recent studies showed that, as in males, when DHA was administered to adult gonadectomized females, it strongly reduced the attack reponse (Haug et al., 1991). This anti-aggressive effect of DHA was even more markedly pronounced among females having received either prenatally (in preparation) or neonatally (day 1 of birth) a T treatment.

The mechanism of DHA anti-aggressive action is still unknown. However, the fact that a marked and significant decrease of brain pregnenolone-sulfate (Δ5P-S) is the only change common to DHA and CH3-DHA administration (Young et al., 1991) suggests that DHA may have its aggression-suppressive effect by interacting with the GABA-A receptor. Indeed,

Δ5P-S inhibits muscimol-stimulated chloride uptake in brain synaptosomes at low micromolar concentrations and both Δ5P-S and picrotoxin decrease the opening frequency of the ion channel. It has also been shown earlier that the potentiation of the GABAergic control results in the suppression of the attack response on lactating females (Haug et al., 1980).

REFERENCES

Haug, M., and Brain, P.F. (1979) : Effects of treatments with testosterone and estradiol on the attack directed by groups of gonadectomized male and female mice towards lactating intruders. Physiol. Behav. 23 : 397-400.

Haug, M., Kim, L., Simler, S., and Mandel, P. (1980) : Studies on the involvement of GABA in the agression directed by groups of intact or gonadectomized male and female mice towards lactating intruders. Pharm. Biochem. Behav., 12 : 189-193.

Haug, M., Spetz, J.F., Schlegel, M.L., and Robel, P. (1983) : La déhydroépiandrostérone inhibe le comportement agressif de souris mâles castrées. C.R.Acad. Sci. 296 : 975-977.

Haug, M., Ouss-Schlegel, M.L., Spetz, J.F., Brain, P.F., Simon, V., Baulieu, E.E. and Robel, P. (1989) : Suppressive effects of dehydroepiandrosterone and 3β-methylandrost-5-en-17-one on attack towards lactating female intruders by castrated male mice. Physiol. Behav. 46 : 955-959.

Haug, M., Young, J., Robel, P., and Baulieu, E.E. (1991) : L'inhibition par la déhydroépiandrostérone des réponses agressives de souris femelles castrées vis-à-vis d'intruses allaitantes est potentialisée par l'androgénisation néonatale. C.R.Acad.Sci. 312 : 511-516.

Schlegel, M.L., Spetz, J.F., Robel, P., and Haug, M. (1985) : Studies on the effects of dehydroepiandrosterone and its metabolites on attack by castrated mice on lactating intruders. Physiol. Behav. 34 : 867-870.

Young, J., Corpéchot, C., Haug, M., Gobaille, S., Baulieu, E.E. and Robel, P. (1991) : Suppressive effects of dehydroepiandrosterone and 3β-methyl-androst-5-en-17-one on attack towards lactating female intruders by castrated male mice. II. Brain neurosteroids. Bioch. Biophys. Res. Commun. 174, 2 : 892-897.

Effects of anxiolytic and antidepressant drugs in an animal model of panic

Patrick Martin

Groupe de Recherche AMC, 70, boulevard Bessières, 75017 Paris, France

The panic attack is the central pathologic feature of panic disorder and agoraphobia. Panic is characterised by unexpected anxiety attacks involving symptoms such as tachycardia, dizziness, shortness of breath, flushes, chest pain, trembling and fear of dying or losing self control (DSM-III-R ; Amer. Psychiat. Ass. ; 1987). Whether panic disorders constitute a homogeneous clinical syndrome is still the matter of the debate. During unexpected panic attacks, some patients try to join a safety-zone and others are in expectation with inhibited cognitive and behavioural processes. These two patterns could represent two different aspects of the pathophysiology of panic disorders and could correspond to different biological defects.

There are only few well accepted animal models of the psychiatric disorders. However, in case of depression, a variety of animal models have been proposed (such as the learned helplessness paradigm) and generally constitute an adequate approach compared with the relevant psychiatric disorders in man. In contrast, the situation is more problematic when considering animal models of panic attacks. In this context, I recently set up a new experimental paradigm where there is homology in the induced behaviours with those observed in panic attacks, particularly in patients who are inhibited in cognitive and behavioural processes.

The experiments were performed in three days. On day 1, groups of rats are exposed to a briefly uncontrollable and aversive situation.
In the morning of days 2 and 3, rats are subjected to an avoidance task in a shuttle-box. The required response was to move from one compartment to the other to escape the aversive situation. Absence of passage (AP) refers to the failure of the animal to change compartment during the shock delivery. AP were recorded for each group.

On the other hand, on day 1, before uncontrollable situation, rats are treated either with water (H_2O) or drugs which are panicogenic in human patients (e.g. caffeine, lactate, yohimbine, mCPP - Experimental groups).

On the third day, 30 min before the shuttle-box session, experimental rats are treated with drugs which reduce panic attack in man (e.g. imipramine, phelnezine, alprazolam).

The results obtained indicate that : at days 2 and 3, during the shuttle-box session, control rats pre-treated with H2O, caffeine or lactate and experimental rats without pre-treatment exhibited the same behaviour to escape the aversive situation.
At days 2 and 3, experimental rats pre-treated with caffeine, lactate, yohimbine or mCCP exhibited a behavioural deficit (absence of Passage) (Figure 1).

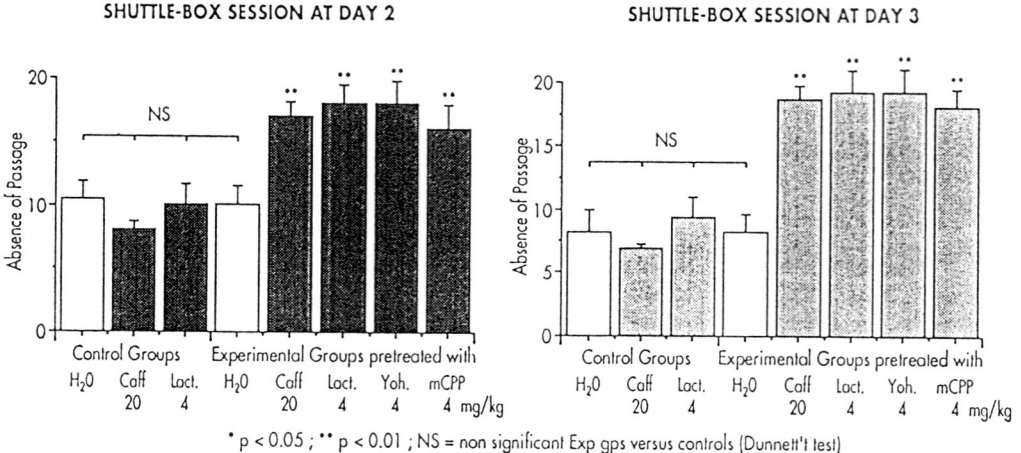

$* p < 0.05$; $** p < 0.01$; NS = non significant Exp gps versus controls (Dunnett't test)

In experimental caffeine-pretreated rats, imipramine, phelnezine, alprazolam and buspirone reverse the behavioural deficit induced by aversive situation at day 1 (Figure2).

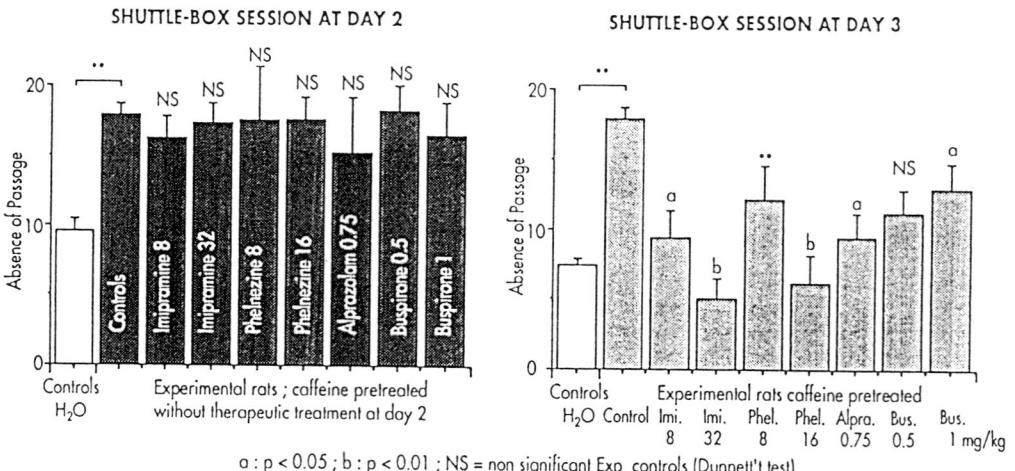

$a : p < 0.05$; $b : p < 0.01$; NS = non significant Exp controls (Dunnett't test)

In conclusion, these experimental conditions might constitute an animal model for studying panic attack and drugs active on this disorder.

Acknowledgment : These investigations were performed in collaboration with BIOTRIAL, Preclinical Studies Department , CHRU, 20 rue Pr J Pecker, 35000 Rennes, France.

A gene on mouse chromosome 4 is involved in anxiogenic processes

Benoît Martin, Yan Clément, Patrice Venault and Georges Chapouthier

Génétique, Neurogénétique et Comportement, URA 1294 CNRS, UFR Biomédicale des Saints-Pères, Université Paris V-René-Descartes, 45, rue des Saints-Pères, 75270 Paris Cedex 06, France

ß-carbolines, such as ß-CCM (methyl ß-carboline-3-carboxylate), classically known for their promnesic, anxiogenic and convulsive effects, constitute an original tool for the genetic analysis of anxiogenic and mnesic processes: since the same molecule is able, depending on the dose, to progressively induce all three of the effects mentionned above, it is consequently easy to suppose that they affect common physiological pathways. This hypothesis presumes that the genetic system involved in any of the three effects could be also involved in the two others. The chosen approach was the following: since it is easier to evaluate convulsive effects rather than anxiogenic or mnesic effects, the localisation of genes involved in these two latter effects in mice was carried out by comparison of the convulsive activity to ß-CCM. All candidate genes were also tested for their involvement in anxiogenic and/or mnesic processes. Genetic analysis of linkage-testing strains (strains carrying a mutation easily identifiable by eye) allowed an association between the *jerker* gene (*je*) on chromosome 4 and seizures induced by ß-CCM to be established. This result could be specific to some ß-carbolines since no association has been found between this gene and strychnine- or pentylenetetrazol-induced seizures. A T-maze learning test, with or without ß-CCM at anxiogenic dose, has also revealed an association between the *jerker* gene and a decrease in learning capacity. These results suggest that a gene carried on the distal part of mouse chromosome 4 is involved in anxiogenic and convulsive processes. Present work is attempting to clarify the possible involvement of this gene in mnesic processes.

Isolation and ACTH induced muricidal behavior in male Wistar rats

Simone Miachon

Laboratoire de Neurochimie Fonctionnelle, INSERM U.171 and CNRS URA 1195, Centre Hospitalier Lyon-Sud, Pavillon 4H, 69310 Pierre-Bénite, France

After 13 weeks of isolation, the majority (69% ; n=40) of male Wistar rats become muricidal. Monoamine metabolism was studied in different brain regions of these animals ; their blood levels of ACTH and corticosterone were also measured. Isolation evoked a large increase in catecholamine turnover in hippocampus, cortex and cerebellum. A modest augmentation in 5-hydroxytryptamine turnover was also seen in cortex and cerebellum. These results are at variance with previous reports using shorter isolation duration (Valzelli & Garattini, 1972). We also observed, for the first time in this model, modifications of the hypothalamo-pituitary-adrenal axis suggesting complex regulatory mechanisms after this long isolation period. Basal levels of corticosterone were lower in isolated rats as compared to group-reared animals: (159 ± 15 ng/ml vs 208 ±17 ng/ml ; n=39, $p<0.05$) ; these changes were concomitant with a significant rise in basal ACTH levels (148 ± 22 pg/ml vs 102 ± 7 ; n=27, $p<0.05$).

Since ACTH was seen to induce pro-agressive and anxiogenic effects in other animal models, we investigated whether it could induce muricidal behavior. Interestingly, we observed that ACTH administration (7.5 µg/100 g body weight, i.p.) reproduced the behavioral effect of long term isolation: it induced muricidal behavior in 60% of male Wistar rats which did not spontaneously express this behavior (n=40). This effect is strain specific since only 14% of Sprague-Dawley male rats became muricidal after the injection of ACTH. This change in behavior was a long lasting phenomenon being still present in 40% of the Wistar rats after 6 weeks, 17% after 12 weeks, 2.5% after 33 weeks. It was prevented by a pretreatment with dexamethasone (350 µg/kg, i.p., three hours before ACTH). Adrenalectomy also induced muricidal behavior in 59% of the animals (n=44), ten days after surgery.

REFERENCE

Valzelli,L. & Garattini,S. (1972) : Biochemical and behavioral changes induced by isolation in rats. Neuropharmacology 11,17-22.

The effect of CCK-4 and L 365.260 on cortical extracellular 5-HT release on exposure on the elevated plus Maze

Andre Rex, Heidrun Fink and Charles A. Marsden*

*Institute of Pharmacology and Toxicology, Humboldt University of Berlin, PF 140, 10117 Berlin, Germany and * Department of Physiology and Pharmacology, University of Nottingham Medical School, Queen's Medical Centre, Nottingham, NG7 2UH, United Kingdom*

The elevated Plus maze is a well established animal model of anxiety and has been widely used in rats (Handley & Mithyani, 1984), in mice (Lister, 1987) and also recently in guinea-pigs (Rex et al., 1993). An "anxiolytic" or "anxiogenic" effect is evaluated by the increase or decrease of the ratio of entries into the open arms and the time spent in the open arms of the elevated plus maze compared to the same parameters of the controls (Pellow et al., 1985). Behavioural studies have indicated that serotonin (5-hydroxytryptamine, 5-HT) is involved in the modulation of anxiety. Wise and coworkers (1972) found that central 5-HT injections had aversive effects, whereas administration of 5-HT antagonists (Graeff and Schoenfeld, 1970) had "anxiolytic" effects in a conflict test. The neuropeptide cholecystokinin (CCK) seems to be also involved in the development of anxiety with induction of panic reactions after administration of the CCK-B receptor agonist CCK-4 in man (Bradwejn, 1992) and "anxiolytic" actions induced by CCK-B antagonists (Ravard & Dourish, 1990).

Previous studies have demonstrated that extracellular 5-HT can be detected in perfusates from the prefrontal cortex of the guinea-pig using intracerebral microdialysis (Lawrence and Marsden, 1991).

Aims of the present study were the usage of the elevated plus maze in combination with the *in vivo* microdialysis in freely moving guinea-pigs to monitor changes in extracellular cortical 5-HT in response to aversive conditions and to investigate the effects of CCK-B receptor agonists/antagonists on cortical extracellular 5-HT release and the accompanying behaviour under aversive and home cage conditions.

Methods: Female coloured-BFA guinea-pigs (Charles River, Germany) $420 \pm 25g$ were group housed under a 12 hr light-dark-schedule with food and water freely available. All animals were handled daily from the day after birth until a week before the experiment.

A day before the experiment a microdialysis probe was implanted into the prefrontal cortex (coordinates: AP 4.0 mm, ML 3.5 mm from bregma and depth 3.0 mm from brain surface). The probe was perfused continously using artificial CSF. The animals were allowed to recover overnight in single cages. Dialysate samples were collected every 20 min and the content of 5-HT and 5-HIAA determined immediately using HPLC with electrochemical detection.

The basal release of 5-HT and 5-HIAA was determined the next morning using three subsequent samples. The animals then received an injection of either vehicle (saline + 1 per cent Chremophor EL) or L 365.260 (100 µg/kg i.p.). After 30 minutes the guinea-pigs were injected with either vehicle, CCK-4 (10 µg/kg i.p.) or L 365.260 (100 µg/kg i.p.). Forty min later the animals were placed in the centre of the elevated plus maze for the subsequent 20 min and the microdialysis continued. The behaviour of the animals on exposure to the elevated plus maze was recorded. The parameters measured were: the total entries, the number of entries into the open arms, the time spent in the open arms and the time spent in immobiliastion after placing the guinea-pig in the centre of the elevated plus maze. After 20 min (one perfusate sample) the guinea-pigs were returned to their home cages and the microdialysis continued for the next 140 min. The experiment was then terminated.

Behavioural results: Guinea-pigs treated with vehicle spent only 25.2 ± 5.4 seconds in the aversive open arms of the elevated plus maze and 11.8 ± 1.7 per cent of all entries into the open arms. An acute single injection of the tetrapeptide CCK-4 (10 µg/kg) decreased the time spent in the open arms and also the entries into these more aversive arms of the elevated plus maze. The immobilisation time increased three fold. Administration of the CCK-B antagonist L 365.260 (100 µg/kg) induced an increase in the time spent in the open arms and increased the percentage of entries into the open arms. The time of immobilisation after placing the animals on the elevated plus maze was decreased. The same dose L 365.260 also blocked the behavioural effects induced by CCK-4 completely (Table 1.).

Table 1. Behaviour of the guinea-pigs on exposure to the elevated plus maze

	vehicle	CCK-4 10µg/kg	L 365.260 100µg/kg	L 365.260 100µg/kg + CCK-4 10µg/kg
entries total	19 ± 0.8	18 ± 1.9	23 ± 2.3	14 ± 7.5
entries open	11.8 ± 1.7 %	5.6 ± 1.5 %	23.5 ± 3.5 %	23.6 ± 6.3 %
time open	25.2 ± 5.4 s	10.7 ± 2.7 s	179.8 ± 10.9 s	204 ± 36.7 s
immobilisation	140.4 ± 14.7 s	443 ± 29.6 s	78.0 ± 17.7 s	45.0 ± 13.5 s

Neurochemical changes: Exposure of the guinea-pigs to the elevated plus maze resulted in an increase in terminal extracellular 5-HT release in the cortex to 142 ± 7 per cent in the sample obtained on the elevated plus maze compared to basal level. When the animals returned to their home cage the release of extracellular 5-HT returned to preexposure level within 40 min.
Administration of 10 µg/kg CCK-4, a potent CCK-B receptor agonist, did potentiate the rise in extracellular 5-HT to 377 ± 108 per cent observed when the animals were placed on the plus maze. On return to the home cages the levels of cortical extracellular 5-HT came back to normal baseline after 80 min. A single dose of 100 µg/kg L 365.260 induced a long lasting decreased basal level (-35 ± 10 per cent) measured during the stay in the home cage and prevented the rise in 5-HT seen on exposure to the elevated plus maze. The same dose of the CCK-B antagonist L 365.260 given 30 min before the CCK-4 (10 µg/kg) injection totally blocked the neurochemical changes induced by CCK-4 alone. Levels of the metabolite 5-HIAA did not change during the exposure to the elevated plus maze and after treatment with CCK-4 or L 365.260.
CCK-B receptor stimulation and blockade induce changes in central extracellular 5-HT levels associated with "anxious" and "anxiolytic" behaviour. Interaction of substances acting at the central CCK-B receptor with drugs acting directly at different 5-HT receptors such as the 5-HT_{1A} receptor and their influence on the behaviour and the extracellular 5-HT release are still to be determined.

References:

Bradwejn, J., Koszycki, D., Couteoux du Terre, A., Bourin, M., Palmour, R. & Ervin, F. (1992): The cholecystokinin hypothesis of panic and anxiety disorders: a review. *J.Psychopharmacology*.6, 345-351

Handley, S.L. and Mithyani, S. (1984): Effects of alpha-adrenoceptor agonists and antagonists in a maze-exploration model of "fear"-motivated behaviour. *Nauyn Schmiedeberg Arch.Pharmacol*.327,1-5

Lawrence, A.J. and Marsden, C.A. (1992): Terminal autoreceptor control of 5-hydroxytryptamine as measured by *in vivo* microdialysis in the conscious guinea-pig. *J.Neurochem*. 58, 142-146

Lister, R.G. (1987) The use of a plus-maze to measure anxiety in the mouse. *Psychopharmacology* 92, 180-185

Pellow, S., Chopin, P., File, S.E. and Briley, M. (1985): Validation of open:closed arm entries in an elevated plus-maze as a measure of anxiety in the rat. *J.Neurosci.Meth*. 14, 149-167

Ravard, S. & Dourish, C.T. (1990):Cholecystokinin and anxiety. *TiPS*. 11, 271-273

Rex, A., Marsden, C.A. & Fink, H. (1993): Effect of diazepam on cortical 5-HT release and behaviour in the guinea pig on exposure to the elevated plus maze. *Psychopharmacology* 110, 490-496

Recent life stress and the corticotropin releasing factor test in panic disorder

D. Servant, D. Bailly, D. Dewailly, R. Beuscart and P.-J. Parquet

Laboratoire de Recherche sur l'Anxiété, Centre Hospitalier Universitaire, 57, boulevard de Metz, 59037 Lille, France

Recently the neuropeptide corticotropin-releasing factor (CRF) has been hypothesized to play a role in the pathophysiology of stress and anxiety (BUTLER et al, 1990). Animal studies support the theory that endogenous CRF mediates the stress response. Preclinical studies indicate that when injected directly into the brain of laboratory animals, CRF produces a number of behavioral effects commonly seen in anxiety. Futhermore CRF produces anxiogenic effects in animal models of anxiety. Clinical data also suggest the etiological role of CRF in anxiety disorders. Two studies documented a blunted ACTH response and enhanced ACTH/Cortisol ratio in response to intravenous CRF in panic disorder (PD) (ROY-BYRNE et al, 1986, HOLSBOER et al, 1987). However a recent study failed to find a significantly attenuated ACTH response to CRF (RAPOPORT et al, 1989). Abnormalities of HPA in PD may be inconstant and modulate by different variables. In human, stressful conditions may alter CRF functioning. In view to explore the CRF function in PD, we studied the ACTH and Cortisol response to ovine CRF in relation to life events.

Seventeen drug free patients with acute panic disorder episode according DSM III - R criteria and 17 matched normal controls received a IV injection of 100 µg synthetic o - CRF. Blood was collected every 15 minutes for 1 hour then every 30 minutes for 1 hour. Plasma was assayed for ACTH and cortisol using specific radioimmunassay. Clinical variable and life events were recorded using multiple semi-structured interview.

There are no difference in baseline Cortisol and ACTH levels and in Cortisol and ACTH response (compared by calculating the net area under the curve : AUC) between panic patients and controls.

We found a negative correlation between number of life events and weighted score occured in the 12 month period preceding the onset of acute panic episode and basal ACTH level and AUC for ACTH. The subgroup of panic patients who had experienced a severe life event before the onset of acute episode (N = 8) showed a blunted ACTH response compared with 8 sex and age matched controls (AUC ACTH : 2340 $\pm$ 619. 6 vs 4612. 5 $\pm$ 1838. 2 : z = - 2.57, p < 0.05). There was no significant different in all measures of Cortisol in relation to life events before acute episode.

Our study fails to demonstrate a blunted ACTH response to CRF in panic disorder as made by previous studies. Our data suggest that stressful event occurring before acute episode may reflect in part HPA dysfunction found in some patients with panic disorder but not in all cases. Severe life events may interact with other genetic or biological vulnerability factors and led to a separation into biologically distinct panic disorder groups. It is possible that in PD severe stressful events may be associated with an episode of CRF cortisol secretion which reflects a brief HPA axis hyperactivity detected under some conditions. It may be that PD patients show heightened HPA response to stress. Futher studies are needed to explore the HPA response to stress in panic and healthy subjects.

References

BUTLER, P.D, NEMEROFF, C.B. (1990): Corticotropin-Releasing Factor as a possible cause of comorbidity in Anxiety and Depressive disorders. In: D MASER and CR Cloninger (Eds) Cormorbidity of Mood and Anxiety Disorders.*American Psychiatric Press. Washington DC pp. 413 - 435.*

HOLSBOER, F., VON BARDELEBEN, U., BULLER R., HEUSER I., STEIGER, A. (1987): Stimulation response to corticotropin-releasing hormone (CHR) in patients with depression, alcoholism and panic disorder. *Horm Metab. Res. ; 16 (suppl.) ,80 - 88.*

RAPOPORT, M.H, RISCH, S.C, GOLHAN S, GILIN J.C. (1989): Neuroendocrine effects of ovine corticotropin-releasing hormone in panic disorder patients. *Biol. Psychiatry. 26, 344 - 348.*

ROY-BYRNE, P.P, UHDE, T.W, POST, R.M, GALLUCI, W, CHROUSOS, G.P, GOLD, P.W.(1986): The corticotropin-releasing hormone stimulation test in patients with panic disorder. *Am. J. Psychiatry. 143, 896 - 899.*

Dopamine transmission and anxiety in mice

Philippe Simon and Jean Costentin

Unité de Neuropsychopharmacologie Expérimentale, CNRS URA 1170, Faculté de Médecine et de Pharmacie de Rouen, B.P. 97, 76803 Saint-Etienne-du-Rouvray, France

Using three tests assessing the anxiety level in mice we have investigated about the influence of the dopamine transmission and the type (s) of receptors involved. These tests were (i) the elevated plus-maze, (ii) a black and white box test, where was measured the latency for entering the white compartment from the black one, in which mouse was introduced, (iii) the thigmotaxis in an open-field, at which animals were exposed for the first time. The two last tests were validated as able to reveal an anxiety with several reference anxiogenic drugs: dexamphetamine (2 - 4 mg/kg s.c.), pentylenetetrazole (12.5 - 25 - 50 mg/kg s.c.), yohimbine (2 - 4 mg/kg s.c.). In addition to dexamphetamine and cocaine (20 mg/kg s.c.), the pure and specific dopamine uptake inhibitor GBR 12783 (5 - 25 mg/kg s.c.) as well as the direct D1 dopamine agonist SKF 38393 (10 mg/kg s.c.) elicited an increase in anxiety. On the test considering thigmotaxis, administration of increasing doses of RU 24926 (125 - 250 - 500 - 1000 µg/kg s.c.), which stimulates for low doses only dopamine autoreceptors and for high doses postsynaptic D2 dopamine receptors, induced respectively a decrease and an increase in thigmotaxis. This suggests that stimulation of D1 receptors is not sufficient to elicit an anxiety, but induces it when postsynaptic D2 receptors are simultaneously stimulated. In the same way, on the black and white box tests we observed that a D2 selective antagonist (± sulpiride 10 mg/kg IP), administered at doses claimed to block preferentially dopamine autoreceptors and therefore to increase dopamine transmission, exerted an anxiogenic effect which was suppressed by the blockade of D1 dopamine receptors SCH 23390 (25 µg/kg SC).

In conclusion, it appears that an increase in dopamine transmission, through the simultaneous stimulation of D1 and D2 receptors mediates an increase in anxiety level.

Author index
Index des auteurs

Abadie P., 129
Adelbrecht C., 197

Bailly D., 187, 209
Balster R.L., 177
Barbaccia M.L., 53
Baron J.-C., 129
Baulieu E.-E., 201
Belotti M., 189
Belzung C., 193
Béracochéa D.J., 191
Beuscart R., 187, 209
Beuzen A., 193
Bickerdike M., 75
Biggio G., 53
Bontempi B., 191
Bouhou E., 193
Boulenger J.-P., 3
Bourin M., 15
Bradwejn J., 15
Brocco M., 153
Buhot M.-C., 195

Cadogan A-K., 75
Chapouthier G., 197, 205
Clément Y., 197, 205
Concas A., 53
Costentin J., 211
Cuccheddu T., 53

Dantzer R., 97
Daugé V., 167
Dekeyne A., 198
Depaulis A., 39
Derrien M., 167

Destrade C., 191
Dewailly D., 187, 209
Durieux C., 167

Fink H., 75, 207
Floris S., 53
François-Bellan A.-M., 83

Galey D., 189
Gozlan H., 141
Griebel G., 200
Grino M., 83
Guernier M., 198

Hamon M., 141
Haug M., 201
Héry F., 83
Héry M., 83

Jaffard R., 191
Joly D., 119

Krazem A., 191

Ladurelle N., 167
Lavallée Y.-J., 3
Lüddens H., 107

Mano M.-P., 189
Marsden C.A., 75, 207
Martin B., 197, 205
Martin P., 203
Miachon S., 206
Millan M.J., 153
Misslin R., 200

Naïli S., 195
Nixon M.K., 15

Oberlander C., 198
Oliver C., 83

Parquet P.-J., 187, 209
Patra S.K., 195
Perche F., 201
Pineau N., 193

Rex A., 75, 207
Robel P., 201
Roques B.-P., 167
Roscetti G., 53

Sanger D.J., 119
Sanna E., 53
Serra M., 53
Servant D., 187, 209
Simon P., 211

Tassin J.-P., 65
Thiébot M.-H., 25

Venault P., 197, 205
Vogel E., 200

Weibel L., 200
Wiley J.L., 177
Wright I., 75

Young J., 201

Zivkovic B., 119

Colloques **INSERM**
ISSN 0768-3154

Other *Colloques* published as co-editions by John Libbey Eurotext and INSERM

133 Cardiovascular and Respiratory Physiology in the Fetus and Neonate. *Physiologie Cardiovasculaire et Respiratoire du Fœtus et du Nouveau-né.*
Scientific Committee : P. Karlberg,
A. Minkowski, W. Oh and L. Stern;
Managing Editor : M. Monset-Couchard.
ISBN : John Libbey Eurotext 0 86196 086 6
 INSERM 2 85598 282 0

134 Porphyrins and Porphyrias. *Porphyrines et Porphyries.*
Edited by Y. Nordmann.
ISBN : John Libbey Eurotext 0 86196 087 4
 INSERM 2 85598 281 2

137 Neo-Adjuvant Chemotherapy. *Chimiothérapie Néo-Adjuvante.*
Edited by C. Jacquillat, M. Weil and D. Khayat.
ISBN : John Libbey Eurotext 0 86196 077 7
 INSERM 2 85598 283 7

139 Hormones and Cell Regulation (10th European Symposium). *Hormones et Régulation Cellulaire (10e Symposium Européen).*
Edited by J. Nunez, J.E. Dumont and R.J.B. King.
ISBN : John Libbey Eurotext 0 86196 084 X
 INSERM 2 85598 284 7

147 Modern Trends in Aging Research. *Nouvelles Perspectives de la Recherche sur le Vieillissement.*
Edited by Y. Courtois, B. Faucheux, B. Forette, D.L. Knook and J.A. Tréton.
ISBN : John Libbey Eurotext 0 86196 103 X
 INSERM 2 85598 309 6

149 Binding Proteins of Steroid Hormones. *Protéines de liaison des Hormones Stéroïdes.*
Edited by M.G. Forest and M. Pugeat.
ISBN : John Libbey Eurotext 0 86196 125 0
 INSERM 2 85598 310 X

151 Control and Management of Parturition. *La Maîtrise de la Parturition.*
Edited by C. Sureau, P. Blot, D. Cabrol, F. Cavaillé and G. Germain.
ISBN : John Libbey Eurotext 0 86196 096 3
 INSERM 2 85598 311 8

Colloques **INSERM**
ISSN 0768-3154

153 Hormones and Cell Regulation (11th European Symposium). *Hormones et Régulation Cellulaire (11e Symposium Européen).*
Edited by J. Nunez and J.E. Dumont.
ISBN : John Libbey Eurotext 0 86196 104 8
INSERM 2 85598 324 X

158 Biochemistry and Physiopathology of Platelet Membrane. *Biochimie et Physiopathologie de la Membrane Plaquettaire.*
Edited by G. Marguerie and R.F.A. Zwaal.
ISBN : John Libbey Eurotext 0 86196 114 5
INSERM 2 85598 345 2

162 The Inhibitors of Hematopoiesis. *Les Inhibiteurs de l'Hématopoïèse.*
Edited by A. Najman, M. Guignon, N.C. Gorin and J.Y. Mary.
ISBN : John Libbey Eurotext 0 86196 125 0
INSERM 2 85598 340 1

164 Liver Cells and Drugs. *Cellules Hépatiques et Médicaments.*
Edited by A. Guillouzo.
ISBN : John Libbey Eurotext 0 86196 128 5
INSERM 2 85598 341 X

165 Hormones and Cell Regulation (12th European Symposium). *Hormones et Régulation Cellulaire (12e Symposium Européen).*
Edited by J. Nunez, J.E. Dumont and E. Carafoli.
ISBN : John Libbey Eurotext 0 86196 133 1
INSERM 2 85598 347 9

167 Sleep Disorders and Respiration. *Les Evénements Respiratoires du Sommeil.*
Edited by P. Lévi-Valensi and D. Duron.
ISBN : John Libbey Eurotext 0 86196 127 7
INSERM 2 85598 344 4

169 Neo-Adjuvant Chemotherapy. *Chimiothérapie Néo-Adjuvante.*
Edited by C. Jacquillat, M. Weil, D. Khayat.
ISBN : John Libbey Eurotext 0 86196 150 1
INSERM 2 85598 349 5

171 Structure and Functions of the Cytoskeleton. *La Structure et les Fonctions du Cytosquelette.*
Edited by B.A.F. Rousset.
ISBN : John Libbey Eurotext 0 86196 149 8
INSERM 2 85598 351 7 .

Colloques INSERM
ISSN 0768-3154

172 The Langerhans Cell. *La Cellule de Langerhans.*
Edited by J. Thivolet, D. Schmitt.
ISBN : John Libbey Eurotext 0 86196 181 1
INSERM 2 85598 352 5

173 Cellular and Molecular Aspects of Glucuronidation. *Aspects Cellulaires et Moléculaires de la Glucuronoconjugaison.*
Edited by G. Siest, J. Magdalou, B. Burchell
ISBN : John Libbey Eurotext 0 86196 182 X
INSERM 2 85598 353 3

174 Second Forum on Peptides. *Deuxième Forum Peptides.*
Edited by A. Aubry, M. Marraud, B. Vitoux
ISBN : John Libbey Eurotext 0 86196 151 X
INSERM 2 85598 354 1

176 Hormones and Cell Regulation (13th European Symposium). *Hormones et Régulation Cellulaire (13e Symposium Européen).*
Edited by J. Nunez, J.E. Dumont, R. Denton
ISBN : John Libbey Eurotext 0 86196 183 8
INSERM 2 85598 356 8

179 Lymphokine Receptors Interactions. *Interactions Lymphokines-récepteurs.*
Edited by D. Fradelizi, J. Bertoglio
ISBN : John Libbey Eurotext 0 86196 148 X
INSERM 2 85598 359 2

191 Anticancer Drugs (1st International Interface of Clinical and Laboratory responses to anticancer drugs). *Médicaments anticancéreux (1re Confrontation internationale des réponses cliniques et expérimentales aux médicaments anticancéreux).*
Edited by H. Tapiero, J. Robert, T.J. Lampidis
ISBN : John Libbey Eurotext 0 86196 223 0
INSERM 2 85598 393 2

193 Living in the Cold (2nd International Symposium). *La Vie au Froid (2e Symposium International).*
Edited by A. Malan, B. Canguilhem
ISBN : John Libbey Eurotext 0 86196 234 9
INSERM 2 85598 395 9

Colloques INSERM
ISSN 0768-3154

194 Progress in Hepatitis B Immunization. *La Vaccination contre l'épatite B.*
Edited by P. Coursaget, M.J. Tong
ISBN : John Libbey Eurotext 0 86196 249 4
INSERM 2 85598 396 7

196 Treatment Strategy in Hodgkin's Disease. *Stratégie dans la maladie de Hodgkin.*
Edited by P. Sommers, M. Henry-Amar,
J.H. Meezwaldt, P. Carde
ISBN : John Libbey Eurotext 0 86196 226 5
INSERM 2 85598 398 3

198 Hormones and Cell Regulation (14th European Symposium). *Hormones et Régulation Cellulaire (14e Symposium Européen).*
Edited by J. Nunez, J.E. Dumont
ISBN : John Libbey Eurotext 0 86196 229 X
INSERM 2 85598 400 9

199 Placental Communications : Biochemical, Morphological and Cellular Aspects. *Communications placentaires : aspects biochimique, morphologique et cellulaire.*
Edited by L. Cedard, E. Alsat, J.C. Challier,
G. Chaouat, A. Malassiné
ISBN : John Libbey Eurotext 0 86196 227 3
INSERM 2 85598 401 7

204 Pharmacologie Clinique : Actualités et Perspectives. (6e Rencontres Nationales de Pharmacologie clinique).
Edited by J.P. Boissel, C. Caulin, M. Teule
ISBN : John Libbey Eurotext 0 86196 225 7
INSERM 2 85598 454 8

205 Recent Trends in Clinical Pharmacology (6th National Meeting of Clinical Pharmacology).
Edited by J.P. Boissel, C. Caulin, M. Teule
ISBN : John Libbey Eurotext 0 86196 256 7
INSERM 2 85598 455 6

206 Platelet Immunology : Fundamental and Clinical Aspects. *Immunologie plaquettaire : aspects fondamentaux et cliniques.*
Edited by C. Kaplan-Gouet, N. Schlegel,
Ch. Salmon, J. McGregor
ISBN : John Libbey Eurotext 0 86196 285 0
INSERM 2 85598 439 4

Colloques INSERM
ISSN 0768-3154

207 Thyroperoxidase and Thyroid Autoimmunity. *Thyroperoxydase et auto-immunité thyroïdienne.*
Edited by P. Carayon, T. Ruf
ISBN : John Libbey Eurotext 0 86196 277 X
INSERM 2 85598 440 8

208 Vasopressin. *Vasopressine.*
Edited by S. Jard, R. Jamison
ISBN : John Libbey Eurotext 0 86196 288 5
INSERM 2 85598 441 6

210 Hormones and Cell Regulation (15th European Symposium). *Hormones et Régulation Cellulaire (15e Symposium Européen).*
Edited by J.E. Dumont, J. Nunez, R.J.B. King
ISBN : John Libbey Eurotext 0 86196 279 6
INSERM 2 85598 443 2

211 Medullary Thyroid Carcinoma. *Cancer Médullaire de la Thyroïde.*
Edited by C. Calmettes, J.M. Guliana
ISBN : John Libbey Eurotext 0 86196 287 7
INSERM 2 85598 440 0

212 Cellular and Molecular Biology of the Materno-Fetal Relationship. *Biologie cellulaire et moléculaire de la relation materno-fœtale.*
Edited by G. Chaouat, J. Mowbray
ISBN : John Libbey Eurotext 0 86196 909 1
INSERM 2 85598 445 9

215 Aldosterone. Fundamental Aspects. *Aspects fondamentaux.*
Edited by J.P. Bonvalet, N. Farman, M. Lombes, M.E. Rafestin-Oblin
ISBN : John Libbey Eurotext 0 86196 302 4
INSERM 2 85598 482 3

216 Cellular and Molecular Aspects of Cirrhosis. *Aspects cellulaires et moléculaires de la cirrhose.*
Edited by B. Clément, A. Guillouzo
ISBN : John Libbey Eurotext 0 86196 342 3
INSERM 2 85598 483 1

217 Sleep and Cardiorespiratory Control. *Sommeil et contrôle cardio-respiratoire.*
Edited by C. Gaultier, P. Escourrou, L. Curzi-Dascalora
ISBN : John Libbey Eurotext 0 86196 307 5
INSERM 2 85598 484 X

Colloques INSERM
ISSN 0768-3154

218 Genetic Hypertension. *Hypertension génétique.*
Edited by J. Sassard
ISBN : John Libbey Eurotext 0 86196 313 X
INSERM 2 85598 485 8

219 Human Gene Transfer. *Transfert de gènes chez l'homme.*
Edited by O. Cohen-Haguenauer, M. Boiron
ISBN : John Libbey Eurotext 0 86196 301 6
INSERM 2 85598 497 1

220 Medicine and Change: Historical and Sociological Studies of Medical Innovation. *L'innovation en médecine : études historiques et sociologiques.*
Edited by Ilana Löwy
ISBN : John Libbey Eurotext 2 7420 0010 0
INSERM 5 85598 508 0

221 Structures and Functions of Retinal Proteins. *Structures et fonctions des rétino-protéines.*
Edited by J.L. Rigaud
ISBN : John Libbey Eurotext 0 86196 355 5
INSERM 2 85598 509 9

222 Cellular and Molecular Biology of the Adrenal Cortex. *Biologie cellulaire et moléculaire du cortex surrénal.*
Edited by J.M. Saez, A.C. Brownie, A. Capponi, E.M. Chambaz, F. Mantero
ISBN : John Libbey Eurotext 0 86196 362 8
INSERM 2 85598 510 2

223 Mechanisms and Control of Emesis. *Mécanismes et contrôle du vomissement.*
Edited by A.L. Bianchi, L. Grélot, A.D. Miller, G.L. King
ISBN : John Libbey Eurotext 0 86196 363 6
INSERM 2 85598 511 0

224 High Pressure and Biotechnology. *Haute pression et biotechnologie.*
Edited by C. Balny, R. Hayashi, K. Heremans, P. Masson
ISBN : John Libbey Eurotext 0 86196 363 6
INSERM 2 85598 512 9

Colloques INSERM
ISSN 0768-3154

228 Non-Visual Human-Computer Interactions. *Communication non visuelle homme-ordinateur.*
Edited by D. Burger, J.C. Sperandio
ISBN : John Libbey Eurotext 2 7420 0014 3
INSERM 2 85598 540 4

230 From Research in Oncology to Therapeutic Innovations. *De la recherche oncologique à l'innovation thérapeutique.*
Edited by P. Tambourin, M. Boiron
ISBN : John Libbey Eurotext 2 7420 0016 X
INSERM 2 85598 542 0

231 Human Ochratoxicosis and its pathologies. *Ochratoxicose humaine et ses pathologies.*
Edited by E.E. Creppy, M. Castegnaro, G. Dirheimer
ISBN : John Libbey Eurotext 2 7420 0017 8
INSERM 2 85598 543 9

LOUIS-JEAN
avenue d'Embrun, 05003 GAP cedex
Tél. : 92.53.17.00
Dépôt légal : 620 — Août 1993
Imprimé en France